Avian Medicine and Surgery

D0851069

LIBRARY OF VETERINARY PRACTICE

EDITORS

J.B. SUTTON JP, MRCVS
S.T. SWIFT MA, VetMB, CertSAC

LIBRARY OF VETERINARY PRACTICE

Avian Medicine and Surgery

Second Edition

B.H. Coles BVSc MRCVS

Blackwell
Science

© 1985, 1997, by
Blackwell Science Ltd
Editorial Offices:
Osney Mead, Oxford OX2 0EL
25 John Street, London WC1N 2BL
23 Ainslie Place, Edinburgh EH3 6AJ
350 Main Street, Malden
  MA 02148 5018, USA
54 University Street, Carlton
  Victoria 3053, Australia

Other Editorial Offices:

Blackwell Wissenschafts-Verlag GmbH
  Kurfürstendamm 57
  10707 Berlin, Germany

  Zehetnergasse 6
  A-1140 Wien
  Austria

First edition published 1985
Second edition published 1997

Set in 10 on 12pt Palatino
by DP Photosetting, Aylesbury, Bucks
Printed and bound in Great Britain
at the University Press, Cambridge

The Blackwell Science logo is a trade mark of
Blackwell Science Ltd, registered at the
United Kingdom Trade Marks Registry

DISTRIBUTORS

Marston Book Services Ltd
PO Box 269
Abingdon
Oxon OX14 4YN
(*Orders:*   Tel: 01235 465500
             Fax: 01235 465555)

USA
  Blackwell Science, Inc.
  Commerce Place
  350 Main Street
  Malden, MA 02148 5018
  (*Orders:*   Tel: 800 759 6102
               617 388 8250
               Fax: 617 388 8255)

Canada
  Copp Clark Professional
  200 Adelaide Street, West, 3rd Floor
  Toronto, Ontario M5H 1W7
  (*Orders:*   Tel: 416 597-1616
               800 815-9417
               Fax: 416 597-1617)

Australia
  Blackwell Science Pty Ltd
  54 University Street
  Carlton, Victoria 3053
  (*Orders:*   Tel: 03 9347-0300
               Fax: 03 9347-5001)

A catalogue record for this title is available
from the British Library

ISBN 0-632-03356-8

Contents

Preface to the First Edition

There is an increasing public interest in birds. More people are keeping aviaries and ornamental waterfowl. Membership of bird-watching societies is increasing. Falconry has seen a considerable revival, and conservation groups are encouraging captive breeding of wild species for re-stocking.

For these reasons veterinarians in practice are increasingly being consulted on avian problems. Apart from some instruction in the specialised field of poultry science, the veterinary graduate receives little or no formal instruction in the medicine and surgery of general avian species.

The purpose of this handbook is to give some guidance to the busy general practitioner presented with a medical or surgical problem concerning birds, with which he may not be very familiar. The book may also be of some value to those undergraduates who feel that this area of veterinary science has not been adequately covered during their training.

A volume of this size cannot pretend to be comprehensive and it is inevitable that it will not be detailed or specific enough on certain subjects. It is assumed that the reader will have a basic knowledge of the anatomy and physiology of the domestic fowl.

The various diseases are not dealt with in the more usual academic method by organ systems, but rather in the form of principal diagnostic signs as presented to the clinician. In this form it is hoped that the handbook will be more readily usable by the veterinary practitioner.

I should like to thank all those colleagues who, by referring their clinical cases to me and by discussing their avian problems, have expanded my knowledge of disease in birds.

I am grateful to Professor A.S. King for advice regarding some aspects of respiratory physiology in the chapter on anaesthesia. My thanks go to Dr John Baker who read Chapters 2 and 3 and gave valuable advice. My thanks also to Miss Underwood who read and gave helpful advice on Chapters 4, 5 and 9. I am particularly grateful to Ted Chandler for reading and editing the whole book and for his continual encouragement. My thanks go to Jane Ratcliffe for permission to print the schedule of bird releases obtained from her meticulously kept records. I thank the editor and publishers of the *Journal of Small Animal Practice* for permission to print large sections of my paper on 'Nursing birds'. Also I thank the editor, the authors and publishers of the *Journal of Anatomy* for permission to adapt the diagram used here as Fig. 4.1. My thanks to the publishers of *Veterinary Clinics of North America* for permission to use Table 2.1.

I am grateful to Mrs J. Padmore and to Mrs S. Postlethwaite for sharing the typing and for helpful criticism of the manuscript. Finally my thanks go to my wife, Daphne, for showing considerable patience and constant encouragement during this task.

Brian H. Coles

Preface to the Second Edition

Since the initial publication of this book, in parallel with the rapid expansion of medical and information technology, veterinary knowledge overall has increased considerably. Fuelled by the global extension of the Association of Avian Veterinarians and the foundation of the European College of Avian Medicine and Surgery, a simultaneous world-wide exchange of information on avian medicine and surgery is occurring. This second edition endeavours to update the basic subject matter together with giving some indication of its breadth. The author's aim is to present the essential facts in a readily accessible form.

Much of the chapter on 'Aids to Diagnosis' has been rewritten and expanded since without accurate diagnosis logical therapy cannot be pursued. Similarly, the formulary and the sections on infectious disease have been updated. An additional chapter has been added on anatomical and physiological diversity with the purpose of indicating the multiplicity of factors that must be taken into consideration when the clinician is presented with an unfamiliar species.

Again, I express my grateful thanks to the many colleagues, both in the UK and abroad, who continue to refer cases and to discuss their clinical problems with me. By so doing they have helped to formulate my thoughts on the subject.

I am indebted to Dr Roger Wilkinson for his very helpful advice on certain parts of the book and in particular for checking the new chapter. I am grateful to Sara Postlethwaite for a great deal of work in transcribing my handwritten notes into a form suitable for publication. My thanks go to Richard Miles of Blackwell Science Ltd for his patience during the prolonged preparation of this second edition. I am very grateful to Dr Kris Grodecki for reading and advising on the additional text to 'Aids to Diagnosis'. I also very much appreciate the meticulous copy editing carried out by Sheila Jones. Again my grateful thanks go to my wife, Daphne, who has shown considerable forbearance during the updating of this work. My thanks go to Mrs L.C. Tuckey for helping to correct the proof copy.

Chapter 1
Diversity in Anatomy and Physiology: Clinical Significance*

There are approximately 8900 species of living birds compared with only about 4200 species of mammals. In this chapter it is not possible to consider all aspects of anatomy and physiology; only those variations in the more clinically important parts of avian anatomy and physiology will be discussed.

To the casual observer there are many obvious differences in size, ranging from humming birds to the ostrich (Struthio camelus) in the varying forms of the bill, and in the colour and profusion of the plumage occurring in different species of birds. However beneath this great variety of body form there is a much greater degree of uniformity in the basic anatomy and physiology of the class Aves than there is in many single orders of other types of vertebrate. Even in the case of the large flightless birds, all present-day living birds have originally evolved from a flying ancestor and the capacity to be able to become airborne imposed quite severe restrictions on the basic anatomy and physiology which have been retained by their descendants. It is because of their ability to fly that birds have been able to quickly (i.e. in evolutionary time) reach and exploit a wide variety of habitats which has in turn resulted in the evolution of many different anatomical forms all with the same overall basic pattern. The field observations of Charles Darwin on the variations in body size and bill shape which adapted the bird to different habitats and sources of food, exhibited by otherwise apparently closely related finches in the Galapagos Islands helped him formulate his theory of the origin of species. However Darwin was primarily concerned with the process of divergent evolution while we now know that convergent evolution also takes place. Apparent externally recognised similarities are not always an infallible guide. For instance the martins, swallows and swifts all look quite similar and all behave similarly and occupy similar habitats. However while martins and swallows are taxonomically placed in the order Passeriformes or perching birds, the swifts are more closely related to the humming birds, both being

* Originally one of a series of lectures given at the Institute of Zoology and the University of London, 1995.

1

placed in the superorder Apodimorphae. Unlike most other birds the skeleton is not well pneumonised in Apodiformes.

The Victorian biologists were great anatomists and much of today's taxonomy is based on their observations, such as those of T.H. Huxley 1867. Consequently we know quite a lot about the detailed anatomical variations between species. We still do not know a lot about the physiological differences.

Some Victorian based taxonomy has been and is being overturned by present day laboratory investigation using DNA analytical techniques (Sibley and Ahlquist, 1990). New World vultures, for example, are now considered more closely related to the storks than to the Old World vultures. Most of our physiological knowledge has been derived from experimental work on domestic poultry (ducks and chickens) and particularly on the domestic fowl which originated from the red jungle fowl (*Gallus gallus*). This particular species is not really typical of birds as a whole.

Since the underlying skeleton of the bird largely influences the external appearance and anatomy these two topics will be considered together.

THE SKELETAL SYSTEM AND EXTERNAL ANATOMY

When carrying out radiography it is important to know what is normal for a particular species so that an inaccurate diagnosis is not made.

The skull

In all birds the cranial part of the skull is remarkably uniform. However that part of the skull associated with the mouth parts, as might be expected, does show considerable variation. In fact one aid in classifying birds used by the Victorian anatomists was to use the relative size and presence or absence of the vomer, the pterygoids and the palatine bones.

In hornbills (Bucerotidae) and cassowaries (Casuariidae) the frontal and nasal bones contribute to the horn covered casque. In the cassowary this is used to push the bird's way through the thick undergrowth of tropical rainforest. In most hornbills the casque is very light and cellular in texture but in the helmeted hornbill it is solid. The many different types of articulation of the maxilla, premaxilla and mandible with the skull are illustrated in Fig. 1.1(a) and 1.1(b). When considering the surgical repair of a traumatised or fractured beak it is important to take into account these interspecific variations.

The sheath of keratin overlying the skeleton of the bill also varies in thickness, composition and sensitivity. In ducks and geese (Anatidae) only the tip is hard, while in waders (Charadriides) the bill tends to be soft, leathery and flexible, extending distally well beyond the underlying bone. Different races of redshank (*Tringa totanus*) have developed different lengths of beak dependent on their preferred diet. In most species of parrot and most raptors the beak is hard and tough. Hardness depends on the content of orientated hydroxyapatite crystals. The hard tip of the bill of the Anatidae contains a tactile sensory structure/the bill tip organ, while herbst capsules, sensitive mechanoreceptors are well distributed over the whole of the beak of waders. The beak of toucans is also a very sensitive structure being well supplied by branches of the Vth cranial nerve. Fig. 1.2 shows the variation in beak form of a closely related group of cockatoos.

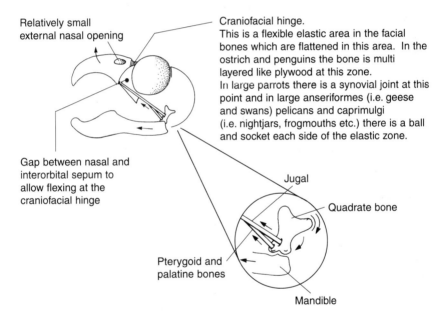

Relatively small external nasal opening

Craniofacial hinge.
This is a flexible elastic area in the facial bones which are flattened in this area. In the ostrich and penguins the bone is multi layered like plywood at this zone.
In large parrots there is a synovial joint at this point and in large anseriformes (i.e. geese and swans) pelicans and caprimulgi (i.e. nightjars, frogmouths etc.) there is a ball and socket each side of the elastic zone.

Gap between nasal and interorbital sepum to allow flexing at the craniofacial hinge

Jugal

Quadrate bone

Pterygoid and palatine bones

Mandible

Fig. 1.1 Kinesis of the avian jaw (simplified and diagramatic).
(a) The prokinetic (hinged) upper jaw. (Adapted from an illustration by King and McLelland (1984)). This type of jaw articulation is found in most species of birds including the parrots.

As the quadrate bone rotates clockwise horizontal forces are transmitted via the jugal arch (laterally) and the pterygopalatine arch (medially) to the caudal end of the ventral aspect of the upper jaw causing this to rotate dorsally pivoting on the craniofacial hinge.

Injury to the cere is common in many birds and may involve the underlying craniofacial hinge. Fractures of the jugal, pterygoid and palatine bones occasionally occur and need good quality radiographs for diagnosis. All the injuries affect prehension of food.

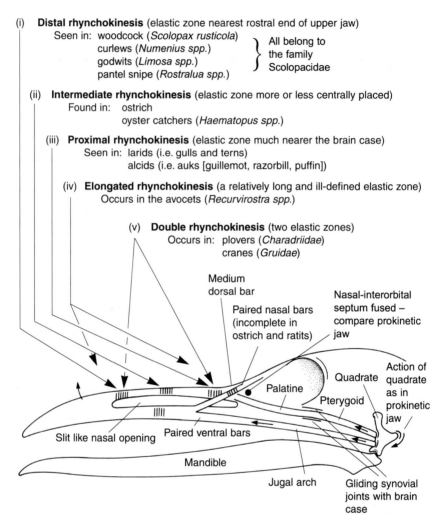

(i) **Distal rhynchokinesis** (elastic zone nearest rostral end of upper jaw)
Seen in: woodcock (*Scolopax rusticola*)
curlews (*Numenius spp.*)
godwits (*Limosa spp.*)
pantel snipe (*Rostralua spp.*)
} All belong to the family Scolopacidae

(ii) **Intermediate rhynchokinesis** (elastic zone more or less centrally placed)
Found in: ostrich
oyster catchers (*Haematopus spp.*)

(iii) **Proximal rhynchokinesis** (elastic zone much nearer the brain case)
Seen in: larids (i.e. gulls and terns)
alcids (i.e. auks [guillemot, razorbill, puffin])

(iv) **Elongated rhynchokinesis** (a relatively long and ill-defined elastic zone)
Occurs in the avocets (*Recurvirostra spp.*)

(v) **Double rhynchokinesis** (two elastic zones)
Occurs in: plovers (*Charadriidae*)
cranes (*Gruidae*)

Medium dorsal bar

Paired nasal bars (incomplete in ostrich and ratits)

Nasal-interorbital septum fused – compare prokinetic jaw

Quadrate

Palatine

Pterygoid

Action of quadrate as in prokinetic jaw

Slit like nasal opening

Paired ventral bars

Mandible

Jugal arch

Gliding synovial joints with brain case

Fig. 1.1 *(Cont)* (b) The rhynchokinetic jaw. Most of the movement of the jaw occurs rostal to the junction of the upper jaw and the brain case within the area of the 'nose'. With the many forms of rhynchokinetic articulation, proximal rhynchokinesis (see (iii) below) most nearly resembles prokinetic articulation, giving these birds (gulls, terns and auks) a wide gape to swallow their prey. Rhynchokinetic articulation overall is found mostly in the order Charadiiformes (i.e. waders and shore birds) which mostly feed on inverbebrates and other aquatic organisms. Many species of these birds probe for their food in sand or soft earth.

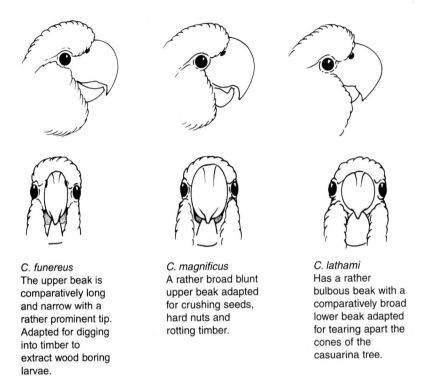

C. funereus
The upper beak is comparatively long and narrow with a rather prominent tip. Adapted for digging into timber to extract wood boring larvae.

C. magnificus
A rather broad blunt upper beak adapted for crushing seeds, hard nuts and rotting timber.

C. lathami
Has a rather bulbous beak with a comparatively broad lower beak adapted for tearing apart the cones of the casuarina tree.

Fig. 1.2 Variations in the form of the beak among the genus Calyptorhynchus i.e. the black cockatoos. (After W.T. Cooper in Forshaw, 1978.) Although C. funereus and C. magnificus inhabit parts of south-western Australia, all three species co-exist in parts of south-eastern Australia where because of their different feeding habits they are ecologically isolated.

THE AXIAL SKELETON

The cervical vertebrae

In all species the atlas articulates with the skull via a single occipital condyle but in some hornbills (Bucerotidae) the atlas and axis have fused possibly to support the very large skull. Most birds, even small Passeriformes with an apparently quite short neck, have 14–15 cervical vertebrae compared with the mammalian 7. The swans (genus *Cygnus*), most of the large herons in the family Ardeidae, most of the storks (Ciconiidae) and the ostrich have an obviously long and flexible neck and as would be expected an increased number of cervical vertebra (in swans 25). Usually long necks go with long legs since the bird needs to use its bill to perform many tasks (e.g. manipulating food, grooming and nest building or burrowing) all of which are often carried out by the pectoral (or fore) limb in mammals.

In darters (genus *Anhinga*) there is a normal 'kink' in the neck between the 7th, 8th and 9th cervical vertebrae. This, when suddenly straightened, enables the bird to thrust forward the beak in a stabbing action at the prey.

The thoracic vertebrae

In many birds the first few thoracic vertebrae (2–5) are fused to form a notarium. This is present in Galliformes, Columbiformes (pigeons and doves) Ciconiida (herons, egrets, bitterns, storks, ibises, spoonbills) and Phoenicopteridae (flamingoes).

The notarium may not be very apparent on all radiographs. In all birds some of the posterior thoracic vertebrae together with all of the lumbar vertebrae, the sacral vertebrae and some of the caudal vertebrae are fused to form the synsacrum which is also fused with the ilium, ischium and pubis. The exact numbers of fused vertebrae derived from the various regions of the spine is not possible to define accurately.

The pygostyle (4–10 fused caudal vertebrae) gives support together with the retrical bulb (a fibro-adipose pad) to the rectrices (the tail feathers). This is well developed in most flying birds in which the tail is important to give added lift during hovering (e.g. kestrel *Falco tinnunculus*) or soaring or for accurate steerage as in the goshawk (*Accipiter genitilis*) and woodland species. This area in the flying birds and those which use the tail for display purposes is well supplied with muscles many of which are inserted into the inter-rectrical elastic ligament. The pygostyle and the free caudal vertebrae are well developed in woodpeckers which together with specially stiffened tail feathers help to support the bird when clinging on to a vertical surface. The tail feathers may also support such species as the penguins when standing or pygmy parrots, woodpeckers and tree creepers when climbing.

The *rigid synsacrum* in most birds, unlike the pelvis in mammals, is open on the ventral surface to allow passage of the often quite large shelled egg. However in the large flightless birds it is fused either at the pubic symphysis (in the ostrich) or at the ischial symphysis. This may help to prevent compression of the viscera when the bird is sitting.

In all birds there is an antitrochanter situated dorsal to the acetabula fossa but even both these two anatomical structures vary between quite similar species such as the peregrine falcon (*Falco peregrinus*) and the goshawk (*Accipiter gentilis*) (Harcourt-Brown, 1995). The pelvis tends to be comparatively wide in the running birds compared with the narrower and longer pelvis of the foot propelled diving birds e.g. loons (Gaviidae) and grebes (Podicipedidae) which closely resemble each other in body form and behaviour but are taxonomically unrelated and this is probably another instance of convergent evolution.

The thoracic girdle

In most birds the scapula is long and narrow but in the ostrich it is short and fused to the coracoid. The clavicles are usually fused at the furcula to form a 'wish bone' and they function as bracing struts to hold the two shoulder joints apart during contraction of the supracoracoideus and they also act as a major attachment for the pectoral muscle; they are well developed and widely spaced in the strongly flying birds. As would be expected both the supracoracoid muscle and the pectorals as well as the other wing muscles are reduced in the non-flying birds.

In some birds (pelicans, frigate birds and the secretary bird (*Sagittarius serpentarius*) the furcula is fused to the sternum. In the ostrich the scapulocoracoid bone is not quite fused but has a fairly rigid attachment to the sternum. In the albatrosses and fulmars (Procellariidae) the furcula forms a synovial joint with the sternum. However in some parrots the clavicles and the furcula are absent, being represented by a band of fibrous tissue. The coracoid is well developed in most species but the 'triosseal canal' normally formed between coracoid, scapula and clavicle is completely enclosed within the coracoid in the hoopoe (*Upupa epops*) and hornbills (Buccrotidae).

The ribs and sternum

The uncinate processes are unusually long in the guillemots or murres (Alcinae) and the divers or loons (Gaviidae). This may help to resist the pressure of water on the thorax when the bird is diving. As is the case of the pelvic girdle the thorax in these birds is long and comparatively thin; consequently the sternum is long thus reducing the space between its caudal margin and the pubic bones and so making surgical access to the abdomen more difficult. The keel of the sternum is well developed in the flying birds particularly the swifts and the hummingbirds (Apodiformes). However it is absent or reduced in the ratites (i.e. with a raft-like sternum). It is reduced in many flightless island species in which other members of the same family are flying birds e.g. the kakapo (*Stringops habroptilus*) or the owl parrot of New Zealand which can only glide downhill or again some of the flightless island rails (e.g. *Atlantisea rogersi*). The sternal keel is well developed in penguins and in these birds the supracoracoid muscle is greatly increased in size compared with the pectoral. In some cranes (Gruidae) and the swans this part of the sternum has been excavated to accommodate the coils of an elongated trachea as is illustrated in Fig. 1.3.

The pectoral limb – the wing

The overall layout of the skeleto-muscular system of the wing is similar in all birds. However the relative lengths of the individual bones do vary

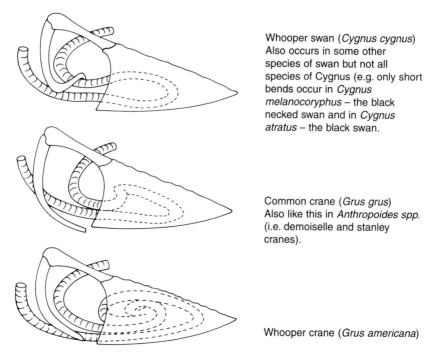

Whooper swan (*Cygnus cygnus*)
Also occurs in some other
species of swan but not all
species of Cygnus (e.g. only short
bends occur in *Cygnus
melanocoryphus* – the black
necked swan and in *Cygnus
atratus* – the black swan.

Common crane (*Grus grus*)
Also like this in *Anthropoides spp.*
(i.e. demoiselle and stanley
cranes).

Whooper crane (*Grus americana*)

Fig. 1.3 Various types of looped trachea partly enclosed in the excavated
sterum. (Redrawn after King and McLelland, 1989, by permission of Academic
Press Limited London.)
Knowledge of these variations is important in the interpretation of
radiographs.

(Fig. 1.4). In most specialised soaring birds (e.g. the gulls (Laridae) the
humerus is short compared with the relatively longer radius and ulna. In
contrast in the albatrosses, which are also soaring birds, the humerus is
longer than the radius and ulna. In the penguins, auks and diving petrels
the humerus and the other bones of the wing have become flattened. The
alula digit (corresponding to the human thumb) is usually well developed
in most flying birds which when abducted from the wing acts as a slot, as
in an aircraft wing, to smooth the airflow over the aerofoil section of the
wing at low airspeeds and when the wing is canted as the airborne bird
comes in to land. During these conditions the airflow tends to break away
from the surface of the wing and the bird or aircraft loses lift. As would be
expected this structure is reduced or absent in some non-flying birds (e.g.
kiwis and cassowaries). In the young hoatzin (*Opisthocomus hoatzin*) there
are claws on the alula and the major digit which the bird uses for climbing
around the nest site. Adult cassowaries, kiwis, emus, rheas and ostrich
also have vestigial non-functional claws on these digits. The varying types
of avian wing are illustrated in Fig. 1.5.

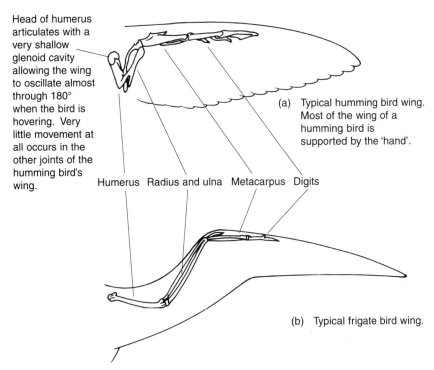

Head of humerus articulates with a very shallow glenoid cavity allowing the wing to oscillate almost through 180° when the bird is hovering. Very little movement at all occurs in the other joints of the humming bird's wing.

Humerus Radius and ulna Metacarpus Digits

(a) Typical humming bird wing. Most of the wing of a humming bird is supported by the 'hand'.

(b) Typical frigate bird wing.

Fig. 1.4 The relative comparable sizes of the wing bones in two different types of birds (*not* drawn to the scale of the two species).

The legs

Again the basic layout of the hind limb is the same in all species with most of the evolutionary changes having taken place in the foot. In the long-legged birds the tibiotarsus and the tarsometatarsus are of approximately the same length. This is essential if the centre of gravity of the bird's body is to remain above the feet when the bird is crouched and the limb is flexed, otherwise the bird would overbalance. In flamingoes there are no menisci in the intertarsal joints. In the grebes (Podicipedidae) and divers or loons (Gaviidae) which are foot propelled diving birds the tibio tarsus lies almost parallel to the vertebral column and the limb is bound to the body by a fold of skin. The cnemial crest in these divers is well developed projecting beyond the stifle joint. In grebes it is fused to the patella thus increasing the area of attachment for the crural muscles. In divers and grebes the gastrocnemius is greatly developed providing the main power stroke of the foot. Quite obviously all the leg muscles are powerful and well developed in the ostrich which can run at 40 mph (64 kph) and can produce a lethal strike forward with its foot.

Type I The elliptical wing

Has fairly low wing loading and a low aspect ratio. Enables bird to take off rapidly and manoeuvre through narrow spaces.

(a) Typical small finch or bunting

This type has a large alula and additional slots in the wing to prevent stalling at slow speed.

(b) Pheasant type

Typical of many galliforms. Adapted for rapid take off often in dense cover.

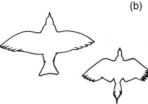

Type II Long wide wing

Enables bird to glide and soar at *relatively low speed*. Has a moderate wing loading and medium type aspect ratio. The alula and wing slots are well developed and obvious, giving bird reasonable manoeuverability.

(c) Typical large eagle

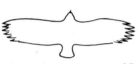

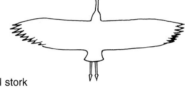

(d) Typical stork

This type also seen in condors, vultures and pelicans.

Type III Long, relatively slim wing

With no wing slots and a tapered end to the wing. Sometimes the alula is large. These birds glide at *high speed* in strong wind. High wing loading, high aspect ratio.

(e) Typical gull

Type of wing also seen in gannets and frigate birds.

(f) Albatross

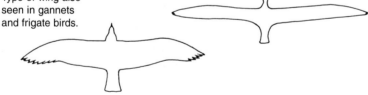

Type IV High speed wing

Long and relatively narrow with no wing slots. Tip of wing pointed and may be swept back. High wing loading, moderate-high aspect ratio enables bird to fly at high speed to chase prey.

(g) Typical falcon

(h) Swift

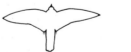

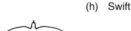

All the major types of avian foot are illustrated in Fig. 1.6.

THE ALIMENTARY OR DIGESTIVE SYSTEM

Brief reference has already been made to the varying types of beak. Within the oral cavity itself there are differences in the anatomy which are not quite so obvious to the casual observer. The palate is often ridged and the pattern of ridges is usually related to the diet. In the Fringillidae group of finches (e.g. chaffinch *Fringilla coelebs* and canary *Serinus canarius*) most of which feed on dicotyledonous seeds (i.e. those of trees, shrubs and most herbaceous plants) there is a lateral palatine ridge between which and the edge of the upper beak the seed is lodged while it is cut by the sharp edged lower bill. Even among the Fringillidae there is considerable variation in bill size and shape. In two other groups of small seed eating birds the Emberizinae (e.g. the cardinal, *Pyrrhuloxia cardinalis* and the snow bunting, *Plectrophenax nivalis*) and the Ploceidae the typical weaver birds (e.g. *Quelea* and house sparrow, *Passer domesticus*) which feed on monocotyledonous seeds (i.e. the grasses and cereal crops) there is a prominence rostral to the choanal gap against which the seed is wedged transversely while it is crushed by the blunt edged lower beak. Many parrots also use the transverse ridge on the rostral part of the palate to hold the seed while it is cracked or manipulated into position by the muscular tongue (the only avian order with intrinsic tongue muscles). The tongues of birds show a lot of variation in relation to the diet and some of these differences are illustrated in Fig. 1.7. Abscessation of the choanal gap and the tongue is common in caged parrots, neoplastic lesions occasionally occur in other species and partial amputation of the tongue or beak owing to a ligature of nylon fishing line is seen in water fowl. All these lesions affect prehension of food.

The *salivary glands*, which mainly secrete mucus, are best developed in birds that swallow dry foods. They are least developed in birds swal-

---

Fig. 1.5 (*Opposite*) Varying types of avian wing (definitely not to scale).

- Any loss of wing extension through fracture trauma or damage to the propatagial membrane is most serious prognostically in birds with a high wing loading although of course if it is extensive enough it is significant in all species of birds. However, see p. 226.
- Trauma to the carpo-metacarpal region resulting in fibrosis or possible ankylosis is most grave in birds with a Type I or Type II wing plan. The author has seen a number of kestrels (*Falco tinnunculus*, type IV wing plan) and gulls (*Larus* sp., Type III wing plan) fly effectively with slight damage to the carpo-metacarpal area.
Clinical importance: assessment for release of wildlife casualties.

Feet with four toes

Anisodactyl i.e. three forward toes and one backward pointing toe. This type of foot is adapted for perching or grasping and is seen in song birds and birds of prey. This is the pattern seen in most birds. The gannets have four webbed toes, so do cormorants.

Zygodactyl i.e. two forwardly directed toes (digits II & III) and digits I & IV are backwardly directed toes. This foot is seen mostly in birds which climb but also grasp with the foot, e.g. parrots, toucans, cuckoos, woodpeckers. In owls, touracos and the osprey the foot is basically of this type but digit IV can easily be moved forwards.

digit IV

Pamprodactyl i.e. all four toes are directed forward. This type of foot is found in the swift. Unable to perch on the ground but clings to a vertical nesting site.

Syndactyl i.e. two digits are partially united, e.g. kingfishers.

digit III & IV

Feet with only three toes, i.e. *tridactyle* feet

This type of foot is seen in running birds (e.g. plovers), wading birds, some climbing birds, some woodpeckers, the emu, diving petrels and auks, cassowaries, kiwis, tinamous and pheasants.

Many birds with webbed feet are like this with a vestigal first digit, e.g. gulls, penguins, loons, albatross, swans and ducks.

Feet with two toes

This is found only in the ostrich. Digits I & II are absent and digit III is much larger than digit IV. The foot is rather like that of the horse where one digit is greatly developed and adapted to running and walking over open country and grassland.

Fig. 1.6 Varying types of avian foot.
Clinical importance: Foot problems in birds are common. As well as obvious trauma digits are sometimes congenitally maldirected so knowledge of what is normal is important.

lowing slippery foods such as fish. In the woodpeckers the mandibular glands below the tongue secrete a sticky fluid for mopping up invertebrates. Swifts secrete an adhesive glycoprotein which after secretion hardens into a nest building material.

Taste buds are variously developed in birds and these are associated with the salivary glands. In most birds there are a few taste buds at the caudal end of the tongue. But in some ducks (e.g. mallard, *Anas pla-*

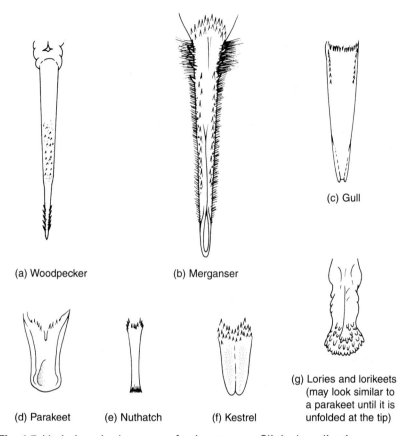

Fig. 1.7 Variations in the types of avian tongue. Clinical application: a completely normal tongue is more important in some species than in others. (Redrawn after King and McLelland, 1979, by permission of Academic Press Limited London.)

tyrhynchos) there are none in this position but they are located near the tip of the upper and lower bill and on the roof of the oropharynx. Parrots have taste buds either side of the choanal opening and just rostral to the laryngeal mound. The acuity of the taste varies between species. Bitter and salt tasting substances are generally rejected.

Some species of birds such as the male of most bustards (Otidae) have inflatable oral sacs on the floor of the mouth which are used for sexual display. In the great bustard (*Otis tarda*) this sac is an oesophageal structure. Those structures also occur in frigate birds, sage grouse (*Centrocercus urophasianus*) and prairie chicken (*Tympanuchus cupido*). In the pelican the sac on the floor of the mouth is large and used rather like a fishing net to catch food.

The oesophagus and crop

This is folded longitudinally and is very distensible in hawks, owls and cormorants but in swifts and some finches feeding on much less bulky food it is quite narrow; a factor to consider if these species have to be gavaged. Just cranial to the thoracic inlet is a storage region, the crop. *Not all birds have a crop.* It is absent in gulls and penguins which store the food along the whole length of the oesophagus. It is also absent in the toucans (Ramphastidae) in many species such as ducks and geese (Anatidae) and also in some species of song birds the oesophagus is only slightly increased in diameter at its caudal end. Swellings at the thoracic inlet which may be occasionally seen in any of these species are not due to an impacted crop.

Crop milk

This is produced by pigeons and doves (Columbidae) to feed the young. Its composition is similar to mammalian milk but lacks calcium and carbohydrates. Both sexes of the flamingoes and the male emperor penguin also produce a nutritive fluid which is regurgitated to feed the young. However in the Columbidae and emperor penguin the crop milk is produced by desquamation of epithelium, whereas that from the flamingoes is a secretion from the merocrine glands of the oesophagus.

The stomach (i.e. the proventriculus together with the ventriculus or gizzard)

Two basic forms of avian stomach are found (1) that in the carnivorous and fish eating birds in which the food requires less trituration and alternatively (2) the more complex avian stomach found in those birds feeding on much less digestible food, which requires to be physically broken up before enzymatic digestion. Such types of bird are granivorous, herbivorous, frugivorous and insectivorous. There are many intermediate forms between these two basic types.

(1) In the simpler stomach the division between proventriculus (fore stomach) and ventriculus (true stomach) is not always easy to discern on external appearance. This type of organ acts largely as a storage zone giving time for the digestive secretions of the stomach to penetrate and act on the food.
(2) In the more complex avian stomach the division between the thin walled proventriculus and the well developed muscular gizzard is easily recognised. Although the distribution of the glands secreting

digestive fluid varies between species, the glands themselves and the composition of the digestive juice containing hydrochloric acid and pepsin does not vary. The foul smelling 'stomach oil' ejected by petrels and fulmars as a means of defence is of dietary origin and not a secretion.

The gizzard itself is lined by a tough cuticle or koilin layer (a material secreted by glands and hardened by hydrochloric acid). This can be stained brown, yellow or quite intense green due to the regurgitation of bile pigment. The intensity of this colour and the extent of staining needs to be noted at autopsy. Sometimes pathological bile staining extends into the proventriculus. Some species (e.g. magpies (*Pica pica*) and common starlings (*Sturnus vulgaris*) normally periodically shed the cuticle. In those species in which the gizzard is less well defined the cuticle is thinner and relatively soft. Erosion and necrosis of the koilin layer can be a sign of gizzard worms in ducks and geese and also a sign of megabacteriosis in budgerigars.

In the carnivorous species particularly, the contractions of the stomach form a regurgitated pellet (called by falconers the casting) from the indigestible parts of the food such as pieces of skeleton, claws and teeth. A healthy hawk should produce these pellets after each feed and they should be firm in consistency and not smell offensive. It is not generally known that many other species of birds besides hawks and owls also sometimes produce pellets (e.g. thrushes (Turdinae), crows (Corvidae) and herons (Ardeidae).

Grit

This is taken in by many species with a well developed gizzard which together with the tough koilin layer helps to grind up food. Although grit is mainly quartz, the size and coarseness of the particles is related not only to the size of the bird but also to the diet. The lesser flamingo (*Phoenicopterus minor*) feeds mainly on algae and diatoms filtered from the water in which it stands so that it ingests a fine sandy grit. The ostrich (*Struthio camelus*) which feeds on coarse vegetation uses pebbles, although ostriches kept in captivity have a habit of swallowing anything which they find and which is unfamiliar to them. The dippers (genus *Cinclus*), some of the diving birds and some ducks which feed on molluscs and crustaceans use a grit derived from molluscan shells. Even when available not all caged birds will take grit into their gizzard and apparently do not suffer any adverse effect.

The pylorus, the duodenum and the intestines

All show quite a lot of variation among different species. In fact the number and the way in which the coils of the intestine are arranged was one method of the classification of birds used by the Victorian anatomists.

In general, as would be expected, the intestines are relatively shorter in carnivores, insectivores and frugivores in which the food requires much less digestion. The alimentary transit time in some frugivores is relatively short (e.g. mynah birds (*Gracula*) $1\frac{1}{2}$ hours, in the common buzzard (*Buteo buteo*) 3 hours). In the granivorous and herbivorous birds the digestive tract is much longer being longest of all in birds feeding on a fibrous diet (e.g. red grouse (*Lagopus lagopus*) which feeds principally on heather (*Calluna vulgaris*). In fact a seasonal change may occur in the length of the intestine in some species in relation to seasonal changes in the diet.

The caeca

Left and right caeca are usually present at the junction of the ileum and the rectum but their shape and size varies considerably as is illustrated in Fig. 1.8. These normal variations should be familiar to the pathologist.

In some species such as the parrots, the swifts, the pigeons and toucans the caeca are either rudimentary or absent. At one time it was thought that the major function of the caeca was primarily concerned with the breakdown of cellulose by the action of symbiotic bacteria. However this theory is now in some doubt and the size of the caeca apparently has little relation to the type of avian diet. However the autochthonous flora of the alimentary canal of those birds with well developed caeca does apparently vary from those birds in which the caeca are absent.

A gallbladder

This is usually present in most species except for most parrots, pigeons and the ostrich. In the cockatiel (*Nymphicus hollandicus*), the rheas, the hoatzin and penguins, its presence is variable. In woodpeckers (Picidae), toucans (Ramphastidae) and barbets (Capitoninae) the gallbladder is exceptionally long in some individuals extending as far as the cloaca.

Fig. 1.8 (*Opposite*) The different forms of caeca found in birds. (After King and McLelland, 1979)
In many species the right and left caeca may not be of equal size with one side being almost vestigial (e.g. Ardeidae – herons), also there are many intraspecific differences in length.

No caeca occur in Psittaciformes (parrots), Apodimorphae (hummingbirds and swifts), some Piciformes (woodpeckers, toucans, barbets, honeyguides etc.) Some Columbidae (pigeons and doves) and kingfishers (Alcedinidae). (Redrawn after King and McLelland, 1979, by permission of Academic Press Limited London.)

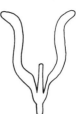

(a) Sparrow hawk
(*Accipter nisus*)

Most falconiforms
(hawks, eagles
and vultures) have
relatively small
caeca.

(b) Marabou stork
(*Leptoptilos
crumeniferus*)

Most ciconiiforms
(herons, storks,
ibis, flamingos)
have short caeca.

(c) Tufted guineafowl
(*Numida
meleagris*)

Caeca are
generally long in
most galliforms.

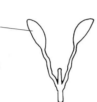
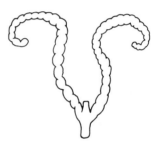

Distal ends
of caeca
usually
expanded in
most owls

(d) Barn owl (*Tyto alba*)

Most strigiforms (owls) have
relatively long caeca.

(e) Great bustard
(*Otis tarda*).

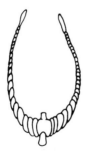

(f) Ostrich (*Struthio camelus*)

Also rather like this in rheas. In
most birds the cacea are directed
cranially, but in the ostrich they are
caudally directed.

(g) Emu
(*Dromaius
novaehollandiae*).

The liver

This varies slightly in the number of lobes present but there is quite a lot of variation in the normal level of liver enzymes even in apparently fairly closely related genera of birds, see Table 1.1. Knowledge about liver enzymes in birds is very patchy but is slowly accumulating. Awareness of these normal variations is important when using this data to make a diagnosis of hepatopathy.

THE RESPIRATORY SYSTEM

There is a lot of interspecific variation in the size and position of the external nares which is useful when masking birds for the administration of a gaseous anaesthetic. In toucans the nares are oval slits placed transversely at the caudal end of the large bill and partially covered by feathers. In the Procellariidae (i.e. the tubenoses or petrels and the fulmar) they are at the rostral end of a small tube which runs along the dorsal aspect of the upper bill. In parrots the external nares are circular holes in the cere. In gulls and cranes the external nares are placed approximately half way along the upper bill and pierce this structure. The gannets (Sulidae) do not have any external nares and breathe through a gap in the corner of the mouth. In kiwis the nostril is on the tip of the long probing beak which the bird uses to smell out its food. Also the surface of the caudal conchal cartilage, which is primarily concerned with olfaction, is extensively increased in conjunction with greatly developed olfactory bulbs in the brain. The sense of smell is also well developed in storm petrels (members of the Procellariidae or tubenoses) which can navigate by smell back to their nesting burrow in darkness. The South American black vulture (*Coragyps atratus*) also uses smell to locate carrion hidden below the tree canopy of the tropical rain forest. In contrast the African vultures searching the open savannah depend mainly on sight to locate their food. In swifts the caudal conchal cartilage is absent as it is in some Falconides and the olfactory bulb of the brain is small.

The nasal cavity of birds in general tends to be rather long and narrow and of the three nasal conchae the middle cartilage is the largest and acts primarily as a heat exchanger and water conservation organ.

The trachea of birds shows quite a lot of variation. As already indicated in the notes on the sternum in some species it is coiled and elongated, Figs. 1.3 and 1.9. Increased length increases the resistance to air flow and increases the dead space. To overcome this disadvantage birds overall have a proportionately greater diameter trachea when compared with mammals of comparable size ($\times$ 1.3), which reduces resistance and the tidal volume is greatly increased ($\times$ 4) together with a rate of breathing which is slower than mammals ($\times \frac{1}{3}$). Very few detailed interspecific

Table 1.1 Differences in the range of normal blood chemistry values of liver enzymes in apparently healthy parrots.

Species	Number of individual birds data based on	Blood chemistry values					
		ASAT (aspartate aminotransferase) (IU/l)	ALAT (alanine aminotransferase) (IU/l)	GGT (gamma glutamyl transferase) (IU/l)	LDH (lactate dehydrogenase) (IU/l)	CPK (creatinine phosphokinase) (IU/l)	Bile acids (µmol/l)
African grey (*Psittacus erithacus*)	103	54–155	12–59	1–3.8	147–384	123–875	18–71
Amazon (*Amazona* sp.)	99	57–194	19–98	1–10	46–208	45–565	19–144
Cockatoo (*Cacatua* sp.)	27	52–203	12–37	2–5	203–442	34–204	23–70
Macaw (*Ara* sp.)	16	58–206	22–105	<1–5	66–166	61–531	25–71

Because of the variation in the maximum and minimum values of the different enzymes in different genera, within this apparently fairly uniform group of parrots, there is an indication of varying liver physiology.

Clinical significance: Blood chemistry values of liver enzymes should not be relied upon as the only diagnostic indication of a hepatopathy particularly if the data has not been recorded for a particular genus or species. This information is based on the work of Lumeij and Overduin (1990).

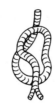

(a) Seen in spoonbills (*Platalea spp.*) and also in the demoiselle crane (*Anthropoides virgo*).
The coils are situated in the thoracic inlet.

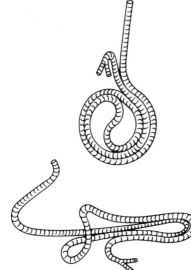

Some species of the birds of paradise for example:

(b) The trumpet bird (*Phonygammus keraudrenii*).
The loops are particularly long in the ♂ bird where there may be 8-9 loops. The trachea can be x21 the length compared with a bird having a more normal length trachea and of comparable body size.

(c) Magpie goose (*Anseranus semipalmata*)
The loop lies between the pectoral muscle and the skin and may reach the cloaca.

Species not illustrated here but which have looped trachea:

The capercaille (*Tetrao urogallus*)

Cracidae (butcher-birds, i.e. crow like found in Australia and New Guinea)

The ♂ *Crax* species (i.e. curassows) trachea extends well into abdomen.

The ♀ painted snipe (*Rostratula benghalensis*).

Guttera species (i.e. crested guinea fowl). Short loops of trachea fit into a hollow cup in the furcula.

The yellow-billed stork (*Ibis ibis*)

Fig. 1.9 The extraordinary shapes of the looped trachea which occur in some species of birds. (Redrawn after King and McLelland, 1989, by permission of Academic Press Limited London.)

In species where the trachea is looped this may only be seen in ♂ birds or if in both ♂ & ♀ it is often more marked in the ♂. It doesn't develop until adulthood and probably has an acoustic function to lower the pitch of the sound of the voice. An elongated trachea may provide an increased area for respiratory evaporative loss.

Clinical significance:

May become important if respiratory rates and tidal volume are gravely depressed during deep anaesthesia when more frequent mechanical ventilation may be required. Also important in the interpretation of radiographs.

physiological measurements have been made but some of those which have been determined are shown in Table 1.2.

In penguins the trachea is divided into left and right segments by a medial cartilaginous septum which also occurs in some Procellariiformes. In hummingbirds the trachea divides into the two primary bronchi in the mid cervical region and in the roseate spoonbill (*Ajaja ajaja*) this division occurs in the caudal two-thirds of the neck. In the male ruddy duck (*Oxyura jamaicensis*) and in both male and female emu (*Dromaius novae-hollandiae*) there is an inflatable tracheal diverticulum. All these facts may be important in correctly interpreting radiographs.

Table 1.2 Diversity in some data on the respiratory system in three different types of bird.

	Starling (*Sturnus vulgaris*)		Pigeon (*Columba livia*)		Black duck (*Anas rubripes*)	
	Rest	Flight	Rest	Flight	Rest	Flight
Body mass (g)	78		380		1026	
Respiratory frequency (min^{-1})	92	180	26	487	27	158
Tidal volume (ml)	0.67	2.80	7.2	6.0	30.2	71.0
Dead space volume (ml)	0.22		2.2		6.4	
Minute volumes (ml)	61.64	504	187.2	2922.0	815.4	11,218

Note: The respiratory frequency at rest is not related to body mass. In small passerines depression of the respiratory frequency, which is often caused by anaesthetic drugs, may be of more concern than in the larger species.

The above information is extracted from King and McLelland, 1989, by permission of Academic Press Limited London. This reference contains a mass of information on respiratory physiology of birds but unfortunately only on a very limited number of species.

The syrinx

Amongst birds as a whole the syrinx shows considerable diversity. Few anatomical structures can have received so much study primarily as an aid to taxonomy and because of the interest in vocalisation and bird song. However an attempt at a logical analysis of this structure's function has often only resulted in greater confusion.

Many male ducks (subfamily Anatidae) exhibit an ossified dilation on the side of the syrinx called the syringual bulba. Again among this group of birds there is some interspecies variation in this structure. This structure can often be seen on radiographs.

The lungs

In most species these extend from the rib carried on the last vertebrae to the cranial border of the ilium. However in the storks, geese and hoatzin it reaches almost to the level of the hip. This results more from the relative increased size of the parts of the skeleton rather than from an actual increase in the size of the lung. The lung is divided into paleopulmo and neopulmo (this part forms 20–25% of the lungs of the more evolutionary advanced birds). The paleopulmo, which allows a continuous unidirectional flow of air through its parabronchii, is considered to be phylogentically the most primitive area of the avian lung and is present in all species. The neopulmo is progressively developed and gradually expands over the dorsal and cranial aspects of the paleopulmo starting on the ventral lateral area of this primordial lung. In penguins the neopulmo is entirely absent so that the whole lung is more triangular in outline than in other species. The neopulmo is minimally developed in the storks and in the emu. It is poorly developed in buzzards, ducks, owls, gulls, cormorants, auks and cranes. In most other orders of birds it is quite well developed including Galliformes, pigeons and Passeriformes. Quite how the neopulmo differs in physiological function from that of the paleopulmo is not clear except that the parabronchii appear to be arranged more in a network than in strict lineal order as in the paleopulmo so that the airflow may not be entirely unidirectional.

The air sacs

These vary considerably in number and size in different orders of birds. Storks have the largest number with each caudal thoracic air sac subdivided into two parts. In song birds the cranial thoracic air sacs are fused into a single large median clavicular air sac. In hummingbirds the caudal thoracic air sac is proportionately larger than in all other species of birds.

The cervical air sac extends up the neck via the tubular extensions running one on each side of the cervical vertebrae with one diverticulum inside the neural canal and another externally running through the transverse foraminae (formed by the head and tubercle of the vestigial rib). In parrots a clinical condition occurs with hyperinflation of this cervicocephalic air sac which has not been seen in other birds. Possibly this structure is more developed in the parrots and it extends round the caudal part of the cranium and connects with the postorbital diverticulum of the infraorbital sinus.

The medullary cavity of some bones of the skeleton (the sternum, the scapula, humerus, femur, pelvis, cervical and thoracic vertebrae) are pneumonised by diverticulate from the air sacs. However in swallows, swifts and some other small birds pneumonisation is minimal. In hummingbirds it is absent. In some aquatic and diving birds including diving ducks, cormorants, loons, rails and penguins pneumonisation of the skeleton is also poor or absent. This may be related to reducing the buoyancy of the bird when diving.

THE FEMALE REPRODUCTIVE SYSTEM

Basic anatomy and physiology is the same for all species. Most species have a left ovary and a left oviduct. However in some species covering some 16 orders of birds among which are the Falconides (i.e. eagles, hawks, buzzards, falcons and the Old World vultures) and also the Cathartinae (the New World vultures) there are both right and left ovaries and also two oviducts. Nevertheless the right oviduct *may* be vestigial and non-functional, occasionally becoming pathologically cyst like. Technicians artificially inseminating birds only recognise the left oviduct but fertility rates do not seem to be affected. In kiwis there are right and left ovaries but only one oviduct with a very large infundibulum extending across the whole body which collects ova from both ovaries.

Breeding maturity in birds

Japanese quail (*Coturnix japonica*) are mature and capable of breeding at 6 weeks. Most seasonal breeders are mature at 11 months and breed in their second year of life. Most medium sized parrots (e.g. Amazon parrots) do not breed until 3–4 years of age (some slightly younger). Macaws are usually at least 5 years old before they breed, while the albatrosses (Diomedeidae) are 8 years of age before reaching maturity.

The number of eggs laid

In general the larger birds lay one egg (e.g. bustards, petrels, gannets, the albatross). However some ostriches may lay up to 48 eggs in a clutch. In general tropical birds tend to lay fewer eggs because when the eggs hatch the birds have fewer daylight hours in which to feed the chicks (i.e. approx 12 hours daylight only). Birds in the more northern or southern temperate seasonal climates lay more eggs and in fact the higher the latitude the longer the daylight hours and the more eggs are laid even among the same species (e.g. European robin (*Erithacus rubecula*).

Some species (e.g. the red jungle fowl from which domestic poultry are derived) are *indeterminate layers*, i.e. they go on laying eggs particularly if the eggs are removed from the nest. A domestic hen is recorded to have laid 352 eggs in a year. However some hens do become 'broody' and stop laying long before this. The yellow shafted flicker (*Colaptes auratus*) has been recorded to have laid 71 eggs and the wryneck (*Jynx torquilla*) has laid 62 eggs. Captive cockatiels (*Nymphicus hollandicus*) sometimes lay large numbers of eggs (up to 80) but this is pathological because they are determinate layers. *Determinate layers* lay clutches of a fixed number of eggs, usually four. Such birds are budgerigars (*Melopsittacus undulatus*), the common crow (*Corvus corone corone*), the magpie (*Pica pica*) and the barn swallow (*Hirundo rustica*). Most birds lay one clutch of eggs a year but some species such as some albatrosses and penguins lay in alternate years. The interval between individual eggs laid in a clutch varies. Usually it is one egg every 24 hours but the eggs will all hatch at the same time. In raptors (e.g. the goshawk (*Accipiter gentilis*)) the eggs are laid at 48 hour intervals and the chicks are also 48 hours apart in age. In the Andean condor (*Vultur gryphus*) the eggs (1–3) are laid 4–5 days apart. In the brown kiwi (*Apteryx australis*) this interval can range from 11 to 57 days. With the exception of the raptors where the age and size of chicks in a clutch are noticeably different, in most clutches of eggs the chicks all hatch at the same time, because they are able to communicate with each other while still in the shell and so synchronise piping times. Pipping or the initial breaking of the shell is usually accomplished by the egg tooth on the dorsal surface of the upper bill but in the ostrich the thick shell (up to 2 mm) is broken by the arching of the powerful complexus muscle which overlies the base of the skull and cranial end of the neck.

The size, colour and shape of the eggs vary considerably between species. What is not generally appreciated is that the texture of the shell surface also varies. Because of this the porosity of the shell varies and this influences the rate at which water is lost during incubation. In cormorants the egg shell surface is chalky, in the flamingo it is powdery, both surfaces being relatively porous and allowing high rates of water vapour exchange in the microclimate of relatively high humidity in which the eggs hatch. Eggs from the same species (e.g. ostrich) laid at the same time but by different individual birds may need to be sorted into batches according to their egg shell appearance before being artificially incubated. The relative humidity of the incubator will need adjusting to suit the egg shell texture of a particular batch. Variation in egg shell texture among farmed ostrich is due to this 'domesticated' bird being derived from a number of original sub-species.

THE MALE REPRODUCTIVE SYSTEM

The most important variations are in the presence or absence of a phallus. Two main types occur.

(1) The intromittent (or protruding) form found in ratites, tinamous, kiwis and Anseriformes (ducks, geese and swans).

(2) The non-intromittent type seen in the domestic fowl and turkey and in some Passeriformes (the Emberizinae).

In type (1) during the resting position the phallus lies on the floor of the cloaca and becomes erected by lymphatic engorgement from left and right lymphatic bodies. Semen is conveyed in an external channel, the phallic sulcus. In the emu, cassowaries, rheas and Anseriformes but not the ostrich, the phallus is filled with a blind ended long hollow tube which when at rest is inverted like the finger of a glove. During erection, also by lymphatic engorgement, the tip of this inversion is protruded. Since the left lymphatic body is much larger than the right, the erected phallus has a spiral twist.

In the non-intromittent phallus (type (2)) there are two lateral folds (the lymphatic phallic bodies) on the ventral lip of the vent. Between these lateral bodies lies a smaller medium body. During ejaculation, which occurs very rapidly, the lymphatic bodies become momentarily engorged with lymph causing the ventral lip of the vent to protrude which is then rapidly applied to the protruding oviduct of the female. Semen is channelled in the groove formed between the two lateral lymphatic bodies.

A third type (3), somewhat intermediate, occurs in vasa parrots (*Coracopsis vasa* and *C. nigra*). In this type the everted and swollen fleshy bag-like protrusion from the male's cloaca is inserted into the relatively large opening of the female's stretched and expanded cloaca. Male and female may remain locked in copulation for up to 100 minutes (Wilkinson and Birkhead, 1995). The cloacal protrusion in the male greater vasa parrot (*C. vasa*) was estimated to be 50–55 mm long by 40–45 mm wide and was freely everted or withdrawn during the breeding season, whether the male was about to mount the female or not. In these circumstances this structure should not be mistaken by the clinician as a pathological prolapse. Although not documented because insufficient research has been carried out, it is possible that phalluses of types (2) and (3) may occur in other species, although tumescence and detumescence may occur so rapidly as to be not practically observable. In all cases if surgery such as partial wedged shaped cloacaltectomy for the resolution of persistent cloacal prolapse is carried out on the ventral area of the male (or female) cloaca this may result in the bird becoming infertile.

Chapter 2
Clinical Examination

HISTORY

Before starting to examine the bird in detail it is important to obtain from the owner as much information as possible. Particular attention should be paid to the following questions:

- What has the owner noticed wrong with the bird? Falconers will often notice a change in a hawk's performance which may be an early sign of disease.
- Are there any other birds kept by the owner and have any of them been ill or died?
- Has the owner bought in any other birds recently?
- How long has the patient been in the owner's possession?
- Has the bird been ill before and has it had any treatment?
- Have there been any changes in the environment which may have put it under stress? Some individuals within a species are more highly strung and therefore more easily distressed than others.
- Has the owner changed the food or bought in a new supply?
- In the case of raptors, was the food fresh? If the food was stored in a deep-freeze was it properly defrosted? Falconers feed their hawks with meat from a canvas bag. This should have a separate, easily cleaned plastic lining. Some falconers become careless and the meat becomes contaminated from a dirty bag. Ask if the droppings (called mutes by falconers) have changed in character.

Other relevant questions will occur to the experienced clinician and the answers should be sought from the client. However, owners vary greatly in their powers of observation and the practitioner may find it rewarding to hospitalise the avian patient so that a more accurate observation can be carried out.

EXAMINATION OF THE CAGE OR SURROUNDINGS

The character of the droppings

Always try to examine some fresh droppings. When the client makes the initial inquiry on the telephone tell them not to clean the cage out before coming to the surgery.

The cloacal excreta usually consist of a dark-coloured central part (from the rectum) and an off-white surrounding portion consisting mainly of urate crystals and also a little clear fluid both from the kidneys. This clear fluid can be collected and tested for specific gravity and the presence of glucose. A tentative diagnosis of diabetes mellitus should be confirmed by blood glucose estimation. For other causes of polydipsia/polyuria see Appendix 9. The consistency and to some extent the colour of the droppings vary with the species and the diet of the bird. Fruit eaters, such as mynahs and starlings, have rather fluid droppings. Even parrots, which normally feed on a seed diet, will develop more fluid droppings if fed with a lot of fruit. On the other hand, geese have a more bulky and rather more formed stool. It is therefore important that the practitioner is familiar with what is normal for each species.

As to be expected in birds with enteritis, the dark, central part of the droppings becomes more fluid; the reverse is true in constipation. An absence of the faecal fraction may be caused by worm impaction (usually ascarids) or by egg binding. In gross worm infestation the bird is thin but often quite bright and eating well whereas an egg bound female is usually dull and anorexic. In contrast in the anorexic bird or one with reduced appetite due to disease other than an enteropathy, the central (faecal) part of the droppings tends to be of a more fluid greenish nature. Birds with pancreatic disease show excessive droppings that are buff grey in colour and waxy in texture (e.g. paramyxo virus in *Neophema* parakeets). Test these for starch with Lugol's iodine. Excessive or decreased urate crystals indicate a renal problem. Urates which are suspicious, of an orange or yellow colour, indicate a biliverdinuria caused by a hepatopathy (be suspicious of *Chlamydia* infection, Appendix 3). Undigested seed or grit in the droppings is always abnormal and indicates a malfunction of the gizzard. Blood in the droppings may come from the rectum, the cloaca, the oviduct or the ureters. Try to decide if this blood is in the faecal or urate fraction. This may indicate ulceration, possibly involving a neoplasm. Sharp foreign bodies, such as pieces of metal, can be ingested and can reach the rectum in some birds such as ducks.

Blood in the cage

Blood spattered round the cage may have come from the cloacal orifice or it may be from an injury to the wings, feet, beak or body. If the blood is widely spread, it is probably from wing trauma, possibly a damaged growing feather.

Regurgitation

With small birds, examine the cage bars, perches, mirrors and other cage furniture for any evidence of adherent small flecks of white material. This may be evidence of regurgitation. Regurgitation is normal courtship behaviour in the male budgerigar. The young are fed in this manner also. However, this normal behaviour can develop into a pathological neurosis and the bird will sometimes even attempt to feed its owner.

Raptors daily produce pellets or castings formed in the gizzard composed of the undigested parts of the diet (skeletal tissues, feathers, fur, etc.). The colour of the castings will depend on the diet but they should be of a crumbly, almost dry texture and have no offensive smell. Liquid or putty-like castings or those with blood or excessive mucus are abnormal. Many other species of birds such as thrushes (Turdidae), crows (Corvidae) and herons (Ardeidae) sometimes produce pellets. Although doubted by some authorities from the author's clinical observations true vomiting occurs in many species of birds and is always a sign of disease.

Other observations to be made on the cage

In the case of seed-eating birds, note whether the seed is being dehusked or simply being scooped out of the feeding dish and on to the floor.

In the case of psittacines note whether the perches or any of the toys are being chewed. The clinician should also observe if there is any sign of rust on the cage structure and see if the paper on the floor of the cage is being chewed.

With a magnifying lens it may be possible to see signs of parasitic mites on the cage fittings. These appear as minute black, red, orange or greyish-white specks, which are seen to move. Some mites hide in cracks and crevices and emerge to feed on the bird at night, so they are best seen with a torch in a dark room or when the electric light is switched on suddenly.

OBSERVATION OF THE PATIENT

If an experienced aviculturist or falconer brings you a bird and says that it is ill, even if you cannot see anything abnormal, the chances are that the bird has something wrong with it. The changes that take place in a bird from one that is completely healthy to one in the early stages of illness are so subtle that it takes an experienced observer to notice them. The problem with most sick birds is that usually by the time someone realises that they are ill, they are very ill. The bird should have a full- rounded, bright eye, with no sign of the membrana nictitans. An eye which is slightly oval means that the bird is not fully alert. Any bird that spends all its time huddled in the bottom of the cage, taking no notice of an observer, is near death.

The plumage of the bird should be sleek and lie flat over the body. If all the body feathers are ruffled, the bird is trying to conserve heat.

Breathing abnormalities

A bird that is obviously dyspnoeic with its mouth open and gasping, may not necessarily have a respiratory condition, but is certainly very ill. Mouth breathing in birds is seen in parrots with blocked nares. These birds may also sneeze. However, geese in flight normally mouth breathe. Tail bobbing in small birds is also a sign of an impaired respiratory system. In both these types of abnormal breathing, a space-occupying lesion of the abdomen may prevent the full expansion and contraction of the posterior air sacs, so that air flow through the lungs is considerably reduced. Cyanosis is sometimes indicated by a blue coloration of the beak and legs. If the part of the neck in the region of the crop slightly inflates with each expiration but breathing is otherwise normal, this may indicate some obstruction of the outlet ostia of the anterior air sacs where these connect with the secondary bronchi. On post-mortem a bird may show gross abscessation of the coelom and yet in life not show any respiratory signs, which indicates the importance of radiography in the initial general examination. A change in the voice, which becomes more harsh, or a change in pitch in the sound from a raptor or parrot could indicate a problem with the syrinx. Hypovitaminosis A with or without secondary bacterial infection and abscessation involving the tissue of the syrinx could be responsible for these signs. A partial blockage of the main airway, particularly the syrinx with a plug of inspissated pus is often an acute and desperate condition particularly in the African grey parrot. Immediate relief by cannulation of the abdominal air sac is imperative (see page 162). Falconers talk of 'kecks' and 'snits' (sneezing) in their birds. An incessant and often irritating high-pitched squeak in the budgerigar is sometimes due to pressure of the enlarged thyroid on the syrinx. This is initiated by an iodine deficiency and a consequent hypothyroidism. A hypothyroidism may also be brought about by suppression of the thyroid gland after prolonged use of thyroid extract subsequent to a misdiagnosis. Clicking or asthmatical noises, which may be almost imperceptible unless carefully listened for, can be caused by viral, bacterial, fungal or yeast infection of the respiratory tract or by the nematode, *Syngamus trachea*, which affects many species of birds. In the latter case, obstruction of the airflow in the trachea is enough to cause gaping typical of the disease.

A change of voice in a bird always indicates a pathological condition of the syrinx and therefore prognosis is much more serious. This contrasts with the situation in the mammal where a change in voice indicates an upper respiratory condition and the outlook is more favourable.

Central nervous system signs

Birds may show any of the following signs: torticollis, opisthotonus, ataxia, circling, paralysis and clonic spasms or fits. All these may be caused by deficiency of B or E vitamins, infectious disease, poisoning, concussion, cerebral vascular disturbances and tumours. A falconer may decide to change the diet, e.g. from dead hatchery chicks to quail. The bird may refuse to eat, which in a thin bird (kept near its so-called 'flying weight') may lead to the acute onset of hypoglycaemia. Such birds may appear 'drunk' or may appear asleep or even dead. Tube feeding these birds with glucose or administration i.v. often leads to a dramatic recovery.

Hypocalcaemia is a well recognised condition in African grey parrots (Rosskopf and Woerpel, 1984). This sometimes starts with a bird which is anorexic and lethargic and progresses to violent seizures. However, some of these birds appear perfectly normal between fits. Confirmation of diagnosis in both hypoglycaemia and hypocalcaemia can be obtained by blood analysis. For the differential diagnosis of fits see Appendix 9.

It is not uncommon for a budgerigar to be presented with the acute onset of a variety of the above signs. Making a specific diagnosis is difficult and the prognosis is always grave. Thrombosis is said by Hasholt (1969) to be uncommon in birds, but atheromata are recorded from a range of species. Hasholt (1969) records the cases of arteriosclerosis of the carotid arteries in three old Amazon parrots. This was believed to have resulted in cerebral ischaemia because the birds kept falling off their perches. Pituitary neoplasia is recorded in a number of species resulting in CNS signs (see pp. 111 and 362).

In diurnal raptors hypocalcaemia and hypoglycaemia are both common causes of fits. Most important among the infectious diseases causing nervous signs is Newcastle disease, which affects all species. The variant of this organism, Paramyxovirus (PMV1), causes nervous signs in pigeons both domestic and feral and some psittacine species, see Appendix 3.

A rhythmic swinging of the head from side to side, particularly in owls, is indicative of vestibular disease and is equivalent to nystagmus in mammals. A flaccid paralysis with an inability to hold the neck up ('limber neck') is seen in botulism and lead poisoning, particularly in swans but also in other birds (Borland et al., 1977). Folic acid deficiency can also cause paralysis of the neck in turkey poults. Bilateral or unilateral paralysis or paresis of the legs may be caused by nephropathy resulting in compression of the lumbosacral plexus, or by Marek's disease (p. 297) or sarcoma/leucosis virus (p. 299).

Wing injuries

A dropped wing may be due to nerve paralysis but is most likely to be due to injury to the bones or muscles. Some idea of the part of the wing that is damaged can be gained from observing exactly how the wing is held. If the injury lies between the digits and the middle of the radius and ulna, the primary feathers are usually trailing on the ground (Fig. 2.1a). Injury to the elbow or the humerus very often results in the wing being held lower than that on the normal side but the primary feathers are held up off the floor (Fig. 2.1b). Injury to the coracoid or shoulder joint causes the wing to be rotated so that, although the whole wing is lower, the primaries are above the level of those on the opposing side (Fig. 2.1c).

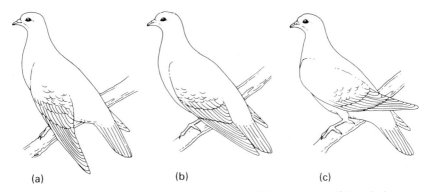

(a)   (b)   (c)

Fig. 2.1 How the wing is held after injury to different parts of the skeleton.

Since there is considerable interspecies variation in the relative lengths of the different sections of the wing and, consequently, variation in the weight of these parts, the signs will not only depend on the nature of the injury (bone, muscle or nerve) but on the species of bird involved. Small birds in particular may sustain quite serious fractures of the wing bones and still look quite normal. An accurate diagnosis can only be made by a detailed inspection and by radiography.

HANDLING BIRDS

Before attempting this in the case of a small and obviously sick bird, it is wise to warn the owner that there is a risk that the bird may suddenly die of heart failure when an attempt is made to catch it. This can occur with apparently healthy birds not used to being handled.

To reduce this risk, the task can be carried out in a dark room using the light from a torch covered with a red filter or in even more cases using blue filtered light. In many species of birds vision is severely restricted at the blue end of the spectrum. In many cases it is then possible to pick the bird straight from its perch. However, some birds see better in subdued light than others.

When handling the larger birds care should be taken to control the feet of raptors, which have a powerful grip, and also to watch the beaks of the larger parrots which can cause a severe biting injury. Small raptors can strike out rapidly with their feet. A hawk which is hooded is often easier to handle, although some falconers are reluctant to use a hood. Hooding any bird of prey (trained or wild) usually has a sedating effect and the use of a towel or even the cut corner of a large brown paper envelope placed over the head is quite effective.

Birds such as herons (Ardeidae), storks (Ciconiidae), rails (Rallidae), gulls (Laridae) and gannets (Sulidae) can use their beaks as stabbing weapons. Cormorants (Phalacrocoracidae) can attack with the hooked end of the beak.

In all these cases a strong pair of welders or industrial gloves is invaluable. Tamed raptors and parrots can be handled without gloves if the bird is used to being handled, but the clinician would be well advised not to take any chances. For catching and handling parrots (but not macaws or large cockatoos) a small hand towel draped over the out-stretched hand is useful. A padded net with a short handle can sometimes be very useful for catching escapees in a room. For catching swans and other large waterfowl a long-handled crook is sometimes used and for controlling these birds a wrap-round cloth of nylon or other tough material with quick fastening Velcro is very useful.

All the large birds are best cast on a cushion or soft surface before examination. The wings need to be held gently but firmly to the body with no undue pressure placed on the thorax.

PHYSICAL EXAMINATION OF THE RESTRAINED BIRD

In a bird that is not too ill, the clinician might find it easier to carry out a more thorough examination if the bird is under moderately deep sedation or light anaesthesia. Refer to the section on anaesthesia.

Feathers and plumage

The plumage should be of a good, even, dense colour. Barbules should lock together so that the feathering gives a uniform outline to the body form. In the normal bird only the axillae are sparsely covered in feathers. If the areas of skin covering the lumbosacral and sternal regions are thinly covered or are covered in an abnormal greyish fluff instead of the usual contour feathers, the cause may be of nutritional or endocrine origin, e.g. thyroid. Progressive feather loss with a typical white, flaky, but thickened skin may be due to ringworm (*Trichophyton* spp.) infection, particularly if this is seen around the head and neck. In poultry a zinc deficiency has caused dermatitis and failure of feather growth. Sometimes, particularly in parrots, there may be evidence of self-trauma. In this case, apart from skin wounds, the vane of the flight feathers may be chewed or the shaft may be crushed (as distinct from snapped or broken off). Some of the growing feathers may have been plucked leaving bleeding follicles. Plucked feathers are usually replaced quickly and new feathers can be seen emerging. In some cases the lesion may be localised suggesting a subcutaneous or deeper painful lesion. Examine these new feathers to see if they are short and club-shaped. See if they have a circumferential constriction or are curled or deformed. Any of these signs may indicate a viral infection causing psittacine beak and feather dystrophy (see p. 312) or a nutrient deficiency. Self-mutilation may be due to frustration or boredom or stress brought on by isolation (parrots are birds which normally live in flocks) or a change in routine or initiated by over-preening during the breeding season. A cardinal sign of the self-plucking bird is usually while any of the other plumage is damaged, that on the head is normal. Sometimes self-trauma may have been initiated by the handler savagely cutting growing flight feathers to stop the bird flying. It may also be initiated by parasitic infection. Mite infestation may lead to invasion of the feather follicle and damage and loss of the feather. Both mites and lice can cause irritation. A careful search of the plumage will show any lice situated along the feather shaft or on the skin surface. Healthy birds groom themselves to keep infestation in check, sick birds do not. Examination of the skin or of the powdery remains of a feather shaft with a magnifying lens will be necessary to identify any mites present. The initiating cause of self-feather-damage may have been eliminated but the habit becomes established and it is difficult to break. Use may have to be made of Elizabethan collars or human antidepressant drugs (see page 277). Feather picking or even more severe injury by an incompatible or dominant cage mate is not uncommon. This may be worse during the breeding season.

Malformed and curled flight feathers or those without proper vane formation are usually the result of faulty nutrition (inadequate essential amino acids or vitamin deficiency), but may also be the result of chewing by lice or other infection. In parrots the yellowing of green feathers may be due to a deficiency of the amino acid lysine. Feathers that are frayed or have the shaft cleanly broken or snapped off are the result of careless handling or inadequate caging. In the budgerigar and some other psitti-cines the condition called french moult, in which fledglings lose some of their primary wing and tail feathers, has been shown to be due principally to two viral infections (see pp. 312 and 313). Some original work by Pass and Perry (1984) on wild Australian cockatoos and by others more recently indicates this may be one of a number of viral infections affecting many species of psittacines. The condition described by Pass and Perry was originally called cockatoo beak and feather syndrome but is now known to infect many species and so is known as psittacine beak and feather syndrome. In these cases the emerging feather is club shaped and does not open up properly. Feathers are not moulted normally and the bird's whole plumage including the head is very unkempt. Large areas become devoid of feathers. The beak looks abnormally shiny in cockatoos due to lack of powder and has a tendency to accelerated growth. In cockatoos skin pigmentation is subtly increased but in lovebirds (*Agapornis*) the skin coloration remains normal. In all cases there is pruritis. In the black vasa parrots (*Coracopsis* sp.) the normal black feathers pro-gressively become white and this is thought to be due to the same virus. In all the above mentioned cases the condition is eventually fatal (see Appendix 3).

The minute structure of feathers may be permanently damaged after contamination with mineral oil, even after this has been completely removed. The barbules may not hook together properly. In aquatic birds where integrity of the feather covering is incomplete due to barbule damage, inability to preen due to beak damage or with disease of the preen gland, the bird may not be able to float properly in water. A well recognised condition known as 'wet feather' of ducks has the same effect. The aetiology is obscure. Lines of decreased density and weakness across the vane of the feather, known variously as 'fret', 'hunger' or 'stress' marks, are recognised by falconers but are also seen in other birds. These are believed to be caused by a check in growth of the proliferating cells of the epidermal papilla during the formation of the feather in its follicle and may be accompanied by other feather defects. Moulting or feather replacement takes place in most birds at well defined intervals – once, twice or three times a year. In a few species such as cranes and eagles moulting may be every two years. However, in parrots the process is continuous. Nutritional or infectious conditions that cause feather abnormalities often have similar effects on the germinative cells of the beak and claws.

Occasionally a developing feather will fail to emerge properly from the feather sheath. The follicle continues to enlarge pushing its way below the surface of the skin and a feather cyst is formed – a condition most com-monly seen in canaries but also seen in other breeds. The cyst is often associated with an inflammatory condition of the skin and causes marked irritation to the bird, so that the bird picks at the cyst and may rupture it.

Tick bites can sometimes be responsible for subcutaneous oedema and haemorrhage and result in acute death (Forbes and Simpson, 1993).

The head region

After detailed examination of the plumage it is best to continue with an examination of the head region starting with the eye.

The eye

The observer may see a variety of conditions. Keratitis, oedema of the eyelids and blepharospasm due to a foreign body are relatively common. Matting of the feathers around the eye can be evidence of epiphora which may be unilateral or bilateral. If bilateral, this could be due to lesions blocking the opening of the nasolacrimal ducts, where they are situated close together in the posterior part of the choanal opening (Plate 5). Swellings just above or below the eye may be evidence of sinusitis of the supraorbital and infraorbital sinuses which may have progressed to abscessation. These are often initiated by hypovitaminosis A. Brown, crusty eruptions around the eyelids and commissures of the beak may be due to avian pox. In budgerigars the powdery white encrustations of cnemidocoptic mange mite infestation may extend from the cere to the areas around the eye and the commissures of the beak. This may also be seen in other species. Retrobulbar neoplasms of the orbit and tumours of the nictitating membrane have been recorded. Examination of the anterior chamber of the eye may reveal evidence of hypopyon, or hyphaema, or damage of the iris. Fluorescein should be instilled on to the surface of the cornea to detect any scars or ulcers. All these lesions are not uncommon, particularly in owls, and may be due to fighting or to road traffic accidents. Also they may be a sign of systemic infection, e.g. Picornavirus (p. 308; see also Plate 3).

Examination of the eye reflexes is generally difficult but is somewhat easier in raptors, because of the proportionately larger-sized eyes. The pupillary light response is difficult to elicit, because the muscle of the iris is striated and partially under voluntary control. It is also affected by emotional disturbance of the bird. A rapid pupillary light reflex indicates central blindness because conscious control may have been removed due to damage to the brain. Pupils may be widely dilated after concussion resulting from an accident. Consensual pupillary light reflexes do not take place in birds because all optic nerve fibres completely cross over at the optic chiasma and representation on the cortex of the optic tectum is contralateral. Touching the cornea produces a pupillary response and a consensual response is shown in the other eye. If a bird is not too frightened, it will sometimes show a fixation reflex towards an interesting object. This can be shown by using food (for a raptor) or a glittering object (for a corvid) moved from side to side in front of the eyes.

A blink reflex of the eyelids or nictitating membrane reflex may be stimulated by a threatening gesture. This should preferably be carried out from behind a transparent screen.

Cataracts are not uncommon and can be seen with or sometimes without an ophthalmoscope. Examination of the posterior chamber with the ophthalmascope is less rewarding. There is no reflective tapetum in birds. The optic disc is obscured by the large vascular projectory of the choroid, known as the pecten. The shape and size of this structure varies in the different species. The retina appears as a uniform granular tissue usually grey or brownish red in colour. Hyper-reflectivity and synchisis scintillans is reported by Greenwood and Barnett (1980) in a wild tawny owl. (Note use of vercuronium to examine eye, p. 269.)

For a more detailed discussion of the functional normality of the avian eye the reader should refer to Greenwood and Barnett (1980). Another useful reference is Lawton (1996) which has an extensive bibliography. Many systemic infectious diseases, for instance, those due to *Chlamydia*, *Salmonella*, mycobacteria and a variety of viruses including the paramyxoviruses are manifested by ocular lesions. These may include epiphora, conjunctivitis, keratitis and iridocyclitis. Conjunctival oedema has been reported as a sign of plasmodia infection in over 40 species of birds.

The ear

This is not obvious in birds since there is no pinna. In most birds the external orifice is covered by modified contour feathers. In owls the ears are large and placed asymetrically, a condition which improves directional sensitivity. Because of its nearness to the eye, the ear may be involved in trauma affecting the eye. Attention is drawn to otitis externa by the feathers being matted around the external ear. Small (1969) reports the protrusion of the tympanic membrane through the external orifice but this is a rare condition.

The skin of the head

This should be examined for any sign of subcutaneous haemorrhage due to accidents or wounds that may be caused by fighting.

The cere and external nares

Look for any discharges which may vary from catarrhal to dried exudate. Nasal exudate is often due to hypovitaminosis A and superimposed microbial infection. This is an indication of upper respiratory disease. Swabs should be obtained for microbiology and antibiotic sensitivity testing. A more representative specimen can be obtained from the choanal slit where there are often associated abscesses. Staining of the feathers above the cere is evidence of nasal discharge. This may be blood stained. Excess growth of the cornified tissue of the cere, a condition often seen in budgerigars and called brown hypertrophy is of no clinical significance unless the nares become blocked (Fig. 2.2).

In the male pigeon there may be a similar exuberant growth of the cere. In the budgerigar, the cere is pink in the immature bird, blue in the male and brown or buff-coloured in the female. Birds that show some blue and brown colouring may be intersexes with both one ovary and one testes present in the abdomen. Reversal of colour may indicate chronic illness.

Knemidocoptic mange infection is not uncommon in budgerigars and can affect other species. It is shown by a greyish, scabby, crumbling texture of the cere often accompanied by excrescences around the commissures of the beak and the eye. The burrowing tracts of the mite can sometimes be seen in the horn of the beak. Associated lesions are sometimes found on the scaley part of the leg. The debris shed from these lesions contributes to the dust of breeders' bird rooms and helps in the maintenance of a high incidence of this condition. Diagnosis can be confirmed by scraping the lesion. After clearing the scrapings with 10% potassium hydroxide, examine under a microscope. Trauma to the cere can be the result of a collision during flight or from a caged bird flying at the mesh work of its cage. Damage to this area may involve the cranial facial hinge situated between the premaxilla, nasal and frontal bones. Occasionally a neoplasm may involve this region (see Fig. 1.1).

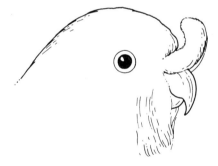

Fig. 2.2 Brown hypertrophy of the cere.

The beak

Examine the beak for any evidence of cracking or splitting, which may be a sign of underlying fractures of the premaxilla or mandible. Care should be taken when examining some birds such as gannets and some ducks in which the edges of the beaks are quite sharp. Toucans (Ramphastidae) and mergansers (*Mergus*) have a serrated edge to the beak. Cracking of the horny beak may be traumatic or a sign of vitamin A deficiency or infection. Overgrowth or distortion of the beak may be due to a neoplasma (e.g. osteosarcoma) or trauma to the proliferating epidermal cells or due to knemidocoptic mite infection. Deficiency of vitamin D, calcium, biotin and B vitamins are all said to cause abnormal beak formation (Altman, 1982). Raptors fed on an artificial diet that does not need very much tearing of the food before swallowing, can develop a marked overgrowth of the upper beak. Parrots can develop beak abnormalities brought about by wear on their cage bars by constant climbing. The beak is a constantly growing and changing structure. Some wild birds, e.g. oystercatchers (Haematopodidae) have a comparatively rapid growing beak which can develop a different shape adapting the beak to different feeding habitats. Those feeding on cockles develop a spatulate shaped beak, whilst those feeding on earthworms develop a more pointed beak (pp. 2 and 3).

The mouth and oropharynx

In aquatic birds a piece of fishing line protruding from the pharynx may be attached to a fish hook embedded lower down the alimentary canal. Diagnosis can be confirmed by radiography or by endoscope. Fish hooks may damage other birds and the author has even seen one case in a blackbird (*Turdus merula*).

To examine the mouth of a conscious powerful bird some sort of speculum may be necessary. A pair of artery forceps can be placed between the two beaks and then opened, or the speculum of a canine auroscope can be utilised.

Abscesses are seen sometimes on the surface of the tongue and small pin-point lesions of candidiasis may be observed also. Both these conditions may be brought on by vitamin A deficiency. This leads to a hyperkeratosis of the epithelium of the mucus-secreting glands (Gordon and Jordan, 1977; Jones, 1979). Abscesses may also be seen anywhere on the mucous membranes of the mouth, particularly around the choanae where they may block the nasolacrimal opening. Closer inspection of the nasal mucous membrane can be carried out by endoscope examination through the choanal space. Abscesses in the mouth may be bacterial in origin or they may be the early signs of trichomoniasis. This is seen more usually as an extensive cheese-like diphtheritic membrane covering the oropharynx and sides of the mouth. This disease occurs in a number of species but is particularly common in pigeons (Columbidae) when it is called 'canker' by pigeon owners and has also been known for many years by falconers to occur in raptors, when it is called 'frounce'. Again, hypovitaminosis A may predispose to this condition. The lesions of both trichomoniasis and candidiasis look very similar and may occasionally be confused with capillaria infection.

Avian pox lesions may be seen at the commisures of the beak, in all species particularly in Passeriformes, Columbiformes, raptors and psittacines. However, they are not seen in Anseriformes.

The glottis is a slit like opening into the larynx and trachea lying on the floor of the mouth usually just posterior to the root of the tongue. In some species such as herons (Ardeidae) it lies farther back. Neoplasms and exudative lesions can affect this area resulting in partial obstruction of the airways. Sinusitis of the infraorbital sinuses can lead to a gross swelling, filled with catarrhal exudate, on both sides of the oropharynx. This condition can be caused by mycoplasma and has been seen in a number of species including parrots (psittacines), gulls (Laridae), mynah birds (Gracula) and raptors. Cooper (1978) advocates digital examination of the mouth and oropharynx and laboratory exploration of any exudate obtained.

The neck

This should be palpated for any swelling which may indicate a foreign body impacted in the oesophagus (e.g. a bone wedge in a raptor's throat) or an impaction of the crop, which can occur in most species. A fluid swelling may be due to the condition of 'sour crop', when there may also be excessive gas present. The crop in the budgerigar may swell also due to thyroid enlargement obstructing the organ. This is sometimes accompanied by regurgitation. Neoplasia of the thyroid, although rare, may be responsible for similar symptoms (Blackmore, 1982; see also p. 161).

Many seed eating birds temporarily store seed in the crop but this should not feel hard to the touch. Gulls (Laridae), penguins (Spheniscidae) and cormorants (Phalacrocoracidae) store food in the oesophagus and can easily regurgitate this food.

Examination of the body

After the thoracic inlet at the base of the neck has been examined, the clavical and coracoid bones should be palpated for evidence of fractures. In the latter case observe how the wing is held when the bird is free standing (Fig. 2.1(c)). Skin wounds around the thoracic inlet are commonly seen in pigeons (Columbidae) as a result of collision with telegraphy wires during flight. They sometimes involve the crop and associated air sacs. Subcutaneous emphysema around the thorax may indicate a ruptured air sac, particularly rupture of the cervical or interclavicular air sacs. Ruptured air sacs often resolve spontaneously.

The condition of the pectoral muscles should be assessed by palpation. They should be symmetrical but one side may be found to have undergone atrophy, in which case the bird's flying ability will be affected. The condition of the pectoral muscles is an important guide to the overall nutritional state of the bird. The carina of the sternum can be felt but should not be very prominent. Decubitus of this region is common in heavy birds such as geese and swans that are unable to walk. Accumulation of fat and lipomas are common over this region of the pet budgerigar.

The ribs and scapulae should be carefully palpated for fractures. Auscultation of the lateral thorax or at the thoracic inlet may reveal abnormal sounds, though it may be difficult to pinpoint these. Heart murmurs are sometimes detectable in the larger birds. Cooper (1978) describes some cardiovascular conditions encountered in raptors at post-mortem.

The use of electrocardiography in birds has been described by a number of authors among which the following reports are most useful for the practitioner: Lumeij *et al.*, 1993 and 1994.

The region of the thoracic vertebrae and the syncrosacrum

These areas should be carefully examined for wounds caused by predators or fighting among cage mates. The preen (or uropygial) gland should be examined for impaction or neoplastic changes (see p. 153).

The abdomen

In the larger birds it may just be possible to palpate the tip of the liver beyond the edge of the sternum. Should the liver be easily felt it is probably enlarged. This can be confirmed by radiography or the use of ultrasound.

The ease with which the abdominal contents can be palpated will obviously depend on the size of the bird. In birds smaller than a budgerigar this is almost impossible to carry out safely without putting too much pressure on the air sacs. In some species, e.g. auks (Alcinae), there is very little room between the sternum and the pelvic bones. However, even in budgerigars it is possible to distinguish a fairly large, rather irregular neoplasm from a regular, smooth and rounded retained egg in the female. The female often has a history of laying several eggs, then has suddenly stopped and the bird is often noticeably unwell. Occasionally a solitary egg may form and cause obstruction (see p. 167).

In slightly larger birds (e.g. pigeons, *Columba livia*) the thick-walled gizzard is easily palpated as firm and globular with angular margins and its retained grit can be felt to grate between the fingers.

In raptors the full or impacted stomach can be distinguished as a rather fusiform softer-walled structure.

Softer and more fluid enlargements of the abdomen which can become quite pendulant in the perching bird, sometimes without apparent ill effect, may be due to either ascites or rupture of the abdominal muscles. Ascites can be confirmed by very careful paracentesis. This is carried out in the midline at the most pendulant part of the swelling. The ascites is often due to neoplasia of the liver or gonads. In female birds, a soft abdominal swelling may be due to an enlarged oviduct caused by salpingitis, or an impacted soft- shelled egg both of which may result in an egg peritonitis. Contrast radiography or the possible use of ultrasound can help in the differential diagnosis.

Large cyst-like swellings over the abdomen can be differentiated from true ruptures by radiography. The cloaca should be palpated. It may contain a calculus of impacted urate crystals or show a prolapse. Cooper (1978) recommends digital exploration of the cloaca in the larger bird, with a well-lubricated, gloved finger and microscopical examination of the evacuations. An auriscope speculum or endoscope inserted into the emptied cloaca can sometimes be helpful to examine the mucosa. Matting of the feathers around the cloaca together with excoriation of the surrounding skin can indicate either an alimentary or urinary problem. If the adherent mass is mainly composed of faecal material and the surrounding feathering is stained green, then the problem is probably due to diarrhoea. If the concretions are white, and especially if this is accompanied by an impacted cloaca, then the bird has a kidney problem. Since the urodeum is the posterior part of the cloaca in which the urates from the kidney and ureters collect, any impaction in this region due to a urate calculus will necessarily hold up the evacuation of faecal matter in the anterior part of the cloaca or coprodeum and the bird will become constipated. Paralysis and prolapse of the penis may occur in some ducks where two or more male ducks are kept together. This is due to bullying and damage to the nerve supply (Humphreys, P.N., 1984, personal communication). However, see duck plague, p. 297.

The body temperature of a bird can be taken via the cloaca, but since there is such a great interspecific variation as well as a normal diurnal variation in individuals, this is not especially helpful in clinical examination. The body temperature of most birds falls within the range 40–42°.

The wings

Examine each wing bone separately for any evidence of fractures, or luxations of the joints. Excessive mobility of the shoulder joint compared with the other side, together with a wing that is slightly dropped at the shoulder could indicate a rupture of the tendon of supracoracoid muscle (deep pectoral) which can be only confirmed by surgical exploration. Swellings of the bones may be due to old fractures or to tumours or infections. In pigeons (Columbidae) swellings and suppuration of the joints may be due to *Salmonella* causing a chronic arthrosynovitis (Gordon and Jordan, 1977). In raptors injury to the carpal joints may result in a bursitis (called 'blain' by falconers). Wing-tip oedema and dry gangrene in raptors has been described by a number of authors, Forbes 1991; Forbes and Harcourt-Brown 1991; Lewis, Storm and Greenwood 1993. In the opinion of Forbes, the condition is most likely caused by tethering a raptor within a metre of the ground in sub-zero temperatures at night. Forbes also suggests an unidentified virus or toxic factor may be involved.

In young birds, deformation of the bones may indicate metabolic bone disease due to calcium/phosphorus imbalance in the diet.

Waterfowl fed on a diet too high in protein (over 18%) can develop an outward rotation of the carpal joint (valgus or 'slipped wing') – the primary feathers are relatively too heavy, because they grow faster than minerals can be laid down in the bone.

The mobility of all joints should be checked and compared in the two wings. Comparison should be made of the swelling and development of the muscles for signs of atrophy. Examine the propatagial membranes, which stretch between the shoulder and carpal joints and form the leading edge of the wing when this is fully extended. These are often damaged in flight and may show evidence of scar tissue formation. This results in the wing not being fully extensible or the proximal attachment of the membrane being displaced more posteriorly. In both cases the bird's flying capability may be affected. However, some birds can still fly, but they veer off to the normal side (see Figs 1.5 and 10.1).

Feather cysts and neoplasms are commonly found in the carpal areas. They are not always easy to differentiate except by biopsy and/or surgical incision. Tumours in this area are easily damaged and may bleed profusely.

The legs and feet

Each of the bones of the leg should be examined for any evidence of fractures or luxations. This may be difficult with the femur in small birds or in such birds as auks (Alcinae) where this bone is well covered by muscle and dense feathering.

In fledgling raptors the tarsometatarsal bones are inwardly rotated in a 'hand-holding' position. As the bird grows and begins to take weight on its legs, the feet rotate outwardly to the normal position. In some young birds with metabolic bone disease this does not happen and the gastro-cnemius tendon becomes permanently displaced medially. The bird becomes a cripple. In some artificially reared waterfowl fed on a too high protein ration (i.e. over 18%) the tibial cartilage can become displaced. The bird grows too fast and becomes too heavy for the rate at which calcium and phosphorus can be incorporated into the bone of the leg. A similar condition called perosis occurs in poultry and has been seen in parrots (Smith, 1979). This is caused by manganese deficiency. This mineral activates several enzymes required for the formation of chondroitin sulphate concerned in bone growth (Butler and Laursen-Jones, 1977). The scales of the legs should be examined for any evidence of swelling, ulceration or scars caused by excoriation of identification rings. In the budgerigar, captive raptors and parrots swelling due to a tight ring can become suddenly an acute problem – restriction to the blood supply to the foot can lead to ischaemic necrosis or gangrene. The feet should be examined for any evidence of abscesses. This condition, known as 'bumblefoot', is seen in cranes, penguins, waterfowl, domestic fowl and especially in raptors; the heavier birds are at greater risk. Bumblefoot abscesses may extend as far as the hock and may erode the bones of the foot. This can be confirmed by a radiograph. Smaller birds such as budgerigars or cockatiels may show abscesses on the feet that may be difficult to distinguish from the tophi of gout due to accumulations of urate crystals.

If the suspected tophi are opened and the contents placed on a slide, confirmation that urates are present can be attained from the following test: the crystals are mixed with a drop of concentrated nitric acid and carefully evaporated to dryness over a Bunsen burner. A drop of ammonia is then added. If urates are present a mauve colour will develop.

Knemidokoptic mange mite infestation can occur on the legs of many Passeriformes, particularly crossbills (*Loxia curvirostra*) and also in other species of birds causing the nails to slough. In canaries the condition has long been called 'tassle foot' (Fig. 2.3). Although the infection is common on the head of budgerigars it is not often seen on the feet. In Passeriformes the lesions on the legs can be confused with avian pox lesions and papillomas. Claws that are overgrown through 'tassle foot' and other causes can easily become broken and bleed. Frostbite has been reported in a number of raptor species and in some aviary birds through clinging to frost-covered wire mesh.

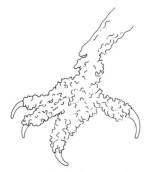

Fig. 2.3 'Tassle foot' as seen typically in canaries.

Chapter 3
Aids to Diagnosis

HAEMATOLOGY, BLOOD CHEMISTRY AND SEROLOGY EXAMINATION

The examination of blood samples is an important aid in the routine diagnosis of avian disease. The veterinary clinician having already taken into account the value of a particular case to the owner and offset this against the potential cost of the anticipated laboratory procedures, should note that one laboratory test or one radiograph by itself is usually of little diagnostic or prognostic value. Serial blood samples taken over a period of time offer a greater degree of diagnostic precision. Some suggested diagnostic routines (incorporating haematology) for the investigation of particular avian syndromes are given in Appendix 9.

The collection of blood samples

Anticoagulant and equipment

A variety of suitable paediatric tubes and micro-containers are available and can often be obtained free of charge from the laboratory which is to carry out the tests. In the opinion of most haematologists, to get the best staining results for the examination of blood cells EDTA is the most suitable anticoagulant. Heparin can sometimes affect the staining of the leucocytes. However, in some species (Corvidae, currasows, crowned cranes, hornbills and the eagle owl) EDTA can cause haemolysis of the erythrocytes so that heparin is preferred. In the opinion of Lumeij (1987, p. 10) one heparinised blood sample can be sufficient for most routine haematology and blood chemistry profiles. The author has followed this advice for the last seven years and had no problems. Nevertheless if the bird is large enough and 1.5–2 ml of blood can be harvested half the blood can be placed in a tube with anticoagulant while the other half is immediately centrifuged and the plasma used for blood chemistry examination. Usually in the smaller birds a 23–25 gauge five-eighth inch

(0.65–0.5 × 16 mm) hypodermic needle bent at a slight angle (approx. 10°) and attached to a 2-ml syringe is found to be satisfactory. The bevel of the needle point is kept uppermost. The walls of avian veins are fragile and haematoma formation easily occurs so that digital pressure should be immediately applied over the puncture site when withdrawing the needle. Too much negative pressure applied to the syringe plunger when withdrawing blood and the vein collapses onto the needle orifice and blood flow stops.

The volume of blood which can safely be collected

In birds generally the circulating blood volume is usually between 6 and 12 ml/100 g body weight (i.e. approximately 10% of body weight). In a 40 g budgerigar the total blood volume may be 2.5–3.0 ml. Consequently in a healthy bird, if a state of shock is not to ensue, 0.5 ml is the maximum volume which can safely be withdrawn from a bird of this size. In the Amazon parrot or an African grey parrot weighing 250–400 g, 2 ml of blood can safely be obtained. Overall birds can tolerate a greater degree of blood loss in relation to size than can mammals. However, splenic contraction in response to blood loss does not occur in birds (see p. 150).

Suitable sites for blood collection

(1) The right sided jugular vein
This is often the easiest place from which to collect blood in most birds including budgerigars, raptors, penguins, flamingoes and the ostrich (however, in this case the operator should take great care not to get injured). This site is not suitable in pigeons due to the presence in the neck of an extensive vascular plexus (particularly in the male). Unlike in mammals the jugular vein in birds is much more mobile and can be found subcutaneously anywhere over the right side of the neck without its lying in a definite furrow. The jugular vein is often covered by a featherless tract of skin and can be made more visible by wetting the area with antiseptic (quaternary ammonium compound) or alcohol. If a finger is placed under the neck with the bird's head extended the skin can be tensed over the site and the thumb can be placed in the thoracic inlet to raise the vein.

(2) The subcutaneous ulnar and brachial veins
To visualise this vein it is often necessary to first pluck a few feathers and then to wet the site with antiseptic (Fig. 3.1). This vein can be utilised in most birds including the ostrich; again the operator must take great care not to get injured when working with this bird or any of the larger ratites. In small birds particularly this vein is very liable to haematoma formation.

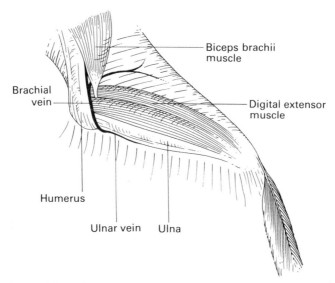

Fig. 3.1 The position of the wing veins used for venipuncture.

(3) The medial metatarsal (caudal tibial) vein

Use of this vein was first described by Murdock and Lewis (1964) for blood collection from ducks. Although perhaps not the most easily visualised of subcutaneous veins it can be utilised in a variety of species apart from duck. It has been used in raptors, pigeons and is particularly useful in the conscious swan (*Cygnus olor*). Digital pressure over the caudal part of the medial surface of the tibial tarsal bone, wetting and rubbing the area with alcohol or diethyl ether usually enables the operator to raise the vein coursing beneath the scaly skin. Because this vein is well supported by surrounding tissue haematoma formation is uncommon and repeated sampling can be carried out from this blood vessel.

(4) Cutting a claw

This method is the most useful for very small birds (i.e. small finches of 10 g or less) or for untrained personnel (Fig. 3.2). The claw and foot are first thoroughly cleansed with a suitable antiseptic (e.g. quaternary ammonium compound) since blood samples taken from this area are quite easily contaminated with the bird's droppings, soil, etc. The blood from the cut claw should be allowed to drip or be drawn into a capillary tube (i.e. a microhaematocrit tube). It should on no account be squeezed out of the foot, since this alters the characteristics of the sample. Blood samples obtained from this site are from capillary blood and may contain cellular artifacts and will affect cell population. Bleeding can be staunched after blood collection by the application of a silver nitrate pencil or ferric sulphate.

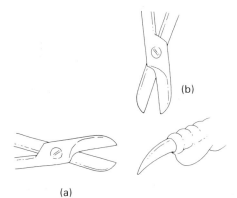

(b)

(a)

Fig. 3.2 Clipping the claw for collection of a blood sample. (a) This is the correct way to clip the claw for collection of a blood sample. (b) This tends to compress the blood vessel.

(5) Other sites for blood collection

Nicking of the external thoracic vein (i.e. running dorsal to the shoulder joint, direct needle puncture of the heart and from the occipital venous sinus have all been used for blood collection mainly in research establishments (Campbell, 1988).

Haematology

The haematocrit or packed cell volume (PCV)

By using microhaematocrit heparinised centrifuge capillary tubes, determination of PCV is quick and easy. The result provides valuable information. In most birds normal values for PCV can be 35–55%. In the adult ostrich the PCV is 32–47% while in ostrich chicks it is 25–45%. More precise details are given in standard texts such as those edited by Petrak (1982), Fowler (1978), Harrison (1984), Harrison and Harrison (1986), Campbell (1988 and 1994) and Hermandez (1991). After determination of the PCV the serum can be drawn off with a micropipette and used for obtaining biochemical information.

Blood smears

Only one drop of blood is needed for a smear that can provide information on blood parasites, cell morphology and differential white cell count. Slides can be stained with Leishman's, Wright's or Giemsa stain. However, avian blood does need a somewhat longer staining period than mammalian blood, at least 5 min, and the third buffer stage of Wright's staining used for washing the slide after staining needs to be more acid, pH5 instead of pH7, and should be left on the slide for at least 5 min. Nevertheless the same routine as used for mammalian blood often yields good results (Grodecki, 1996, personal communication). Avian white cells can be more difficult to find than the corresponding mammalian cells. Apart from the fact that the avian red cell is nucleated, the leucocytes in the blood smear are scattered throughout the slide and not aggregated at the edges of the smear as in the case of mammals. There is also much more variation in the appearance of leucocytes in avian blood. Unless a practitioner is carrying out a lot of avian work, it is probably better to just air dry the smear and send it to a specialist laboratory for examination. The overall interpretation of the haemogram will depend on the laboratory and the expertise of the technician examining the sample. Notwithstanding this, the fact is that the fresher the blood sample is at the time of examination, the more consistent and reliable the results. Useful illustrated references for avian haematology are Campbell and Dein (1984), Campbell (1988 and 1994, p. 181–195) and Hawkey and Gulland (1988).

The clinically significant numerical and morphological changes in the erythrocytes

The reader should note the avian red blood cell (RBC) is nucleated, contrasting with the non-nucleated mammalian erythrocyte. Erythrocyte counts can be obtained by using standard blood cell counting techniques. The figures for a range of species are given in standard texts edited by Fowler (1978), Wallack and Boever (1983), Hawkey and Gulland (1988), Harrison and Harrison (1986) and Ritchie *et al.* (1994). As a general rule, although the normal erythrocute count varies between species, the values for *PCV* (40–55%), *haemoglobin* (12.2–20.00 g/dl) and *mean corpuscular haemoglobin concentration* (28–38 g/dl) are constant within fairly narrow limits across the taxonomic range. Also as a general rule immature birds, particularly those not fully fledged, tend to have lower values for PCV, total erythrocyte count and mean corpuscular haemoglobin concentration than adult birds (Hermandez, 1991 (p. 426) and Garcia del Campo *et al.*, 1991). They may also show large numbers of fairly mature polychromatic RBC precursory cells in the circulating blood. Blood values in wild birds also vary with seasonal activity and depending on whether they migrate and fly at high altitudes and low oxygen tension. As a guide, the values for *total red cell counts* range from 2.1 to 5.5 $\times$ 10^{12}/litre with a mean value of 3.9 $\times$ 10^{12}/litre.

The mean corpuscular erythrocyte indices

These values can be calculated from PCV, haemoglobin total concentration and total RBC count and when used together with the erythrocyte morphology and the total serum protein can give an indication as to the type of an anaemia and may also suggest the ethiology of the disease process.

Mean corpuscular volume (MCV) =
(Expressed in Femtolitres (fl))

$$\text{MCV} = \frac{\text{PCV (\%)} \times 10}{\text{Total RBC count (i.e. millions/}\mu\text{l or } 10^6/\text{mm}^3}$$

For most birds the value lies between 121 and 200 but for small psittacines it can be as low as 99 and in the cassowary it can be as high as 286.

An increase in this value is most useful for indicating a regenerative (i.e. macrocytic or increased cell volume) anaemia. In a non-regenerative anaemia (i.e. normocytic or microcytic) the cells are either normal or reduced in size.

Mean corpuscular haemoglobin concentration (MCHC) =
(Expressed as a percentage or g/dl)

$$\text{MCHC} = \frac{\text{Hb (g/100 ml)} \times 100}{\text{PCV (\%)}}$$

A reduced value (i.e. a hypochromic anaemia) usually indicates an iron deficiency anaemia or the reticulocytes do not have a full complement of haemoglobin. An increase in this value does not occur since RBCs do not become supersaturated with haemoglobin.

Mean corpuscular haemoglobin (MCH) =
(Expressed in micro-micrograms
(i.e. $\mu\mu$g) or picograms (pg))

$$\text{MCH} = \frac{\text{Hb (g/100 ml} \times 10}{\text{Total erythocyte count (i.e. millions/}\mu\text{l or}10^6/\text{mm}^3)}$$

This is not such a useful index as the MCHC.

The polychromatic index (PI) =

$$\text{PI} = \frac{\text{polychromatic RBCs} \times 100}{\text{mature RBCs}}$$

This is the ratio of polychromatic or immature erythrocytes to fully mature RBCs and is expressed as a percentage. This index gives some indication of the rate of turnover of the RBCs and is a useful parameter together with the MCV for indicating if an anaemia is regenerative or non-regenerative and how well the bone marrow is responding. Hermandez (1991) indicated that in various raptors in a regenerative anaemia the values are all above 3.5.

Anaemias

It should be stressed that anaemia as such is only a sign of underlying disease. Anaemias can be classified as follows:

- Haemorrhagic (both acute and chronic) ⎫ regenerative
- Haemolytic (both acute and chronic) ⎭
- Depression anaemia (i.e. non-regenerative).

Regenerative anaemias

These are so named because the body's haematopoietic tissues are endeavouring to replace depleted numbers of normal RBCs. These anaemias are indicated by changes in the morphology of circulating erythrocytes. There may be an increased polychromasia (with new methylene blue stain A, reticulocytosis) together with an increase in size of the RBCs (i.e. macrocytic anaemia) or there may be an excessive variation in the size of the RBCs (i.e. anisocytosis). Reticulocytes are precursor RBCs stained with new methylene blue which stains RNA and which are equivalent to the polychromatic cells produced by Wright's stain. Polychromatic cells, the precursors of mature RBCs occur normally in the blood in small numbers (1–5%). They are slightly larger more rounded cells (Campbell, 1994, pp. 188 and 196) than the mature ovoid RBC and have a more basophilic cytoplasm containing a more rounded and less condensed nuclear chromatin. These cells are often more evident in the normal blood of the large raptor species (Hermandez, 1991, p. 426). Birds tend to develop chronic anaemias more rapidly than mammals because of the shorter RBC lifespan.

Acute, subacute haemorrhagic and haemolytic anaemia

This type of anaemia is usually indicated by normal cell morphology (i.e. normocytic = normal MCV and normochromic) but the RBC count, PCV and total haemoglobin are reduced if the blood sample has been taken within a few hours of the acute incident. When, however, the sample is taken some days later i.e. >72 h), which in practice is often the case, the haemopoetic tissue will have had time to respond and the RBC morphology will become macrocytic (i.e. increased MCV) due to the presence of polychromatic cells or reticulocytes. However reticulocytes increase in the bone marrow within 6–24 h of an acute incident. Possible causes of these anaemias are:

(1) Road traffic accidents or other violent trauma such as a gunshot wound, an attack from a predator, a cage mate or even severe self-trauma.
(2) Ulceration or rupture of an internal organ (e.g. rupture of a friable neoplasm of liver).
(3) Bacterial and viral infection resulting in gastrointestinal haemorrhage (e.g. septicaemic salmonellosis resulting in haemolysis, colibacillosis, conure haemorrhagic syndrome, yersiniosis, megabacterial proventricular ulceration (seen in small birds and also diagnosed in ostriches), trichomoniasis in budgerigars occasionally results in ulceration, campylobacteriosis in juvenile ostriches,

Pacheco's virus in parrots and some other avian herpes virus infections.

(4)   Acute toxaemias (mycotoxins, lead).

Chronic haemorrhagic and haemolytic regenerative anaemias

Anaemia develops slowly and hypovolaemia does not occur. Both the PCV and the total haemoglobin levels are decreased but the MCV is increased and there is a polychromasia or reticulocytosis (indicating the haematopoetic tissues are responding). The causes of this type of anaemia can be:

(1)   Blood parasitism (e.g. microfilaria, *Plasmodium, Atoxoplasma, Aegyptianella, Haemoproteus* and *Leucocytozoon*). There may be some inter-species variation since the latter two parasites are often found in Spanish raptors without causing anaemia (Hermandez, 1991).

(2)   Gastrointestinal parasitism (e.g. *Capillaria,* ascarids, caecal worms, coccidiosis, histomoniasis, giardiasis, *Hexamita*). Often gastro-intestinal parasitism is associated with a nutritional deficiency or actual starvation which results in a chronic non-regenerative anaemia.

(3)   External parasites (e.g. red mite, *Dermanyssus* sp.; Northern fowl mite, *Ornithonyssus* sp.; hippoboscids (louse flies) and ticks).

(4)   Some bacterial infections.

Chronic non-regenerative or depression anaemias

This form of anaemia can be either normochromic or hypochromic. The cell morphology can be either normocytic or microcytic (i.e. the MCV value may be normal or depressed). The number of polychromatic cells or reticulocytes are reduced or absent (i.e. non-regenerative). Possible causes:

(1)   Chronic infectious disease (e.g. mycobacterium avian, often leading to a chronic debilitating disease, is said to be a common cause of anaemia in Spanish wild raptors (Hermandez, 1991). Other possible chronic infectious diseases are *Chlamydia*, toxoplasmosis, aspergil-losis, salmonellosis, yersiniosis, colibaccillosis, campylobacteriosis in juvenile ostriches (this is usually acute or subacute). Chronic forms of viral diseases such as polyoma disease, duck plague, Marek's disease, papillomatosis and avian sarcoma/leucosis complex.

(2)   Toxaemias (e.g. to lead, copper, zinc, rat poisons (warfarin) (can also be regenerative), chloramphenicol, pesticides (DDT, carbamates), aflatoxins, oak leaves and some other toxic plants).

(3)   Nutritional deficiencies of haemopoetic factors (e.g. iron, copper, vitamin B_{12}, folic acid). Overall malnutrition and starvation,

secondary nutritional hypoparathyroidism, hypothyroidism (iodine deficiency).

(4) Hepatopathies and coagulopathies.
(5) Debilitating malignant neoplasms.

The definition of some terms used by haematologists

Anisocytosis:	A variation in the size of RBCs (results in macrocytes and microcytes).
Aplastic anaemia:	A disease of the multi potential stem cell resulting in pancytopenia. A pure red cell aplasia causes a selective loss of erythroid precursors in the bone marrow.
Crenation:	Collapse of the normal cell resulting in an irregular outline, usually as a result of poor drying of the smear, i.e. an artefact.
Smudge cell or ruptured cell:	Cytoplastic rupture of the cell membrane usually the result of a faulty method in making the blood smear or the presence of fragile cells (e.g. neoplastic lymphocytes)
Howell–Jolly bodies:	Small round densely staining inclusions in the cytoplasm which are remnants of the nucleus. Large numbers are the result of malfunction of the mononuclear–phagocytic system.
Hypoplastic anaemia:	Aplastic anaemia as above.
Poikilocyte:	An abnormally shaped RBC.
Polychromasia, polychromatic, polychromatophilia:	The cytoplasm of the RBCs, shows a variable bluish colour, which is evidence of a regenerative response.
Reticulocyte:	(= Polychromatic cell stained with a vital stain (e.g. new methylene blue)). Immature RBC rather more rounded in shape than the ovoid shape of the mature RBC. The cytoplasm shows a darker staining reticular pattern. (New methylene blue stains the RNA content of the cell.)
Erythroplastids:	Abnormal avian RBCs without a nucleus, i.e. anucleated cytoplasmic fragments.

The leucocytes

In birds the equivalent to the mammalian neutrophil is the heterophil. The cytoplasmic granules of the heterophil are eosinophilic and often fusiform in shape. Although in some species the cytoplastic granules may be round. The heterophil has a partially lobed (2–3 lobes) and usually eccentrically situated nucleus.

Interpretation of the avian leucocyte count

Identification and differentiation of the avian white cells can be difficult for the inexperienced observer. The primary purpose of this section is not only to aid the field worker in the interpretation of laboratory reports but also to help that person to make any necessary requests for a more detailed further examination of the sample. Those persons wishing to carry out their own haematological examinations are advised to refer to more detailed text with colour illustrations, e.g. Campbell, 1988 and 1994, and Hawkey and Gulland, 1988.

There is some interspecies variation in the morphology of the avian leucocyte and *also quite a wide diversity in the normal numerical value not only between species but also within a particular species.* Consequently it is often more helpful to the clinician, if it is practical and economic, when using leucocyte counts in assessing a particular case to compare the changes taking place in serial blood samples spaced out over several days. Also this routine is helpful if the range of normal numerical values for a particular species is unavailable. As a *very general guide* values for the total white cell count range from 1.0 to 32.00 × 10^9/litre with percentages for heterophils 20–75%, lymphocytes 20–65%, monocytes 2–5%, basophils 2.5–6% and eosinophils 1–4%.

Changes in the leucocyte picture indicative of certain disease processes

- *Leucopenias:* i.e. an overall decrease in the number of all types (or just one cell line) of circulating leucocytes. This usually occurs with severe toxaemia by itself or associated with an overwhelming septicaemia or viraemia. Toxic drugs or chemical poisons can cause this situation.
- *Leucocytosis:* i.e. an overall increase in the number of circulating white blood cells which is usually well in excess of 10^9/litre. This can be caused by:
  - (a) infection with bacteria, fungi or parasites;
  - (b) trauma resulting in massive tissue necrosis;
  - (c) neoplasia with extensive tissue necrosis;
  - (d) lymphoid leukosis complex. In the opinion of Gerlach (1994) differential leucocyte counts are rarely of any help in diagnosis. The lymphocytes are usually mature and there can be an overall leucocytosis.
  - (e) A marked leucocytosis with a relative heterophilia (i.e. a bias towards the heterophils) often indicates a recent inflammatory

change (e.g. *Chlamydia, Mycobacterium avium* or aspergillosis). Leucocytosis may result from the use of glucocorticosteroids or as the result of a stress response. However, in this case the leucocytosis is usually only slight to moderate. However, if the heterophilia is dominated by large numbers of very immature heterophils, this could indicate a severe infection which has destroyed large numbers of the mature heterophil population resulting in the rapid mobilisation of immature cells from the haematopoetic tissues in the medullary cavities of the bones. A true shift to the left is not often recognised because the heterophil nucleus is already segmented before leaving the bone marrow and the granules obscure the nucleus so that normally immature forms are difficult to recognise, but can sometimes be recognised.

The presence of toxic heterophils (i.e. loss of granulation, vacuolisation and a change in cytoplasmic staining to basaphilia) which are graded by Campbell (1988 and 1994) as stages 1–4 also indicates a severe systemic illness and a poor prognosis.

- *Heteropenia:* This may occur as a very early reaction to a viral infection, or an overwhelming septicaemia.
- *Lymphocytosis:* This usually indicates chronic antigenic stimulation which is often viral in origin but can also be bacterial or parasitic. However it could possibly indicate a lymphoid leukaemia with neoplastic cells and their precursors. Gerlach (1994) is of the opinion that this does not often occur although there may be an overall leucosis exhibiting mature lymphocytes. The presence of reactive lymphocytes (identified as medium to large circular WBCs with a large round nucleus in which both cytoplasm and nucleus are deeply staining) indicates an active immune response and these cells are often referred to as immunocytes.
- *Lymphopenia:* this usually indicates an acute viral infection but could be caused by continuous stress or the use of corticosteroids.
- *The avian thrombocyte:* Small ovoid nucleated cells about the size of small lymphocytes but with a colourless cytoplasm, but frequently with a few small red-purple granules in the cytoplasm. Like mammalian platelets they tend to clump in blood films and they are involved in blood coagulation. They are also phagocytic and the normal count for most birds is $20–30^9$/litre.
- *Thrombocytosis:* This is possibly a response to a bacterial infection or as a result of excessive haemorrhage. Campbell (1994) describes early and late immature thrombocytes and also reactive forms.
- *Thrombocytopenia:* This is usually the result of a severe septicaemia or poor blood collection techniques.
- *The avian monocyte:* These are the largest of the leucocytes and are believed to be the precursors of tissue macrophages. Chemically attracted to such infections as *Chlamydia* and mycobacteria.

- *Monocytosis:* This indicates a successful host response to a chronic bacterial infection or to tissue necrosis or parasitism. Monocytosis is often associated with chronic inflammatory disease resulting in granulomatous lesions. A monocytosis usually takes 4–5 days to initially develop. But in acute infection it may be manifest in as little as 12 hours after induction of inflammation. Monocytes are relatively long lived cells and can survive 45 days. *Chlamydia* (and some other pathogens) which may have been phagocytosed by these cells remain viable within them for the whole 45 day period and this necessitates at least a 45 day treatment for birds infected with *Chlamydia*.
- *The avian eosinophil:* An increase in eosinophils in avian blood samples may not necessarily indicate a parasitic infection since the function of these cells may be different from that in mammals. It is thought that an eosinophilia may indicate a delayed hypersensitivity reaction. However changes vary widely and should be interpreted with caution.
- *The avian basophil:* This leukocyte is believed to carry out the same function in birds as in mammals being involved in the early acute inflammatory reaction, in anaphylaxis and in reaction to neoplasms with significant tissue necrosis.

The selection of biochemical data as an aid to diagnosis

Only those enzymes, metabolites and electrolytes which are of most value to the avian diagnostician are mentioned in this text. However, additional information may become available on the usefulness of other blood chemistry constituents.

The advised routine for the collection of blood chemistry samples

If the clinician is going to take the trouble to collect a blood sample from a bird and is to obtain meaningful information then it is imperative that the collection procedure and the subsequent handling of the sample should be faultless.

(1) The venipuncture site, the needle and the syringe must all be clean and the equipment should be new and unused. Water droplets in a resterilised syringe invalidate the result.
(2) The correct type of microcontainer containing either no or an appropriate anti-coagulant should be selected.
(3) Preferably use plasma obtained after *immediate* centrifrugation of freshly drawn unclotted blood. Before centrifugation the plasma is best placed in a microcontainer with a neutrally reactive gelatine serum separator.

The sooner the cellular element of the blood is separated from the plasma the better, since nucleated RBCs continue metabolism apace. The level within the cell of adenosine triphosphate (ATP) drops, the cell cannot maintain its ion pumps, the cell becomes hypoglycaemic and starts to leach lactate dehydrogenase (LDH) and aspartate amino transferase (AST) into the plasma even before haemolysis is apparent, so effecting the assay of plasma enzymes.

(4) If an anticoagulant is used lithium heparin (not the potassium or sodium salt) should be used for most biochemical estimations but it should not be used for estimations of glucose or calcium.

(5) To mix the sample with the anticoagulant, the container should be rolled along the work surface. It should not be shaken violently which may result in haemolysis so invalidating some results.

(6) Serum can be used after the blood has clotted and the clot has been allowed to contract which will take a minimum of 20 min. Speeding the clotting process by placing the sample above a radiator only produces erroneous data.

(7) Whether serum or plasma is obtained, the sample should preferably be tested immediately but if this is not practical and it has to be posted to a laboratory, it is better to first freeze the sample and then pack in insulated wrapping.

How much reliance can be placed on the results?

It is important for the avian practitioner to appreciate that the biochemical data obtained from a particular bird *can only be a rough guide* to a final diagnosis. It is a mistake to base a definitive diagnosis solely on the information obtained about one or two biochemical constituents after checking these against the values on the data base taken from so-called 'normal' healthy birds. This is because there is a wide variation in both the physiological (i.e. age, gender, moulting, egg laying, possible migratory behaviour and circadian rhythm) and environmental conditions (i.e. whether the bird is wild or captive, husbandry, nutrition, varying weather conditions, also possible exposure to undiagnosed subclinical viral infection), imposed on these so-called 'normal' birds. A variety of other factors which may influence the level of plasma enzymes has been reviewed by Lumeij (1987, pp. 52 and 53).

Another important factor affecting the validity of the result will be the laboratory. Different commercial laboratories will use variously different methodologies when estimating for the same enzyme. All the methods used have been developed for use and comparison on humans and domestic mammals. The net result is that the final figures obtained from the same sample from a particular case may vary slightly from one laboratory to another.

During the last decade an abundance of data has been collected on those elements of biochemistry mentioned in this text. Nevertheless often the information published by different groups of workers in this field differs to a greater or lesser degree; consequently here only a broad guide to the 'normal' levels of blood biochemical elements is given together with an indication of when these values for a particular species are known to be outside the normal pattern. All values are also expressed in SI units (i.e. Systeme International d'Unites, 1977) (conversion factors to SI units are given).

All biochemical data can only indicate a trend towards a particular clinical condition and to be of any significant value most results (particularly in the case of the enzymes) should show a result of at least a twofold increase above the 'normal' data base. All diagnosis is a matter of obtaining as much available evidence from as many varied sources as possible (i.e. haematology, biochemistry, imaging and all the other different aids mentioned in this chapter) after which using one's clinical acumen to assess the balance of probabilities in favour of a specific diagnosis. In addition to this the practitioner will have to consider the economic cost of the various tests of the time and cost of laboratory fees, etc. in direct relation to the value of a particular case to the client.

The plasma proteins

These can provide important information on the overall state of health of the bird

Total serum protein

For most species this will lie between 3 and 5 g/l. Note the level of plasma protein will be approx. 0.15 g/dl above the value for serum protein because the fibrinogen will have been removed during coagulation. However normal levels of fibrinogen do vary, e.g. cockatoos 0.09–0.33 g/dl, macaws 0.1–0.32 g/dl. In the past many avian clinicians have used a hand held refractometer, a method which was quick and convenient. Unfortunately the results so obtained have been shown to be unreliable. Both haemolysis and lipaemia are only two of a number of factors affecting the result.

Assessment of total protein values is probably of most use when used in conjunction with protein electrophoresis.

Hypoproteinaemia

Since most of the serum proteins are produced by the liver a reduction in total serum protein is one indicator of the severity and progression of hepatopathy. Other possible causes of reduced serum protein level are any disease associated with an anaemia, haemorrhage, malnutrition, starvation, malabsorption consequent upon gastrointestinal disease, gastrointestinal parasitism, glomerulonephritis, severe trauma, prolonged stress, acute lead poisoning, chronic infectious disease and Pacheco's disease, etc.

Hyperproteinaemia
This may be due to dehydration (PCV is also elevated), shock or acute infection (globulins are elevated). There is also a rise in the total serum protein just before egg laying due to the transport of the globulin yolk precursors to the ovary (Lumeij, 1987, p. 83). Serum protein tends to be higher in older birds. Very high levels of serum protein may be encountered with the leukosis complex.

Albumen
This is usually between 1.0 and 2.2 g/dl for most species of birds. This is the major protein produced by the liver and forms most of the plasma protein so that a hypoalbuminaemia is usually responsible for a drop in the total serum protein. Since albumen is important in the transport of anions, cations, fatty acids and thyroid hormone a drop in the serum level of albumen has overall serious consequences.

Globulins
This fraction of the serum protein comprises the α, β and γ globulins together with the globulin precursors of the yolk proteins. As Hochleithner (1994, p. 238) has indicated α and β globulins (one of which is fibrinogen) are acute phase proteins and tend to rise with acute nephritis, with a severe hepatitis and with trauma including surgery. The γ globulins are the immune globulins which increase with both acute and chronic infection. Their increase should be compared with any simultaneous lymphocytosis, which may or may not be present.

Hyperglobulinaemia
This usually is the result of subacute or chronic infectious disease, alternatively it can occur as a result of trauma including surgery.

Fibrinogen
For psittacines levels greater than 0.3–0.5 g/dl are significant. This is one of the significant β globulins and since it is concerned with the blood coagulation mechanism it has to be determined in plasma. EDTA must be used as the anticoagulant not heparin. As Hawkey and Gulland (1988) indicated this plasma protein is an important guide to an acute inflammatory response.

The albumen : globulin ratio
For many birds the normal values are between 1.4–4.9. As Lumeij (1987, pp.

80–86) has indicated serial determinations of the A : G ratio are a valuable guide to the progress of a disease process. The ratio tends to decrease (the globulins rise and the albumen falls) during both acute and chronic infections (e.g. *Chlamydia*, aspergillosis, mycobacteriosis and egg peritonitis). As recovery proceeds the globulins tend to fall while the albumen level rises and the ratio returns to normal. A persistent low A : G ratio together with an overall reduction in total protein indicates liver failure.

The metabolite fraction of the plasma biochemical elements

These substances tend to provide more organ-specific information regarding the functional condition of some of the body's tissues.

Glucose

For most birds serum glucose lies between 200 and 500 mg/dl (to convert mg/dl to mmol/l multiply by 0.05551). In the emu the normal level can be as low as 158 mg/dl. For a rapid estimation the Dextrostix (Bayer Diagnostics) is a useful indicator.

When collecting avian blood samples for glucose estimation it is not necessary to use fluoride as an anticoagulant provided the plasma sample has had the red cells immediately removed. In any case fluoride can have an inhibitory effect on some enzyme test samples.

In general avian serum glucose levels are much higher than in mammals but as with many other biochemical constituents of avian blood the level does tend to vary with age, diet, breeding season, stress and also diurnally. For most birds the level falls during daylight hours and rises at night. The reverse may be true in the nocturnally active birds. In the moulting mallard duck the normal level of serum glucose is rather on the low side at 185 mg/dl. Depending on the laboratory technique used lipaemia may invalidate the result.

Hyperglycaemia
This state can occur during stress, including hyperthermia. It has been recorded in Amazon parrots with lead toxicosis. Also it may be seen in some cases of peritonitis where there is an associated pancreatitis.

Diabetes mellitus
This has been recorded in some granivorous birds, budgerigars, cockatoos, Amazon parrots, macaws and cockatiels, also in toco toucans (which are not granivorous), Lewandowski *et al.* (1986). In these cases the serum glucose levels can be above 750 mg/dl and can reach 1000–2000 mg/dl. However this hyperglycaemia may not be due to an insufficiency of insulin (in these granivorous birds) since the hormone gluca-

gon is more important in the regulation of blood glucose levels. In carnivorous birds insulin may be a more important regulator of blood glucose as is the situation in mammals. However this subject in birds has not been well researched (see p. 361).

A transient hyperglycaemia occurs for the first 72 hours after the withdrawal of food in pigeons (Lumeij, 1987) in consequence of which, except in the case of the very small (i.e. below 100 g) birds pre-surgical fasting has a positive advantage especially when gastrointestinal surgery is anticipated.

Hypoglycaemia

Glucose levels below 100 mg/dl indicate a grave prognosis. Hypoglycaemia occurs in cases of starvation and particularly in immature raptors and can result in hypoglycaemic convulsions after only a few days of anorexia. How long this state of affairs takes to develop will depend on the size of the bird and on the species. Some inexperienced falconers in an attempt to reduce a bird's weight to its so-called flying weight will take the reduction of food intake too far and produce relative starvation.

Hypoglycaemia may be induced by malnutrition, possibly by hypovitaminosis-A, by toxaemias resulting from bacterial and viral septicaemias, and by neoplasia, aspergillosis and Pacheco's disease.

Uric acid

For most birds the normal value lies between 2 and 15 mg/dl (to convert mg/dl to μmol/l multiply by 59.48; to convert mmol/l to mg/dl multiply by 0.0168). Levels of uric acid vary with age and species (they are generally 50% lower in granivorous birds than in carnivorous birds).

Birds excrete 60–80% of their nitrogenous waste as uric acid (synthesised in the liver but excreted through the kidney) in a form which is almost independent of the rate of the flow of fluid urine through the kidney. Of this uric acid 90% is excreted dynamically via active cellular secretion from proximal renal tubules and glomeruli. A much smaller amount is derived from actual glomerular filtration. The avian kidney has at least 50% reserve capacity so that extensive nephrosis must have occurred before the amount of uric acid in the plasma exceeds normal, providing of course other factors affecting the level of uric acid remain normal. Abnormally high amounts of uric acid in plasma occur in starvation (due to catabolism of the body's tissues), in extensive trauma, in gout (often uric acid rises before clinical gout is seen), in toxicosis of the kidney with aminoglycosides particularly gentamycin, excessive vitamin D_3 (causing nephrocalcinosis) and some other medicaments such as occasionally sulphonamides or the azole antifungals.

Uric acid can rise after the use of corticosteroids, in dehydration, toxaemia from some bacterial and viral infections and with gastrointestinal haemorrhage, also, possibly, due to chronic hypovitaminosis-A resulting in damage to the epithelium of the kidney tubules. To keep the uric acid and urate crystals in colloidal suspension large amounts of mucus have to be secreted by the healthy cells of the renal collecting tubules.

Because of the multiplicity of causes which can result in a rise of the uric acid level, plasma uric acid is not a very useful *single* indicator of kidney disease.

Urea

Normal levels for most birds are between 2.4 and 4.2 mg/dl (to convert mg/dl urea nitrogen to mmol/l of urea multiply by 0.3510; to convert mmol/l to mg/dl multiply by 6.0). In the ostrich the normal is 1.8–3.00 mg/dl and in the cassowary it is 8.7–9.9 mg/dl.

Urea, which forms 20–40% (the actual amount varies between species) of avian nitrogenous waste, is excreted by glomerular filtration. In normally hydrated birds a little is reabsorbed in the distal renal tubules but in dehydrated birds nearly all of the urea is reabsorbed. The urea is in aqueous solution so that its excretion unlike that of uric acid is entirely dependent on the rate of flow of fluid through the kidney. Consequently any factor which impairs this flow such as dehydration, cardiopathy, or postrenal obstruction (e.g. cloacal impaction, a neoplasm or blocking of the oviducts with an egg which may cause pressure on the ureters) or possibly the careless surgical placement of a purse string suture around the vent to reduce a prolapse, or impaction of the renal tubules with urate crystals as happens in cases of salt poisoning, can all cause a rapid rise of the urea in the plasma in 2–3 days. This rise can be as much as 15-fold particularly if there is a concurrent increase in the level of nitrogenous waste production

The urea : uric acid ratio

For pigeons the normal is 1.8 ± 1.8. Experimental work by Lumeij (1987) on the pigeon has shown that this ratio is not only an indicator of the state of dehydration (as also demonstrated by PCV) but may also be an indicator of urinary fluid flow so that in cases of renal failure accompanied by a reduced urinary flow, the urea : uric acid level rises significantly. After 4 days of starvation (i.e. resulting in tissue catabolism and increased nitrogenous waste production) accompanied by 4 days of water deprivation, the ratio rose to 12.0 ± 2.0.

$$\text{Urea} : \text{uric acid} = \frac{\text{urea (mmol/l)} \times 1000}{\text{uric acid (}\mu\text{mol/l)}}$$

To convert uric acid in mg/dl = μmol/l; multiply by 59.48

Creatinine

Normal values in most birds are 0.2–0.5 mg/dl (to convert mg/dl to μmol/l multiply by 88.4). In the present state of knowledge about avian blood biochemistry, estimations of this constituent are not a lot of value to the avian clinician.

Cholesterol

Normal values lie between 108 and 330 mg/dl (to convert mg/dl to mmol/l multiply by 0.02586). In ostriches the normal range is 58.05–162.57 mg/dl.

This substance is the precursor of all steroid hormones (i.e. sex hormones and corticoid hormones) as well as the bile acids. Some cholesterol is obtained from the fats in the diet, its level being higher in carnivores. The remainder of the cholesterol is produced in the liver. Plasma levels of cholesterol are increased in cases of fatty liver and kidney syndrome. Very high levels of plasma cholesterol accompanied by a lipaemia indicate fatty degeneration of the liver. Hochleithner (1994, p. 234) has indicated that the plasma cholesterol may increase together with xanthomatosis in the budgerigar; and the author has seen this in an African grey parrot *Psittacus erithacus*. Hypercholesterolaemia may indicate hypothyroidism.

Lipaemia

This may occur together with a rise in plasma cholesterol and sometimes there is a post-pradial increase in chylomicrons in the blood particularly with a high fat diet. Diets containing seeds such as sunflower, hemp, rape and safflower can produce this effect. Lipaemia also occurs with hepatopathies (not only fatty liver), in hypothyroidism and sometimes with egg peritonitis (egg yolk absorbed from the coelomic peritoneal cavity).

Lipaemia can be recognised by the naked eye in plasma and serum samples. Very often immediately the blood sample is collected it is noticed to be milky in colour. The presence of lipaemia may invalidate or may make the carrying out of some blood biochemical tests impossible.

Bile acids

For psittacines see Table 1.1, p. 19. Bile acids are produced by the liver and excreted in the bile. After acting on the ingesta they are reabsorbed and recycled through the liver. A small amount continues to circulate in the bloodstream. There is normally a post-prandial rise in plasma bile acids. Anything which interferes with the normal recycling process leads to a rise in plasma levels. In hepatopathy there may be an imbalance between the normal quantity manufactured in the liver and the amounts being re-used by the liver (which may drop) so that an inevitable rise in the blood level occurs. Conversely a reduction in liver size resulting from chronic liver disease and fibrosis leads to a gradual reduction in the synthesis of bile acids but the circulating bile acid tends to persist. Bile acids are therefore a good indicator of liver disease and these substances have the great advantage that they are stable compounds unaffected by the handling of the blood sample.

Since birds produce mostly biliverdin rather than bilirubin true icterus does not usually occur in birds although it can occasionally be detected on the face of macaws if the level of bilirubin exceeds 2.36 mg/dl (Hochleithner 1994, p. 233).

The serum enzymes

The enzymes found in serum function normally within the confines of the individual cells of specific organs. Anything which disrupts the integrity of the cell leads to a great increase in the release of enzymes into the blood stream. In consequence their presence and the quantity present give the clinician some indication of the degree of organ or tissue damage.

The amino transferases

This group of enzymes controls the transfer of amino groups in amino acids. None of these enzymes is organ specific. Besides the liver these enzymes are found in the heart muscle, skeletal muscle, the gastro-intestinal cells, the kidney and brain. Of this group of enzymes the most useful to the avian clinician is:

Aspartate amino transferase (AST, SGOT)

Normal plasma values in most birds should normally be below 230 IU/l but can be in the range of 52–270 IU/l. In the ostrich the normal is 100–160 IU/l. As with the biochemistry of many of the blood constituents the level varies with the age and seasonal activity. Although, as already indicated, AST has a wide distribution in the body's tissues and although it is not liver specific it is possibly the single most useful enzyme for indicating liver disease. However, any soft tissue muscle damage including intramuscular injection, particularly with irritant drugs (e.g. doxycycline, occasionally potentiated sulphonamides) can result in an elevation of the plasma AST. Because of this the level of AST should always be compared with that of CK which is specific for muscle trauma and is unaffected by liver damage. Increases of AST occur with any kind of hepatopathy including Pacheco's disease, chlamydiosis, also toxic chemicals (e.g. some pesticides and carbon tetrachloride) and the use of some drugs (e.g. doxycycline injection), besides causing a rise in CPK also can result in a rise in AST. The use of many of the azole antifungal drugs – ketaconazole, fluconazole and itraconazole can also increase AST levels).

Alanine amino transferase (ALT, SGPT)

'Normal' levels in birds vary considerably from 6.5 to 263 IU/l. Changes in the plasma level of this enzyme are *not* a reliable index of hepatopathy in birds.

Lactate dehydrogenase (LD, LDH)

For most birds normal levels are 46–442 IU/l. In the ostrich they can be between 1000.0 and 2000.0 IU/l and in canary finches they are approximately 1582.63 IU/l (Schöpf and Vasicek, 1991). This enzyme is not organ specific; in fact it is found in many tissues of the body. However, increased blood plasma quantities are commonly noticed with hepatopathy and myopathy. Levels of this particular enzyme tend to rise and fall much more rapidly with acute hepatopathy so that in this respect LD has some value in indicating acute liver disease. Nevertheless the value of LDH should always be compared with that of CPK (see p. 19).

Alkaline phosphatase (AP)

Levels for psittacines fall between 42 and 479 IU/l. In the ostrich they lie between 330 and 820 IU/l. This is another non-organ-specific enzyme which is found mostly in the duodenum and kidney (Lumeij, 1987). Some authors consider this enzyme to be a good indicator of osteobalastic activity (i.e., Osteomyelitis, bone neoplasms, fractures, rickets and hyperparathyroidism). Its level is also increased in growing birds and in egg laying birds when calcium metabolism is increased in the medullary bone. It is suggested that AP blood levels may also be increased in some cases of liver disease such as aflatoxin poisoning. However one should also look for concurrent rises in AST and bile acids. Low levels of AP may be seen in zinc dietary deficiency.

Creatinine phosphokinase (CPK, CK)

Normal values in birds lie between 110 and 480 IU/l. In the ostrich they can be 400–900 IU/l. This enzyme is a specific indicator of muscle trauma. It is therefore a very useful guide for the differentiation of muscle and liver damage when levels of AST and LDH may also be raised. It should be noted that intramuscular injections given before blood sampling may help to increase CK values. Also CK values are said to rise with neuropathies associated with convulsions, with lead toxicity, with chlamydiosis, with bacterial septicaemias and vitamin E deficiency (see p. 19).

The blood electrolytes

Maintenance levels of these in the blood plasma are essential for many living processes.

Calcium

Normal levels in most birds are within the range 8–12 mg/dl (to convert mg/dl to mmol/l multiply by 0.25). In the ostrich they are 6.8–10 mg/dl, in budgerigars they are 6.4–11.2 mg/dl and in the chicken 13.2–23.7 mg/ dl.

Blood samples for calcium analysis must be collected in heparinised tubes since all other normal anticoagulants (i.e. EDTA, citrate, oxalate) bind calcium ions in the blood. Because some calcium ions in the blood are bound to protein (principally albumen), the total blood calcium level should always be considered together with the level of albumen. A hypoalbuminaemia can result in a drop in total blood calcium. However, the calcium bound to protein is not in an ionised biochemically active form.

Total blood calcium levels tend to be higher during ovulation (corresponding with increased ALP) and coincident with the transport of protein-bound calcium to the shell gland but the level of calcium ions in the blood remains constant. Immature birds tend to have lower blood calcium levels.

Hypercalcaemia

Serum calcium levels may be raised after use of excessive dosage with vitamin D_3 and also in conjunction with some osteolytic bone tumours. Also possibly dehydration may result in an increase in total blood calcium.

Hypocalcaemia

Normal blood calcium levels of ionised calcium falling below 6.0 mg/dl in most birds lead to loss of muscular condition, muscle twitching and eventually to clonic and tonic muscle spasms. In some species (e.g. African grey parrots and some raptors) the bird becomes hypersensitive so that when suddenly startled it develops a seizure. A hypoalbuminaemia can result in a depression of protein-bound calcium and eventually to a hypocalcaemia. Glucocorticoid therapy can also result in a decrease in the total blood calcium.

Chloride, sodium and potassium determinations

These are of questionable value in the diagnosis of avian disease except for the confirmation of hypernatraemia which may occur in cases of suspected salt poisoning in wild birds after drought conditions or in parrots fed on large amounts of salted peanuts or potato crisps. Normal values for plasma sodium for most birds are between 127 and 170 mEq/l (1 mEq/l = 1 mmol/l) but for the ostrich they are between 113 and 181 mEq/l.

Microbiological investigations

Since bacteria and fungi play an important part in the development of avian disease, the clinician should try to establish what potential pathogens are present. However, it is easy to make a hurried decision and conclude that some innocent micro-organism is the sole cause of the disease process.

Birds pick up a variety of micro-organisms from their contacts such as wild birds, rodents and human handlers. Birds newly introduced into an aviary can bring in disease. The United Kingdom insists at present that recently imported birds undergo a 35-day quarantine period, but this is only to protect national poultry flocks against Newcastle disease. Other diseases such as chlamydiosis (psittacosis), salmonellosis, avian tuberculosis or Pacheco's parrot disease can be introduced at the same time. Also cage and aviary hygiene can sometimes leave much to be desired, and perches, food and water containers become contaminated.

Bacteriological swabs can be taken from a variety of sites such as bumblefoot abscesses, suspected cysts, wounds and natural orifices including the trachea. They can also be taken after paracentesis of abdominal fluid. In the first instance they should be cultured on blood agar plates at 37°C and the organism checked for antibiotic sensitivity.

Faecal swabs are best obtained direct from the cloaca, the vent having first been cleaned and sterilised with a quaternary ammonium antiseptic. If this is not possible the swab can be taken from faecal droppings on a clean surface. When a bird is first handled it will often eject fresh faecal matter from the proctodeum and this can be utilised. A useful method of collecting uncontaminated faeces from small cage birds is to substitute the sand sheet in the bottom of the cage with a piece of X-ray film. Faecal swabs should be routinely cultured on blood agar and MacConkey agar plates.

When Salmonellae are suspected, enriched culture media will be needed and culture is best carried out by a specialist laboratory. Salmonellae are found in most species of wild birds and easily spread to aviary birds by faecal contamination. However, Salmonellae do not appear to be common in the faeces of raptors (Needham, 1981). *Salmonella typhimurium* is by far the most common specific organism in this group isolated from birds.

It should be noted that a wide variety of bacteria are normal commensals in the gut of many birds and these may be pathogenic only if the bird is subjected to stress. A careful assessment of the patient is necessary before one can be reasonably certain that the organism isolated is causing the disease. To some extent the spectrum of avian gut flora is influenced by the diet of the bird. *Escherichia coli* is a normal inhabitant of the gut of most raptors and is probably acquired from the intestine of the prey species (Needham, 1981). Gram-negative bacteria are not normally present in large numbers in the alimentary tract of grain and fruit eating birds but may become more evident when the bird starts eating insects during the breeding season.

Tracheal swabs can be taken in the anaesthetised or sedated bird and a human nasopharygeal calcium alginate swab is very useful for this purpose.

When *Aspergillus* is suspected, swabs should be cultured on Sabouraud's dextrose agar at 37°C for 36–48 hours. Redig (1981) describes the use of air-sac washings in the investigation of respiratory disease. These are obtained by inserting a sterile, flexible catheter, attached to a syringe into the last intercostal space of the bird, and injecting 3 ml of sterile saline (in a large bird 3 kg and above) and then immediately withdrawing this fluid for culture.

Swabs should be taken from any eggs that have failed to hatch. The surface of the egg should be first sterilised with alcohol before a small hole is made in the shell and a swab used to sample the contents. Swabs should be cultured on blood agar and MacConkey agar, because faecal contamination is a common cause of infection of the egg (see Chapter 9, p. 220).

When taking swabs from post-mortem specimens, one should take into account that cultures obtained from birds that have been dead more than 24 hours may not be representative. Some organisms, such as *Proteus*, that are normally present in the gut of some birds (e.g. raptors) may rapidly invade other organs after death and overgrow other pathogens on a culture plate.

Examination of stained smears

This is quick, and although not conclusive, it is a useful guide to examine stained smears of pus, faeces and exudate. These can be stained with Gram stain, methylene blue (for bipolar staining of *Pasteurella*), or where Avian tuberculosis is suspected with Ziehl–Neelsen stain. Liver impressions smears can also be stained for acid-fast organisms. Where *Chlamydia* (psittacosis) infection is suspected these smears can be stained by a modified Ziehl–Neelsen technique to show up the intracytoplasmic inclusion bodies. The modified Ziehl–Neelsen technique is carried out as follows: the slide is flooded with dilute carbolfuchsine stain for 10 min but is not heated as in normal Ziehl–Neelsen staining. The slide is then washed and decolorised with 0.5% acetic acid – not acid alcohol which is normally used. Decolorisation is carried out only for 20–30 s until the slide is very faintly pink. Counterstain with methylene blue in the normal manner. The tissue cells may then be seen to contain clusters of very small red intracytoplasmic inclusion bodies. However, because of the risk of zoonotic infection, investigation of this disease is best left to specialised laboratories that have the necessary air extraction safety cabinets.

Woerpel and Rosskopf (1984) state that it is generally considered that the presence of Gram-negative bacteria is abnormal in caged birds. Routine staining of a sample by Gram's method can help in the interpretation of antibiotic sensitivity testing. The stain will indicate the relative numbers and morphology of Gram-negative and Gram-positive bacteria and also if yeasts are present. This technique may show anaerobic bacteria to be present when there is little or no growth with a routine blood agar culture.

If *Aspergillus* is suspected in a post- mortem preparation, a portion of the lesion can be teased out on a slide and treated with 20% KOH. The alkali clears the other tissues and renders the fungal hyphae more easily seen. If necessary they can be subsequently gently washed, fixed with heat and stained with lactophenol cotton blue. Suspected lesions of *Candida* can be stained with Gram's stain or mixed with Indian ink or nigrosin stain, when the budding yeast like cells may be seen. *Candida* can also be stained with lactophenol cotton blue stain.

Serology, DNA probes and viral culture

The laboratory examination of serum samples can be a valuable aid in assessing if a bird has already been exposed to infection by a specific micro-organism, which particularly in the case of some viruses may remain latent for years. Alternatively by using paired serum samples taken 2–3 days apart the bird can be shown to be actively responding immunologically to the infection by a rising titre. Serology is particularly valuable in making a definitive diagnosis of viral infection where there are often no or few pathognomic signs and viral culture may be difficult and take weeks.

Viruses can be cultured in living cells from a variety of tissues from both ante- and post-mortem cases providing the autopsy specimen is very fresh. However, if viral culture is to be attempted special transport media containing antibiotic (to prevent bacterial overgrowth) is needed and the swab of specimen needs to be frozen (−4°C). When intending to use this aid to diagnosis the clinician is advised to first consult with the laboratory which is to carry out the culture. There are a variety of serological tests available, e.g. complement fixation, virus neutralisation, ELISA, hae-maglutination inhibition, immunofluorescence and others. Some of these serological tests are much more sensitive and specific than others. Which test is to be used for a particular case is best left to the judgement of the laboratory but before a choice can be made, the laboratory will need a good anamnesis and an indication of the clinician's tentative diagnosis. Specific nucleic DNA probes which are extremely sensitive and which are usually carried out on whole blood have been developed for the detection of the presence of some micro-organisms such as polyoma virus and *Chlamydia*. Apart from blood, virus-containing nucleic acid can be detected in a variety of tissues and excretions which have a cellular content. In the detection of *Chlamydia* infection faeces are used. Nevertheless all these DNA probes will only indicate the presence of the infecting micro-organism, they do not give any indication of the activity of the infection. Table 3.1 lists various pathological micro-organisms together with the different serological tests which can be used for the detection of that particular infection.

Table 3.1 Tests for pathogenic micro-organisms.

Micro-organism	Possible laboratory tests for the detection of specific organisms
Aspergillosis	ELISA (enzyme linked immunosorbent assay)
Avian encephalomyelitis virus	Immunodiffusion test or ELISA
Avian influenza virus	Immunodiffusion test or ELISA
Avian reticuloendotheliosis virus	Histological examination only
Avian sarcoma leukosis virus	Virus isolation in culture and histological signs, possibly ELISA
Chlamydia	ELISA, DNA probe (more sensitive) (clearview test, Unipath)
Equine encephomyelitis virus Eastern and Western strains	Haemaglutination, ELISA, haemaglutination inhibition test
Avian herpes viral infections:	
a) Infectious laryngotracheitis	Virus neutralisation, immunofluorescence, ELISA
b) Duck plague virus (duck virus enteritis)	Virus neutralisation
c) Pacheco's parrot disease	Virus neutralisation, ELISA or immunofluorescence, immunodiffusion test
d) Budgerigar herpes virus	Virus neutralisation or immunodiffusion
e) Pigeon herpes (inclusion body hepatitis)	Virus neutralisation, ELISA or immunodiffusion

Table 3.1 Continued.

f) Pigeon encephalomyelitis (contagious pigeon paralysis)	Serological tests are not at present available. Confirmation of diagnosis will depend on histopathology, often using electron microscopy
g) Marek's disease	
h) Amazon tracheitis	
There are many other species specific avian herpes viral infections	No generally available serological tests available. Diagnosis can only be confirmed by histopathology and electron microscopy.
Avian mycobacterium	ELISA, slide agglutination test
Mycoplasma	ELISA
Avian paramyxo viruses (including Newcastle disease and PMV1 pigeon)	Haemaglutination inhibition test, viral culture
Papilloma virus	Histopathology
Parvo virus infection of geese	Virus neutralisation, ELISA or immunofluorescence
Psittacine beak and feather disease virus	DNA probe (need 0.2–1 ml whole blood) with a heparin anticoagulant), haemaglutination inhibition test
Polyoma virus	Virus neutralisation, DNA probe. If budgerigar fledgling disease or French moult is suspected. Also check the differential diagnosis for Psittacine beak and feather disease
Avian pox viruses	Viral culture. Virus can be cultured from the faeces of carrier birds. Virus neutralisation test or immunodiffusion test. Histopathology is best for confirming clinical cases
Salmonella	ELISA
Adeno viruses There are a multiplicity of adeno viruses not all of which may be pathogenic. Some adeno viruses may act as triggers for other pathogens.	Although group specific antibodies are detectable by ELISA and immunodiffusion tests and there are also specific DNA probes for some adeno viruses, diagnosis of these pathogens mostly depends on virus neutralisation, histopathology with a search for inclusion bodies and also on electromicroscopy

For more detailed information on the detection of viruses consult Gerlach (1994, p. 437) and for more information on particular laboratory tests available in the UK: The Central Veterinary Laboratory, New Haw, Addlestone, Surrey KT15 3NB; telephone 01932 34111, fax 01932 347046. Also for information on DNA probes consult: Vetgen Europe, PO Box 60, Winchester SO23 9XN; telephone 01962 880376, fax 01962 881790.

Diagnostic cytology

The microscopical examination of cell morphology in samples harvested from abnormal tissue is a quick and relatively inexpensive method of making a tentative and sometimes a definitive diagnosis. The technique has almost infinite possibilities. Specimens for examination can easily be obtained and examined immediately by the experienced clinician, so that the result is available much more rapidly than when biopsy samples are sent away for histopathology. However, *cytology will only indicate changes in individual cell morphology* and will not show any structural changes in diseased tissue.

Collection of samples

Hyperplastic tissue, swellings and suspected malignancies
The surface of the tissue is first cleaned with alcohol and allowed to dry. Using a hypodermic needle (e.g. 14–22 g × 2.5 cm) attached to a 10-ml syringe, the needle is then inserted into the tissue and a sample aspirated into the syringe. A quantity of tissue is obtained so that it just appears above the hub of the needle in the bottom of the syringe. If too much aspirate fills the syringe then it is difficult to expel. While aspirating the sample it is best to partially withdraw the needle and reinsert it several times in different directions to get a representative sample. The sample is then expressed on to a slide, spread into a thin smear, fixed and stained. When making the smear the aim is to achieve a single layer of cells. This can sometimes best be carried out by squashing the specimen between two glass slides and then sliding these carefully apart so that two smears are obtained, one on each of the opposing faces of the two glass slides. Each can then be stained differently.

Bone marrow samples
Examination of such samples is helpful when the haematology of a blood sample reveals a grossly reduced or absence of one or other of the normal cellular constituents. Alternatively such samples may be helpful in cases of non-regenerative anaemia or suspected leukaemias.

Bone marrow samples can be obtained from the keel of the sternum or more easily from the proximal tibiotarsal bone when approached from the medial aspect *just* distal to the stifle joint. The skin over the sampling area is first cleaned and sterilised with alcohol and a small incision made with a scalpel. A hypodermic needle containing an indwelling stylet is best used (e.g. a paediatric bone biopsy needle or a 23 g spinal needle). Sometimes a normal hypodermic needle can be used with a length of sterile stainless steel suture wire inserted in the lumen or as a last resort a tunnel can be pre-bored in the bone with a suitable diameter Steinmann intramedullary pin and the hypodermic needle inserted through this prepared entrance hole.

Abdominocentesis

Samples of abnormally present abdominal fluid can be carefully aspirated for examination. The sampling needle is carefully inserted in the mid point of the abdomen and directed towards the right hand side of the bird (e.g. the operator's left hand if the bird is in dorsal recumbency) so as to avoid the gizzard (ventriculus). If the needle is inserted too far anteriorly it is liable to puncture the liver and if too far posteriorly it will enter the distended cloaca. Samples for cytology from the abdomen can also be obtained using the laparoscope.

Crop washings

A blunt ended catheter or gavage tube can be used to instil up to 3 ml (depending on the size of the bird) of normal saline into the crop. The fluid is then immediately aspirated but care must be taken not to apply too much negative pressure to the syringe otherwise the mucous membrane is liable to be sucked into and block the catheter.

Tracheal washings

A small diameter (16 g or 1 mm, e.g. a canine i.v. catheter) length of nylon tube, long enough to reach the syrinx which lies just caudal to the thoracic inlet, is passed through the glottis with the neck extended and 0.5–2 ml/kg of normal saline is flushed into the lumen of the trachea and immediately withdrawn for examination. Probably best carried out in the lightly anaesthetised or deeply sedated bird.

Aspiration of infraorbital or paraorbital sinuses

The needle is inserted into the point of greatest distension or through the skin at the commisure of the mouth passing either above or below the zygomatic arch (which can be palpated just below the skin). Great care needs to be taken in directing the needle so that it does not puncture the eye ball or any of the adjacent musculature and so induce profuse bleeding (see pp. 155 and 156).

Impression imprints from autopsy specimens

After incision through a representative area (e.g. liver, neoplasm) the cut surface is blotted gently with paper towel to remove excess blood or fluid. A glass slide is then firmly placed on the surface and then removed. Sometimes indurated tissue is best scraped with a scalpel and the scrapings placed on the slide for examination.

Processing samples

Fluid samples

After collection into the aspirating syringe and before processing, exudates are best first transferred to an EDTA blood collection vial to prevent any tendency to clotting which sometimes occurs. If the fluid is relatively clear and possibly has little suspended cellular content it can be centrifuged at slow speed (1500 rpm) for 10 min to concentrate the cellular content. High speed centrifugation can damage some cells. Alternatively the sample can be placed in a vertically supported tube and allowed to precipitate by gravitation. Another method is to place a piece of filter paper with a suitable size hole (8–10 mm) on top of a glass slide and then hold paper and inverted tube in place with a rubber washer placed over the hole and clamped to the slide. The fluid for examination having been placed in a glass tube placed over the centre of the hole is gradually absorbed by the filter paper leaving the solid cellular content on the glass slide for examination.

Fluid samples should first be assessed for their colour (haemolysis, milky – indicating fat droplets, etc.), clarity, specific gravity and protein content (using a 'dipstick'). A smear is then made, air dried and stained with a Romanowsky or a 'quick' stain. The cellular content of the sample should be analysed for the presence of heterophils, macrophages (containing phagocytosed bacteria), extracellular micro-organisms, normal epithelial cells and cells with signs of malignancy.

Solid samples

If the tissue from which the sample was obtained looks fatty the smear should be stained with Sudan III or IV together with new methylene blue stain (a water-soluble stain). Otherwise the smear can be stained with a Romanowsky stain (Wright's or Giemsa). It is often useful to stain a second companion slide with new methylene blue since some features of cell morphology are seen more clearly with this stain while other aspects of the cell are seen best with the Romanowsky stain. In some cases use of a bacterial stain (Gram or acid fast, etc.) may be appropriate.

Interpretation of samples

Hyperplastic tissue, inflammatory swellings and malignancies

An attempt should be made to identify the various types of cell present in the sample and also their relative proportions. Does the smear contain a high proportion of leucocytes indicating an *inflammatory reaction*? Are these cells mainly heterophils, monocytes or lymphocytes, indicating an acute or chronic inflammatory response? Do any of the heterophils look toxic? *Cell toxicity* is indicated by a degranulated and degenerative rather indistinct staining nucleus. The cytoplasm of the cell tends to stain more basophilic (but compare this with the general background staining of the slide). Also there may be variable granulation and vacuolation in the cytoplasm. Do some of the monocytes (macrophages) contain phagocytosed bacteria? If a sample has been obtained from the surface of a mucous membrane or from fluid adjacent to such (e.g. alimentary canal, trachea) and has been stained with a bacterial stain which indicates a *mixed* selection of extracellular organisms, then these are most likely representative of normal flora. If the stained smear is dominated by one particular organism this is most likely pathogenic.

Neoplastic cells not only show an increase in proportion of cells with mitotic figures in their nuclei (the presence of which is normal in a few bone marrow and liver cells) but also *the overall size of the nuclei* in relation to the cytoplasm is greater than in normal mature cells. Also the cytoplasm tends to stain more basophilic, i.e. bluish. Neoplastic cells overall and their nuclei in particular tend to be much more pleomorphic (i.e. they vary considerably in size and shape).

Bone marrow

On a sample from a normal bird it should be possible to identify the normal maturing stages of erythroblasts. The early, very immature cells, the rubriblasts, like all immature cells, are large round cells containing a nucleus which occupies most of the cell. Although both cytoplasm and nucleus are intensely stained, at this stage the cytoplasm is the more densely stained of the two. As maturity proceeds the overall size of the cell reduces and the nucleus becomes much smaller in proportion to the cytoplasm. Also the intense colour of the cytoplasm gradually fades passing through a polychromatic phase, with varying depths of blue staining, and ultimately acquiring the pale pink of mature erythrocyte. At the same time the nucleus shrinks and its chromatin becomes condensed and more intensively stained.

In normal bone marrow all stages of this developing process should be recognisable and not dominated by one type. The precursor cells of avian granulocytes (myeloblasts) are at first similar to the rubricyte although the cytoplasm is less deeply staining and gradually it will develop the cytoplasmic granules typical of heterophils (fusiform light red eosinophilic), basophils (*deeply* staining basophilic dark blue spherical granules) or eosinophils (round *deeply* staining eosinophilic red granules). Round cells (approximately the same size as erythrocytes) which have a large nucleus and in which the whole cell is very intensely stained are the precursory cells of thrombocytes. These cells gradually reduce in size and take on the shape and characteristics of small erythrocytes except that their cytoplasm is colourless or very faintly blue in colour.

Also normally found in bone marrow samples are small numbers of lymphocytes, monocytes, osteoclasts and osteoblasts. Mitotic figures are normally seen in some of the cells examined in a bone marrow sample.

For those clinicians wishing to pursue this subject the best references with colour illustrations are Campbell (1988) and (1994).

Crop washings

Check the pH of the aspirate which should be around 6.5–7. An increased pH may indicate sour crop. The normal sample of crop washings should show squamous epithelial cells, a mixture of normal symbiotic bacteria (mostly Gram negatives) and a lot of background debris. If the squamous epithelial cells are excessively cornified (use the same stain as when examining canine vaginal mucosa for signs of oestrus) this may suggest hypovitaminosis A. In the case of a candida infection, one may see budding yeast cells together with short length hyphae, both of which stain with methylene blue or the Romanowsky stains. Trichomonads will only be seen in freshly examined wet mounted samples preferably placed on a slightly warmed slide. When present the flaggelated protozoa can be seen to be moving vigorously.

Tracheal washings

The observer should look for signs of bacterial phagocytosis and, if present, stain for chlamydia. Also, look for signs of aspergillosis. The hyphae are long, septate and branch at 45°. Occasionally a conidiophore may be seen. Again, these fungi stain with methylene blue or the Romanowsky stains.

For those who wish to look for further information on the technique of avian cytology the most useful texts are Campbell (1988), Campbell (1994) and Dorrestein (1996). Although written for application to the dog and cat, another very useful publication on cytology is that by Perman *et al.* (1979).

Biopsy

Biopsy specimens can be most easily taken from surface neoplasms. They may also help in the diagnosis of skin lesions such as those caused by avian pox virus when the typical inclusion bodies may be found. Biopsies may be taken also from internal organs under direct vision via a laparoscope. Detailed explanations are given by Taylor (1994). Histology of post-mortem tissues may be necessary to help to confirm a diagnosis of such disease as Pacheco's parrot disease. This often shows few signs except slight mottling of the liver and the typical acidophilic intranuclear inclusion bodies in the liver cells and sometimes the kidney cells.

Histopathology may be the *only* method of confirming a diagnosis in some diseases such as neuropathic gastric dilatation of psittacines or viral induced papillomatosis of Amazon parrots. Liver biopsy samples may be obtained using direct vision via an endoscope or by making a small incision in the abdomen just posterior to the sternum.

Examination of faeces for evidence of helminth infection

Birds carry a variety of helminth parasites. Many birds kept in outside aviaries will easily become infected from the faeces of wild birds which may shed large numbers of parasite eggs. Imported birds may be carrying unfamiliar parasites from their country of origin. Faecal samples should therefore be examined on a routine basis. If the first sample is negative, subsequent samples on alternate days should be examined as some species of helminth parasites shed their eggs intermittently. Also, if the owner has recently but inconclusively wormed his birds, then samples are best not examined for several days as some drugs, especially if used at sub-optimal doses, merely suppress egg-laying rather than completely kill the parasites. Faecal samples can be examined by the standard flotation and centrifugation concentrating techniques.

LAPAROSCOPY

Laparoscopy in one form or another has been used in man and animals since the early part of the twentieth century. However, only comparatively recently, with the development of the human arthroscope, has the technique been applied to birds. It was first used in birds to determine the sex of those species that do not show sexual dimorphism – the so called technique of surgical sexing. Other methods of sexing birds are discussed in Chapter 9, p. 210. However, apart from the direct visual inspection of the avian gonads, it is also possible to evaluate the state of many of the other organs. It is possible to see much of the kidneys, the adrenal glands, the posterior surface of the lungs, the heart, the liver, the proventriculus, the gizzard and the intestines. It is also easy to see parts of the air sac system. Laparoscopy is therefore a useful tool to aid in the diagnosis of many conditions.

The equipment

The endoscopes used for this operation have been designed for the inspection of human joint spaces and range in diameter from 1.7 mm to 2.7 mm. A larger 5 mm instrument can be used on larger birds or sometimes even in birds down to 200 g in weight, when it is necessary to do photography. The apparatus consists of a light source, a flexible light

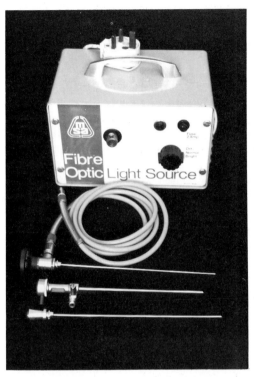

Fig. 3.3 The essential equipment to carry out laparoscopy. The light source, the light guide attached to the 2.7 mm arthroscope, the cannula and the trocar.

guide and the arthroscope, together with a trocar and cannula. The latest systems now use a fluid-filled light guide. The endoscope is made up of an outer bundle of glass fibres, transmitting light into the organ being viewed, which are wrapped around an inner core of lenses forming the viewing telescope. The whole is encased in a stainless-steel sheath. The angle of vision varies with different instruments from direct-forward to retrograde. The direct-forward viewing lens is the simplest to use for avian laparoscopy.

Operative methods

Various entry sites to the bird's body are favoured by different authorities for viewing the gonads and other organs. The author prefers the technique demonstrated to him by Samour *et al.* (1984). The anaesthetised bird is placed in right lateral recumbency with the left side uppermost. The left leg is then drawn forward and held in this position by an assistant or by a restraining tape. In birds below 400 g in weight it is often easier if the operator holds the left leg and left wing out of the way of the incision site. The area of the incision is found in the angle formed just posterior to the proximal end of the femur and anterior to the pubic bones (Fig. 3.4(a)). Methods used by other operators are to pull the left leg posteriorly and to make the incision midway into the space between the anterior edge of the femur and the last rib. Bush (1980) describes using the sternal notch, a landmark in the angle formed between the sternum and where this is joined by the last rib (Fig. 3.4(b)). Böttcher (1980) makes his incision between the last two ribs just above the angulation (Fig. 3.4(c)). Whichever point of entry is used, it is very important, particularly in small birds, to get the bird correctly positioned and to be certain of the anatomical landmarks. Before use, the instrument is sterilised using either ethylene oxide gas or by cold sterilisation with benzalkonium chloride (1:2500). The latter method is more convenient when a number of consecutive surgical sexings are being carried out. After cold sterilisation the endoscope is rinsed in sterile water and dried with a sterile towel. Together with the endoscope it is necessary to have a scalpel fitted with a number 11 blade and useful to have a selection of sterile ophthalmic instruments available.

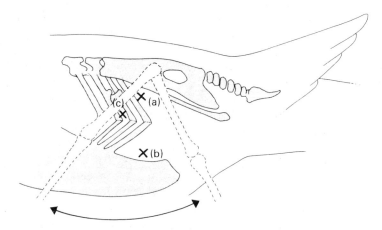

Fig. 3.4 Entry points (a), (b), (c) for laparoscopy in relation to the skeleton.

The operation can be carried out using either a general or local anaesthetic. Local anaesthetic is only really suitable for a quick inspection of the gonads, when a large number of surgical sexings are being carried out consecutively. General anaesthesia allows much easier and safer control of the patient, with much less risk of damage to internal organs by the endoscope. In addition there is more time to carry out a thorough inspection of all viscera.

Having correctly positioned the anaesthetised bird, the operation site is plucked free of feathers. Only the minimum number of feathers necessary to clear the area should be removed. The region is then cleaned and sterilised with a quaternary ammonium antiseptic, taking care not to get the bird too wet. An alcoholic or iodine preparation can be used to complete the process. The operation site is then draped with a transparent plastic or paper drape. Both of these are lighter in weight than cloth drapes and a transparent drape enables the bird's respiratory rate to be seen during the operation. Either type should contain a small central opening.

A small incision 4–7 mm in length is made and any bleeding from the skin vessels is controlled because this is liable to cloud the distal end of the endoscope during insertion and obstruct the view. Also any subsequent leak of air from the air sacs during expiration will cause blood on the surface of the skin to foam and obscure the incision. The cannula, fitted with the trocar, is next inserted through the underlying muscle using controlled pressure and at the same time slightly rotating the trocar backwards and forwards. To minimise trauma and reach the desired area it is most important to aim the trocar and cannula in the right direction. If the site using the angle between the femur and pubic bone is used, the instrument is directed downwards and forwards at a slight angle to the vertical away from the vertebrae so that it is travelling more or less towards the centre of the abdominal cavity. In the other methods the trocar and cannula are directed vertically in a direction parallel to the plane of the thoracic and lumbar vertebrae. If the procedure is carried out correctly, the operator can feel the slight pressure on the trocar suddenly 'give' as it pops through the muscle layer into the abdominal cavity. The trocar is then withdrawn leaving the cannula in position so that the arthroscope can be inserted. Should there be any blood on the trocar when this is withdrawn, the whole operation is stopped immediately. During manipulation of these instruments it is best to be seated and to have the elbows resting on the table. The left hand supports the cannula near the point of entry and the right hand controls and directs the trocar and laparoscope. This position of the operator allows a delicate and careful control of the instruments. In small birds below 60 g and down to 20 g in weight, the arthroscope can be inserted after the initial incision has been made in the muscle, by pushing a pair of mosquito artery forceps into the incision and opening these slightly to expand the incision. Care must be taken not to bend or break the arthroscope when applying this method.

Problems associated with the technique

No method is without hazard. The first site of entry described has the slight risk that the ischiatic nerve and femoral blood vessels may be damaged. In all methods if care is not taken and the instrument is pushed in with too much force or is wrongly directed the viscera could be damaged. Obviously rupture of the heart or of a main blood vessel will prove rapidly fatal. However, slight puncture of the liver or kidney results in haematoma formation which usually resolves within a few days. Penetration of the gizzard is unlikely in the herbivorous birds because of its thick-walled nature, but in carnivorous birds the gizzard has a much thinner wall and is much more likely to rupture, particularly if the bird has not been starved for 12 hours before laparoscopy. However, before starving the bird, the clinician should take account of the bird's nutritional state because of the danger of hypoglycaemia. If the gizzard is punctured this will necessitate a laparotomy and suturing the organ, together with appropriate antibiotic cover. In the case of all sites of entry there is a slight risk of subcutaneous emphysema through air leaking from the air sac system but this usually resolves spontaneously.

Apart from these hazards the technique is not as easy as it might at first appear and much practice is required to develop the necessary skill, particularly in the smaller birds. The practitioner would therefore be wise to learn this art on several freshly-killed cadavers before proceeding to the live bird. One of the first difficulties of an unskilled operator is failure to obtain a clear sighting of the internal organs when looking down the telescope. One may see nothing more than an opaque pale-pink haze. This usually means that the tip of the endoscope is lying against one of the viscera or its view is obscured by air sac or peritoneal membrane or it has not properly penetrated the abdominal muscles. Very slight and slow retraction of the endoscope and cannula or slight withdrawal of the endoscope into the cannula, often results in the view clearing. If nothing happens the instrument should be pulled further back and if there is no improvement then it is likely that the abdominal muscle has not been penetrated. The endoscope should be removed and the trocar reinserted and the direction of the penetration reassessed.

If the internal organs can be dimly seen but they are not clear then the operator is looking through an air sac membrane. Air sacs vary in their clarity and it may be possible for the experienced clinician to identify an ovary or testes without proceeding further. However, to obtain a clearer view, the posterior abdominal membrane will have to be ruptured. It may be possible to do this by simply advancing the endoscope and cannula and at the same time giving a slight twist. However, it might also be necessary to reinsert the trocar.

If the view down the endoscope is obscured by a blood red haze, then a blood vessel has been ruptured or the liver or kidney has been penetrated. It is safer to cease the operation for a short period until the situation can be evaluated. If the endoscope is only partially obscured by blood this can often be wiped free against a suitable internal organ such as the gizzard.

Another problem is excess abdominal fat. This is not uncommonly found in captive, inactive raptors. Also the abdomen may be partly filled with exudate as in the case of an egg peritonitis.

Having penetrated the abdomen and obtained a clear view, the next problem experienced by the unskilled operator is orientation of the various organs in relation to each other. The operator must learn to appreciate that slightly advancing or withdrawing the endoscope makes a relatively rapid change in the magnification of the object being viewed.

Examination of the internal organs

The first organs usually to be seen and which are unlikely to be mistaken by anyone who has carried out a number of avian post-mortems are the lungs. The caudal ventral surface of these structures can be examined and the ostia of the secondary bronchi where these enter the caudal thoracic air sac can be seen. Depending on which site of entry is used, the endoscope may have entered the caudal thoracic or the abdominal air sac. It may be necessary to puncture the division between these two air sacs to see other organs clearly. Lying ventral to the lungs (to the left in the recumbent bird) the pulsating heart can easily be recognised. Moving the tip of the endoscope further to the operator's left, the lobes of the liver can be seen as they approach the heart and partially envelop the gizzard. If the endoscope is then carefully moved to find the medial caudal edge of the left lung, the large rounded dark brownish-red colour of the left cranial division of the kidney can be recognised. This lies posterior but very close to the lung. Immediately ventral and slightly anterior to the kidney is situated the pink-coloured adrenal gland. The gonads lie adjacent but caudal to the adrenal gland, so that the kidney, adrenal and gonads form the three points of a triangle (Fig. 3.5).

Surgical sexing

In the immature male the testis is a rounded, slightly oval structure very little bigger than the adrenal gland but a little more yellow in colour. In some species the testes may be wholly or partly pigmented dark green or black in colour. In the immature bird it may be possible to see both testes lying one on each side of the dorsal aorta and vena cava. As the testis matures, it increases in size and blood vessels become obvious on the surface. The blood vessels become more tortuous with age. In the active testes during the breeding season the organ may become very large and more difficult to recognise. In the aged testis the gonad is more angular in shape. In the immature female the ovary tends to be 'L' shaped and about the same length as the cranial division of the left kidney. The colour is a buff yellow, the surface is flat and the texture slightly granular in appearance. Sometimes the ovary is pigmented. As the ovary matures

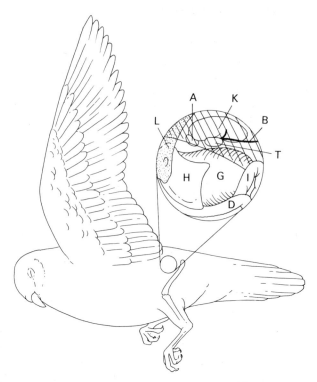

Fig. 3.5 Organs that can be identified by laparoscopy. ▨indicates the extent of the abdominal air sac. A, adrenal gland; B, main blood vessels; D, duodenum; G, gizzard; H, liver; I, intestine; K, kidney; L, lung; T, testis.

follicles become more apparent and these will vary in size. Gradually as the ovary increases in size it begins to obscure the kidney and adrenal gland. In the active ovary during the breeding season some of the individual follicles can become very large, taking up a large part of the abdominal cavity. In the old female bird the ovary has contracted again and while follicles can be recognised much of the ovary is occupied by scar tissue.

At the end of laparoscopy the skin and underlying muscle are brought together with a single suture. Some operators consider this unnecessary. Bush (1980) describes the taking of biopsy specimens under direct vision, using a secondary cannula with biopsy forceps or using a biopsy needle, to aid in the early diagnosis of tuberculosis of the liver. Samples can also be taken from other organs for culture and histopathology. Fluids can be aspirated from an air sac under direct vision or small quantities (3 ml in a large bird) of fluid can be instilled into the air sacs to obtain sample washings.

Other uses for the endoscope

The instrument can also be used to examine the posterior part of the nasal cavity through the choanal opening. The trachea, the syrinx and bronchi may also be inspected. Before the latter is examined the posterior air sacs are cannulated to allow obstructed respiration to proceed. The ease with which all these cavities can be viewed will obviously depend on the size of the bird. It is also possible to visualise the oesophagus, crop and proventriculus of a bird as small in weight as 40 g.

Laparoscopic photography

Special cameras can be used for clinical documentation of the organs viewed through the endoscope. Adaptors can also be obtained so that the telescope eyepiece can be coupled to the standard lens of any single lens reflex camera. The best results are obtained if a xenon flash tube is incorporated in the light source but this increases the initial cost of the equipment. For photography it is better to use a 5 mm diameter endoscope which transmits more light than the smaller diameter instruments – less exposure of the film being necessary. Nevertheless, it is possible to obtain reasonably good results with a 2.7 mm diameter endoscope, using Kodachrome 64 (ISO.64) film, with exposures of the order of 0.25–0.50 seconds. Kodachrome 200 film will produce even better results. One needs a steady hand, good anaesthesia and an assistant to operate the shutter of the camera with a cable release. The camera lens is focused at infinity and set to maximum aperture before coupling to the endoscope. If the camera has interchangeable viewing screens a clear screen is best.

RADIOGRAPHY

This is a useful aid to diagnosis particularly in the case of abnormalities of the skeleton, but also in disease of other organ systems.

Restraint of the avian patient

In the opinion of the author radiography is best carried out under general anaesthesia, preferably using isoflurane. However, other workers have obtained consistently satisfactory results while having the conscious bird restrained in a custom-made radiotransluscent jig. Both methods enable the radiographer to position the bird carefully with correct centring and collimation of the X-ray beam. It is possible to take quick radiographs of the extremities of a hand-held bird, but apart from the risks to the handler, it is almost impossible to adequately and gently restrain a small bird whilst wearing protective lead rubber gloves. Having attained anaesthesia or deep sedation the patient is best maintained in the required position using adhesive plaster or Sellotape placed over the limbs and neck and stuck to a radiolucent, transparent perspex sheet, placed over the X-ray cassette.

Radiographs, to be of maximum diagnostic value, should be obtained only after care has been exercised to obtain a true ventro-dorsal or lateral position of the patient. This is tedious and needs meticulous assessment by the operator to judge by sight and touch that the sternum overlies the vertebrae. If correct positioning is not achieved in the ventro-dorsal position, the two sides of the body cannot be accurately compared. Apparent distortion of various structures and body cavities may be seen which has no clinical significance. The air sacs on one side may look smaller than those on the other side of the body. The shadow of the liver and the position of the gizzard may become distorted. In the true lateral position the two hip joints and the two shoulder joints should overlap. The wings must be held by the tape above the body. The legs need to be held positioned so that their radiographic image does not obstruct any part of the body which is of radiographic interest (e.g. the spleen, the reproductive tract, the intestine).

When X- raying the wings care should be taken, not only to have both wings in a flat position and as close to the X-ray film as possible, but also to make sure that both wings are extended to the same degree. It is very helpful in making a diagnosis to be able to compare the radiographic image of the two wings. As the shoulder joint extends, slight rotation of the humerus takes place and as the elbow joint extends, the radius slides longitudinally in relation to the ulna. Also in extension of the carpal joint, pronation of the metacarpal region occurs.

Radiographs of the skull should be in true ventro-dorsal and lateral positions with the neck fully extended. Left and right oblique views with the head rotated 15° around the long axis of the body line and the X-ray beam centred on the orbit, may also be helpful.

X-ray film and exposure factors

Radiographs may be taken on X-ray film held in the cassettes preferably with fast calcium tungstate or rare-earth intensifying screens. Alternatively, non-screen film may be used to obtain greater detail. Using Ilford red seal film with rare-earth screens at a distance of 36 inches (91 cm), a kilovoltage of 48 and a milliamp/second (m.a.s.) value of 4, is found to be satisfactory for a bird the size of a budgerigar. For somewhat larger birds of about 400 g (e.g. African grey parrot) the kV should be increased to 58. McMillan (1982, p. 330) suggests increasing these kV values by 10 units, and so halving the m.a.s. value.

When using non-screen film, the focus to subject distance can be reduced to 20 inches (50 cm). This will reduce the exposure time necessary and in the case of small birds there will be very little loss of image quality due to distortion.

The radiographer should be aware that there is considerable difference in size in the air sacs between the inspiratory and expiratory phases of respiration. If possible the exposure is best made at the end of the inspiratory pause when the air sacs are at maximum dilation so that optimal use is made of the natural air contrast in the avian body. No grid is necessary since most avian bodies are less than 10 cm in thickness and the total mass of tissues is less than in mammals of comparable size.

Many diseases are multisystemic so that it is good policy to get into the habit of examining whole body radiographs in a systematic manner. One should start with the external outline and work inwards, so that each organ system can thus be considered in detail. A common fault is to fix attention on an obvious lesion and miss less apparent abnormalities

Radiographs of the muscle/skeletal system

Radiography is an aid to avian orthopaedic surgery, and is helpful in assessing the degree of distortion and prognosis in metabolic bone disease. Osteoporosis is most often but not only seen in raptors. It occurs in fledglings which have not received a balanced calcium phosphorous intake which should be about 1.5 : 1.0. This results in folding distortion of the thin and weak cortex of the long bones. Gross distortion of the bones in the wings and legs takes place which often results in the bird becoming a permanent cripple. The disease is most likely to occur in the case of artificially-reared birds of prey fed entirely on a diet of meat, which contains little if any calcium. Also it is not uncommon in fledgling parrots, particularly when hand reared, that one of a clutch of chicks will develop the condition while its siblings are normal. It also occurs in wild birds. Other conditions that can be recognised by radiography include osteo-myelitis, neoplasia, arthritis and tuberculosis. In mycobacteriosis there is often localised osteolysis together with surrounding sclerosis and also accompanied by focal densities in the long bones (Peiper and Krautwald-Junghanns, 1991). These signs in the skeletal tissues are often seen together with soft tissue changes in the lungs (focal densities) together with hepatomegaly and splenomengaly. When an osteomyelitis is present in a long bone, new bone tends to be formed by the cortex of the bone and the endosteum rather than by the periosteum as is the case in mammals. Neoplasia tends to be predominantly osteolytic. This is sometimes seen in pigeons, in the carpal and shoulder joints, with *Salmonella* infection. Radiography of all the limb joints in the bird is easy except in the case of the hip joint where the shape of the ilium makes outlining of the joint difficult.

Another condition, often found incidently during radiography is polystotic hyperostosis. This is not uncommon in the budgerigar and is also occasionally seen in other psittacines. It is recognised by the medullary cavities of the long bones – normally filled with air – becoming filled with solid bone. There is also a general overall increase in bone density throughout the skeleton. This condition normally occurs in hens before egg laying but in the pathological condition the bone appears much more dense on the radiograph and also sometimes involves the bones of the skull. It has been reported by Stauber *et al.* (1990) as occurring in a cockatiel with a neoplasm of the oviduct and has been seen by the author in the male budgerigar with sertoli cell tumours. The disease is believed to be due to excess oestrogen and can be reproduced by a stilboestrol implant (McMillan, 1982, p. 340).

When viewing radiographs of the skeleton in the diagnosis of orthopaedic problems, one should try and get as much information as possible about the muscular system. A reduction in size of one of the pectoralis muscles due to muscle atrophy, can often be seen on a radiograph though it may not be so obvious by palpation. It may be possible to detect slight contraction and swelling of the muscle mass of the supracoracoideus after rupture of the tendon that passes through the foramen triosseum. In the forelimb, the shadows of the biceps and triceps brachii muscles can be identified. A large part of the latter muscle originates from the surface of the humerus and is liable to sustain trauma in fracture of the adjacent bone. The tensor muscles and tendon of the propatagial membrane are often damaged. This may result from collision with such objects as telephone wires. The flexors and extensors of the carpus and digits should be examined.

Signs of injury to muscles are shown by a subtle increase in density when compared with the other wing. Some idea of how recent an injury to the skeleton is, can be gauged by the condition of the neighbouring muscles. In a very recent injury there is a noticeable increase in size and density of the radiographic shadow. This usually decreases considerably, almost returning to normal during the course of the next few days, providing the fracture is not compound and there is no superimposed infection.

Interpretation of soft tissue radiographs

Since the radiograph is a two dimensional shadow of a three dimensional structure, it is essential to take both ventro-dorsal and lateral views when X-raying the internal organs. Whereas the air sacs provide some natural contrast, it is still essential to make a correct exposure if one is to gain the maximum information from the radiograph. Also, if possible the exposure should be made at maximum inspiration.

One of the most obvious features to be seen when first looking at an avian ventro-dorsal radiograph is the 'waist' between the shadow of the heart and that of the liver. In raptors generally, particularly if they have been fasted for sometime, the liver shadow tends to be more elongated and consequently the hour glass outline is less distinct. If the two shadows become indistinct and merge into one uniform outline, this usually indicates hepatomegaly often accompanied by an increase in density of the hepatic shadow. Alternatively a decrease in radio opacity of the liver is indicative of fatty infiltration. However, an apparent increase in size on the left side of the hepatic shadow may be caused by an increase in size of the proventriculus. A thickening of the wall together with an increased density of the proventriculus, seen in both ventro-dorsal and lateral projections, may indicate hypovitaminosis A or neoplasia. A definite enlargement with the organ occupying much of the thoraco-abdominal cavity best seen using barium contrast usually indicates psittacine proventricular dilatation (macaw wasting disease, a condition which has now been identified in many species of parrot (Gerlach, 1991). Candida infection may occasionally cause an enlarged proventricular shadow. Increased density in the oesophagus usually indicates neoplasia. Alternatively, a reduction in size due to atrophy of the liver may be recognised. If the liver is enlarged, in the ventro-dorsal view the gizzard is often seen to be displaced well to the left-hand side and in the lateral view to be displaced caudally and slightly dorsally. The gizzard is easily recognisable in granivorous birds because of the retained grit and normally occupies a position just to the left of the mid-line and just below an imaginary line joining the two hips. In raptors the non-grit-filled ventriculus (or gizzard) is usually just cranial to this level and not so distinct. In granivorous birds, if the amount of grit in the gizzard is excessive, as is rather the case with the parrot illustrated in Figs. 3.6 and 3.7, this tends to indicate malfunction of the gastrointestinal tract. Other signs of gastrointestinal disease are an increased density, leading to greater visualisation of the intestinal loops. This is sometimes accompanied by gas filling and distension. These signs may also be indicative of microbiological or parasitic infection. However, gas filling is normal in some waterfowl and game birds. Foreign body obstruction of the intestine in birds is not usually accompanied by a build-up of gas as is the case in mammals. There may, however, be enlargement and greater visualisation of the intestine. Gastrointestinal disease is also indicated by grit and when using barium contrast, undigested seed in the intestine.

Foreign bodies such as fish hooks, lead shot and nails are not uncommonly seen lodged in the oesophagus, the proventriculus or gizzard of water fowl and are sometimes seen in other species. They may occasionally pass farther along the alimentary canal. If a bird has been given only soluble oyster shell grit, then the gizzard may not be identified

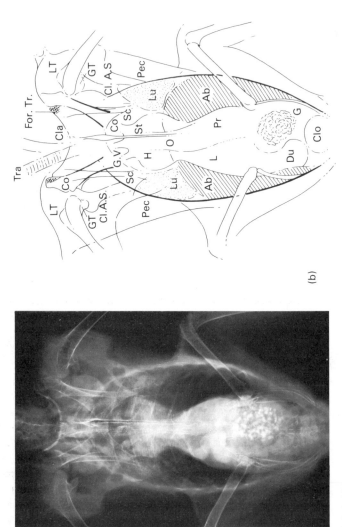

(a)

(b)

Fig. 3.6 (a) Ventro-dorsal radiograph of festive Amazon parrot. (b) Ab, abdominal air sac; Cla, clavicle; Clo, cloaca; Cl.A.S., clavicular air sac diverticulum; Co, coracoid; Du, duodenum and supraduodenal loop of intestine; H, heart; For. Tr., foreamen triosseum; G, gizzard; GT, greater tuberosity for the flexor muscles of the shoulder joint; G.V., great blood vessels – the aorta and its branches; L, liver; Lu, lung; LT, lesser tuberosity for the insertion of the supracoracoideus. Immediately behind the deltoid crest for the insertion of the pectoralis; O, oesophagus; Pr, proventriculus; Pec, pectoralis major muscle; Sc, scapula; St, sternum; Tra, trachea.

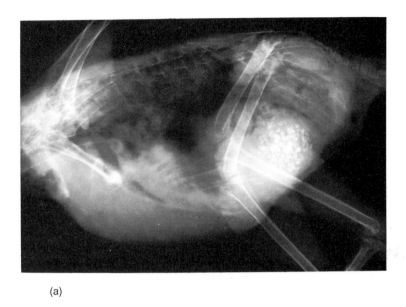

(a)

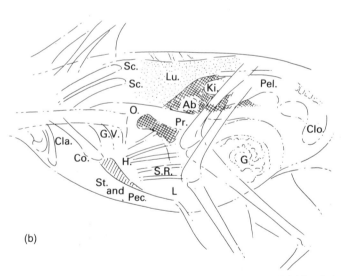

(b)

Fig. 3.7 (a) Lateral radiograph of a festive amazon parrot, (b) Ab, abdominal air sac; Cla, clavicle; Clo, cloaca; Co, coracoid; G, gizzard; GV, great vessels; H, heart; Ki, kidney; Lu, lung; L, liver; O, oesophagus; Pel, pelvis; Pr, proventriculus; Pec, pectoralis muscle; Sc, scapula; St, sternum; SR, sternal ribs.

by this method. Also a bird may have been deprived of grit. Space-occupying lesions may be responsible for displacing the normal position of the gizzard shadow. Enlargement of the gonads, which occupy a position central to the anterior of the kidney and the syncrosacrum, may, if greatly enlarged, displace the gizzard. This is normal in the breeding season. In lesions of the oviduct, such as a gross salphingitis and impaction with inspissated yolk, the gizzard will be displaced ventrally and either cranially or caudally. A collapsed, distorted and impacted egg may damage the oviduct and result in an egg peritonitis. Occasionally dilation of the oviduct may be caused by radiotranslucent, uncalcified soft shelled egg. The renal shadow occupies a similar position to that of the gonads occasionally, but particularly in budgerigars, enlargement together with an increase in density may be due to a neoplasm such as an adenocarcinoma. An increase in density without enlargement may be a sign of lead intoxication. Occasionally a meshwork of delicate tubules filled with urate crystals can be seen in the kidneys. This is more likely an indication of *Eschericia coli* or other infection than visceral gout. This is more apparent if the left kidney is affected. Pathological change in the viscera is often accompanied by a slight increase in density of the radiographic shadow. In species of birds such as raptors where the gizzard is not detectable by its retained grit, the gizzard can be made visible only by using barium sulphate contrast media.

The spleen is best seen on the lateral projection. It shows as a relatively small round or oval (in raptors) shadow situated between the angle of the liver and the gizzard. In Fig. 3.7 its shadow is overlain by that of the distal end of the more ventral of the two femurs. Although in normal birds the spleen may not always be recognisable, when it is enlarged due to infection or neoplasia it is easily seen. In psittacines a great increase in size together with increased visualisation of the air sacs (through striation) accompanied by focal consolidations in the lungs and hepatomegaly is very suggestive of *Chlamydia*. These signs without any signs of air sac involvement tend to suggest mycobacteriosis.

In good quality radiographs the two lungs can be identified by their slight honeycomb appearance. This effect is best seen in the lateral view, and at maximum inspiration. The diagnostician should look for any slight localised increases in density or patches where there is loss of the normal reticular pattern. Such localised densities are more discrete and nodular when caused by aspergillosis. When bacterial infection is the cause the patches of abnormality are more diffuse and very occasionally are accompanied by calcification if the infection has been prolonged. The air sacs should be carefully examined. The extrathoracic diverticula of the clavicular sacs can be seen in the pectoral muscle mass around the proximal end of the humerus. However there is considerable inter-specific variation in these diverticula (McLelland, 1989). In fractures of this bone this part of the air sac system may be damaged as is shown by a change in shape or increase in size or density of the X-ray image. When looking at the abdominal air sacs, absence of their outline may be due to a space-occupying lesion, or more likely due to adhesions or gross air sacculitis. Less severe air sacculitis is recognised by a general haziness of part or all of the air sac spaces. In the lateral view striated dense lines on the radiograph represent the end-on view of thickened air sacs. Enlargement of the abdominal air sacs, which may be unilateral, can be caused by 'air trapping' due to mycotic granuloma or congestion of the mucous membrane lining of the ports of entry and exit from the air sacs. The left and right abdominal air sacs should always be compared for any signs of localised increase in density due to *Aspergillus* infection. In pigeons the abdominal air sacs are often considerably reduced in size due to excessive fat. An overall homogenous 'ground glass' increase in density, of both thoracic and abdominal cavities accompanied by obvious distension of the caudal abdomen is usually due to peritonitis or ascites. In mynah birds, some other passeriformes and toucans a degenerative iron storage hepatopathy is often responsible for ascites. These birds are often in respiratory distress, due to malfunction of the air sac system and are bad anaesthetic risks, particularly if placed in dorsal recumbency. Consequently good X-rays of this condition are not easy to obtain.

If the cardiac shadow is enlarged overall and increased in density this may indicate an increase in pericardial fluid possibly with contained uric crystals. Increased visualisation possibly due to calcification of any of the great vessels of the heart, particularly in very old parrots, indicates arteriosclerosis. On the ventro-dorsal projection, a prominent left atrial shadow together with increased length from base to apex of the heart accompanied by more visually prominent great vessels may indicate cardiopathy. A less obvious (i.e. more blurred) reticular pattern to the lateral lung field also indicates venous congestion.

There are a few interspecies peculiarities of which the avian radiologist should be aware. In some species the cervical air sac extends subcutaneously along the ventral side of the neck. Overall there is a considerable interspecific and sometimes intraspecific variation in the anatomy of the air sacs and also in the pneumatization of the bones. For a good review of the subject, see McLelland, 1989.

In the Anatinae (ducks and geese) there is a normal balloon-like irregular distension of the syrinx. This increases in size with age. In swans, cranes, spoonbills and birds of paradise, the trachea is elongated into coils which lie between the skin and pectoral muscles or within a tunnel in the sternum (King and McLelland, 1975). In penguins the trachea is bifurcated for most of its length (see Figs 1.3 and 1.9 and p. 21).

The use of contrast media

Contrast radiography of the alimentary canal

Barium sulphate suspension can be placed in the crop by an oesophageal tube made from any suitable diameter plastic or rubber tubing fitted to the nozzle of a hypodermic syringe. A rigid metal catheter, smooth at the distal end, can also be utilised for birds such as psittacines which are liable to nip off a softer tube. When using a rigid tube, it should be well lubricated. After extending the bird's head in a vertical direction, allow the tube to slide down under its own weight. The barium sulphate is best diluted with an equal quantity of water and then flushed down with water. A suitable quantity of diluted barium sulphate for a budgerigar is 0.5 ml, followed by another 0.5 ml of water. For a bird the size of an African grey parrot 2 ml amounts would be reasonable. Give the suspension slowly to avoid reflux up into the pharynx. The time taken for the contrast media to reach the various parts of the alimentary canal will depend on any drugs used for premedication and anaesthesia and also on any pathological condition that may be present. On average the barium will have reached the proventriculus and gizzard within 5 min and be in the small intestine within 30 min. Contrast media can help to define the position of the alimentary canal relative to the other viscera. It should reach the cloaca in about 3 h. In some raptors and particularly in frugivores, e.g. mynah birds, the passage time may be considerably shorter. Barium sulphate suspension or one of the iodine contrast agents such as meglumine iothalamate 70% w/v or sodium diatrizoate 45% w/v can be used for an enema to outline the cloaca and rectum. Suitable amounts of the correct agents for this technique in an Amazon parrot would be 1.5 ml of diluted barium sulphate followed by 3.5 ml of water. Air may be used as an alternative in the crop. Approximately 3 ml of air are required for this purpose in the budgerigar. Double contrast techniques are useful for the examination of the proventriculus and cloaca.

Urography and angiocardiography

The iodinised water soluble contrast agents mentioned above can be injected intravenously and will outline the heart and kidneys. For a bird the size of an Amazon parrot 1 ml should be given by slow injection and the radiograph for the heart taken immediately the injection is finished. If it is required to outline the kidney the X-ray should be taken after 5 min.

Cealiography

McMillan (1982, p. 359) describes a method of outlining the viscera in the budgerigar, by injecting 0.2 ml of sodium diatrizoate into the abdomen.

Ultrasonography

Ultrasound is an additional non-invasive diagnostic imaging technique which has been used in veterinary practice for the last 20 years and which with some limitations is applicable in avian clinical practice. It is useful in complementing imaging information gained by radiography. Whereas a radiograph provides a series of superimposed shadows of the external outlines of various internal organs, ultrasonography in some circumstances may give some indication about internal structural changes occurring within soft tissue organs. Pathology such as cysts or nodular tumours within an apparently externally normal liver can be detected. Sometimes an increased density of hepatic tissue may indicate fibrosis. However these changes detected by ultrasonographic imaging will need supplementing by blood biochemistry evaluation and by biopsy. The biopsy needle can even be accurately guided into position using the ultrasound beam.

In the present state of knowledge, unlike radiography, ultrasound is thought to be completely biologically safe for both the operator and the patient. It is painless, quick and can sometimes be used on the hand-held conscious bird without anaesthesia or sedation. However the capital investment in apparatus is expensive (at 1995 prices £12,000–£14,000) but once acquired the running costs are minimal. Because of this the apparatus is unlikely to be acquired solely for use in avian practice although a practitioner may have access to the equipment if it has been purchased for use in other species. The use of ultrasound in birds is limited by several factors. First the presence of the air sac systems produces a number of highly ultrasound reflective soft-tissue–air interfaces which impede the transmission of the ultrasound beam. Second the avian body is relatively better enclosed by a bony skeleton and bone absorbs ultrasound. Third in most birds there is only a small acoustic window (i.e. the area of the body through which the ultrasound beam can effectively be transmitted through the body's tissues) where the liver lies in close contact with the surface tissues just caudal to the xiphisternum and cranial to the bones of the pelvis.

For practical purposes Krautwald-Junghanns *et al.* (1991, 1995) has found that in birds from 10 g to 1 kg in bodyweight the optimum apparatus is one using a mechanical sector scanner (which sweeps out a fan shaped beam of 60°) and with a transducer producing an ultrasound frequency of 7.5 mHz. The working surface of the scanner should be no larger than 1.5 × 2.5 cm. Also the apparatus should be capable of producing an image with a wide Gray scale range (optimum 64 Gray scales) which helps in the differentiation of changes in tissue structure. Using this apparatus through the relatively small acoustic window available, a reasonably large area of the body's tissues can be surveyed. The scanner also has limited use when used through the right lateral flank just caudal to the last rib.

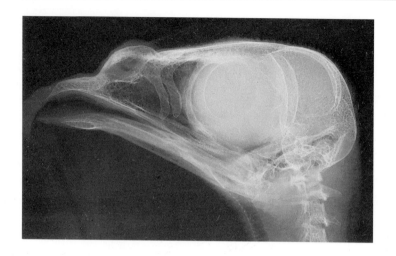

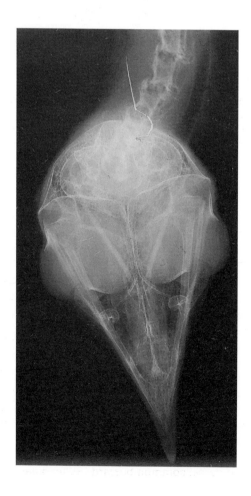

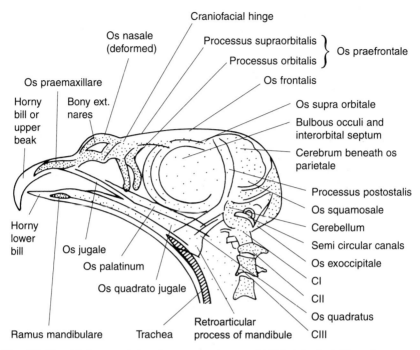

Fig. 3.8 Head laterao – lateral common buzzard (*Buteo buteo*) Showing distorted nasal bone around the external nares and leading to malfunction of the craniofacial hinge resulting in a malfunctioning upper beak, the horny sheath of which has overgrowth. This is a wild casualty bird and was not fit for release (see Fig. 1.1).

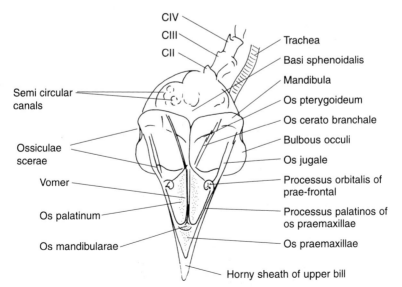

Fig. 3.8 Head ventro-dorsal common buzzard (*Buteo buteo*)

When using the apparatus to achieve the best results, food should be withheld for a suitable period so that the gastrointestinal tract is empty (i.e. unless the observer wants to investigate the GI tract). Also in most birds it is necessary to pluck the area of feathers from where the scanner is to be applied and at the same time to use plenty of acoustic coupling gel (which is water soluble and will not damage the plumage). The operator should not be tempted to use mineral oil or other substitutes which may damage the apparatus.

The avian clinician should get into the habit of working to a fixed routine so that in each area of the body that is examined by the ultrasound beam each organ is recognised and any changes in normal gross anatomy identified. This procedure should be carried out in a routine serial order.

The avian clinician needs to build up practical experience (which can to some extent be learnt by use on vertebrates other than birds) in being able to interpret the visual image produced by the echo of the ultrasound beam as it passes through the different organs in its path. Also the clinician needs to be able to recognise the various imaging artifacts which can occur such as acoustic shadows, acoustic enhancement and reverberation from reflective interfaces.

Some pathological conditions such as the impaction of an egg (even a soft shelled egg, which cannot be seen by radiography) are reasonably easy to identify, while ovarian tumours may not be so easily seen. Ultrasound is not a lot of help in the examination of the normal avian kidney, the quiescent testes or inactive ovary. However, it is possible to detect developing follicles in the ovary as the amount of echogenic yolk increases.

The proventriculus, gizzard and intestines can be seen particularly if water is administered beforehand. Peristalsis can sometimes be recognised. The avian eye is a relatively large structure compared with the body size of most birds so that ultrasonography has been effectively used to diagnose many pathological conditions in this structure. Krautwald-Junghanns *et al.* (1995) have elegantly demonstrated the dynamic imaging of the avian heart and its various internal structures while simultaneously recording the ECG.

Chapter 4
Post-mortem Examination

There is probably no other way in which a clinician's acumen is increased than by post-mortem examination. The post-mortem of patients subsequent to an ante-mortem diagnosis will help increase the practitioner's diagnostic ability and indicate ways in which the diagnostic routine can be improved.

The owner of a single bird, be it a pet cage bird or a falconer's hawk, is often interested in the cause of death and if there was anything he/she could have done to prevent death.

The client who has a flock of wild fowl or an aviary of birds that are chronically sick is often willing to sacrifice one or a few birds to establish the cause of the problem.

To be of maximum value post-mortem specimens should be as fresh as possible. Owing to the high initial body temperature of 40°C and to good body insulation of the feathers, autolysis occurs rapidly in birds. However, sometimes a client will produce a carcass of a bird which died 24–36 hours previously. In this case the carcass should be thoroughly soaked with cold soapy water and placed in a plastic bag with any excess air expressed. The sealed bag should then be put in a refrigerator so that the body is kept at a temperature just above freezing *but not frozen*. The feathering helps to retain body heat, so cooling the body as quickly as possible will help to reduce autolytic changes. If the carcass is deep-frozen the fine cellular structures are ruptured by ice crystals. Such tissues are useless for histopathology.

In those specimens that are up to 3 days old and in which no precautions have been taken to prevent autolysis, some useful information may often still be obtained.

A post-mortem should always be carried out in a systematic and routine order so that nothing is overlooked or forgotten. Having a checklist to hand is invaluable.

The practitioner should realise that the gross lesions seen during post-mortem can only provide a tentative diagnosis. Further laboratory tests will be needed for confirmation in most cases. Therefore it is wise to have certain equipment ready before starting the autopsy.

EQUIPMENT AND LABORATORY TECHNIQUES

(1)   A check-list of all body organs to be examined.
(2)   Scalpel and blades.
(3)   Rat-toothed forceps.
(4)   Sharp-pointed dissecting scissors.
(5)   Spirit lamp or Bunsen burner.
(6)   Bacteriological culture plates, blood agar and MacConkey agar.
(7)   Bacteriological swabs in transport medium. However, do not use transport medium if a swab is taken for a PCR test to detect *Chlamydia*. The use of the transport medium may give a false positive result. All living specimens have a better chance of survival if placed in transport medium.
(8)   Screw-top containers with 10% formol saline that should preferably be neutral buffered. Use of buffered formol saline makes histological examination easier. When harvesting solid organs specimens should not be more than 0.5 cm thick, otherwise the formalin will not fully penetrate the tissue. At least 10 times the volume of preservative as the specimen is required.
(9)   Screw-top sterile containers to contain tissues for bacteriological culture.
(10) Slides. These can be used for:
    (a)   Bacteriological staining; if the slide is sterilised by heating in the flame, the bacteriological swab will remain uncontaminated after the smear has been made on the sterile slide (p. 67).
    (b)   Slides can be used to make impression smears from liver, spleen and air sacs. Liver smears can be stained with modified Ziehl–Neelsen or Macchiavello's stain for *Chlamydia* inclusion bodies or with haematoxylin and eosin for herpes virus inclusion bodies seen in some species.
    (c)   If the bacteriological swab is rolled along the sterile slide instead of smearing across it, it can be stained with Wright's or Leishman's stain and then used for cytological examination.
(12) Strong scissors or even bone forceps for large birds.
(13) Some sterile gauze swabs are sometimes useful if a blood vessel is inadvertently punctured.
(14) Sterile syringes and needles for the sterile collection of heart, blood and intestinal contents for culture. If the ingesta are too viscid, a little sterile normal saline injected into the lumen of the gut will make them more fluid. To collect sterile samples from the interior of unopened hollow organs, first sterilise the surface by searing with a hot spatula before inserting the needle.
(15) At least one pair of sterile petri dishes to collect tissues for virus isolation, as suggested by Harrison and Herron (1984) (p. 68).

(16) Good lighting possibly combined with a magnifying lens is a great help.
(17) A suitable board and dissecting needles for pinning out small birds.

Always wear gloves and a mask. Apart from the risks of *Chlamydia* infection, which is not confined to parrots and is not uncommon in ducks and pigeons, there are many other avian zoonoses.

A photographic camera with a macrolens focusing down to 5–6 cm with an attached ring flash is a very useful aid to record observations.

EXTERNAL EXAMINATION

Before starting the post-mortem it may be helpful to X-ray the carcass, if for instance it was suspected the bird was shot or suffering from metabolic bone disease or was involved in some sort of accident or was ill because of heavy metal poisoning (e.g. fisherman's lead weights, lead chewed from leaded light windows etc.). X-rays will also show if a bird has been microchipped.

Before opening the body a thorough examination should be carried out looking for any of the external signs described in Chapter 2. External parasites are often a lot more obvious on the dead body as they move away from the cooling surface of the skin. The specimen should next be saturated with a quaternary ammonium antiseptic. This reduces the amount of airborne feather debris. Feather dust can carry *Chlamydia* and other organisms and also contaminates the viscera when the carcass is opened.

The body is next pinned out on a board. In large birds the medial adductor leg muscles can be cut and the 'hip' joints disarticulated. Simpson (1996) suggests pinning the legs over the flexed wing tips to keep the wing feathers out of the way. Plucking the whole body is unnecessary. The removal of feathers along the mid-line in densely feathered species, such as ducks and gannets, does help to make it easier to incise the skin cleanly without damaging the underlying viscera.

OPENING THE BODY

The initial incision is made through the skin from the cranial end of the sternum to just in front of the vent. The cut is then extended on each side just along the caudal edge of the sternal plate. By blunt dissection the skin is then eased away from the underlying pectoralis muscle and at the same time the condition of the muscle is observed.

The pectoralis muscle

Both sides should be similar and well-rounded. If the two muscles are not symmetrical it may indicate an old injury or an inspissated and contracted abscess. The muscle should be of normal red colour showing no sign of anaemia, hyperaemia or bruising. The latter may be anything from bluish-black to green (within 24 hours) in colour depending on how long previously the trauma occurred. Discoloration of abdominal muscles may occur if they have had prolonged contact after death with the gut or gallbladder (if this was displaced caudally). Bacterial invasion from the gut into the surrounding tissue can be relatively rapid in the uncooled carcass.

Incise the pectoralis muscle and look for any evidence of petechial haemorrhages in the muscles which could indicate warfarin poisoning (Reece, 1982) or vitamin K deficiency. Note the observations of Fiennes (1969) mentioned in the section dealing with disease of the lower alimentary canal (p. 104). Also look for evidence of pale streaks in the direction of the muscle fibres which may indicate sarocytosis or so-called leucocytozoon infection (Simpson, 1991). If suspected submit a specimen for histopathology.

Exposing the viscera

The skin incisions are now deepened through the muscle and the lateral incisions are now extended to the level of the costochondral junctions which are either cut with scissors or shears if very large birds, or, in small birds, dislocated by pressure from the handle of a scalpel. Do not cut through the coracoids or clavicles at this stage, as this may damage the large blood vessels leaving the heart. The sternum now can be lifted upwards away from the underlying viscera. As this is done examine the underside (anatomically the dorsal aspect) of the sternum together with the general appearance of the organs. If the body cavity is filled with exudate, take swabs for culture. There should be very little fluid in the normal coelomic cavity. Decide if the colour of the tissues looks a normal pink or is hyperaemic indicating a possible septicaemia. Discoloration, due to hypostatic congestion, on one side only, would indicate the bird had been left for some time lying on that side after death.

The carcass may look anaemic. Even if heavy infestation with blood-sucking parasites had been noticed initially, there may also be other less obvious contributing factors. The muscle may look dry indicating dehydration or shrunken indicating cachexia.

Examination of the viscera before removal from the body

The signs of air sacculitis may be seen and will become more evident as the post-mortem proceeds. During the initial stages of air sacculitis the crystal-like clarity of these delicate sheets of tissue is lost. They become increasingly opaque and thickened as exudate begins to collect between their two layers of cells. At first this cloudiness is patchy but later extends through the whole system of air sacs. Yellow caseous material becomes more evident. There may be a varying distribution of discreet 'suede-like' greenish yellow disc-like plaques which show a necrotic centre. These may indicate *Aspergillus* infection and diagnosis should be confirmed by taking a swab for culture and microscopical examination. *Aspergillus* lesions vary in colour from cream to bluish grey etc. Mixed infections of Aspergillus *Mycobacterium avium* can occur. An impression smear can also be taken and stained with Gram stain or lactophenol blue when mycelia and the club-shaped fruiting heads can be seen, particularly at the edge of the specimen. In air sacculitis due to *Escherischia coli*, the thickened parts of air sac and caseation tend to be more generalised and irregular in shape. In egg peritonitis large quantities of yellow inspissated yolk material may cover the intestines.

Occasionally at this stage of the post-mortem the organs can be seen to be covered with a scintillating sheen of urate crystals indicating visceral gout. The minute black mites of the genus *Sternostoma* may be seen in the air sacs particularly of finches. Occasionally in falcons nematodes of the genus *Serratospiculum* may be seen in the air sacs (Cooper, 1978). These have also been seen by the author in an immature herring gull (*Larus argentatus*).

The liver

If the liver is ruptured and is accompanied by a large blood clot this could be due to a blow over the sternum. In this case there will usually be signs of bruising of the overlying muscle and skin. The liver may be bile-stained (in those species which have a gallbladder – it is absent in many pigeons and parrots) due to bile diffusion from the gallbladder through the dead tissue of the bladder wall – a process which takes place within a few hours of death. The patency of the bile duct should be checked by gently squeezing the gallbladder, particularly in Amazon parrots in which there is a high incidence of bile duct carcinoma. These birds also show papillomata of the cloaca and/or oral cavity and oesophagus. The liver may be enlarged, and in fatty livers rupture will occur easily without any external trauma. Enlargement of the liver is indicated by loss of the normal sharp edges which become rounded. If this is accompanied by faint areas of necrosis which are seen at the same time as a fibrinous or serous pericarditis and air sacculitis, death may have been due to *Chlamydia* (psittacosis) infection. An impression smear of the liver stained with either a modified Ziehl–Neelsen stain (see Chapter 3, p. 67) or Macchiavello's stain, may show the pink intracytoplasmic inclusion bodies. Also in *Chlamydia* infection the spleen will usually be enlarged or distorted in shape. In fledgling parrots up to 14 weeks of age hepatosplenomegaly accompanied by subepicardial and subserosal haemorrhage may be due to avian polyoma virus.

Pacheco's parrot disease may cause liver lesions that mimic *Chlamydia* infection. These lesions tend to be more saucer-shaped and cause a faint yellow discoloration which stands out against the mahogany-coloured liver. Other herpes viruses affect other groups of birds and can cause necrotic foci in the liver. Principal among these is the disease in falcons, storks and cranes. Pigeons can also be affected by a herpes virus but this attacks mainly the young birds. In owls, herpes virus liver lesions look more like avian tuberculosis, with small white or yellowish pustules up to the size of a pea and possibly not raised above the surrounding surface. Some of the other organs may be covered by these lesions. Avian tuberculosis or even bovine or human TB in birds should not be confused with the pin head white or yellow necrotic foci of *Salmonella*, *E. coli* or *Yersinia pseudotuberculosis*. A swab stained with Ziehl-Neelsen and Gram stain may identify the organism. Fiennes (1969) describes the liver as being a rich golden colour and somewhat swollen and fatty in the case of septicaemic *Salmonella* infection.

In neonates the liver is normally a pale yellow colour due to lipidosis caused by the metabolism of egg yolk from the yolk sac which is absorbed after several days.

In turkeys and game birds the black, circular lesions of blackhead due to histomoniasis infection may be found. If the liver is mottled with irregular, lighter-coloured areas this may be neoplasia.

If at this initial examination of the viscera there are signs of a septicaemia, and the carcass is fresh, a sterile specimen of heart blood should be taken. The surface of the organ is first sterilised by searing with the blade of a hot spatula. A sterile needle attached to a syringe is then inserted into the heart for the withdrawal of blood.

If the bird has not long been dead it may be possible to make a smear and look for blood parasites. The blood obtained should also be cultured and stained with Gram stain.

In *fresh* specimens it is possible to carry out a vitamin A analysis. A minimum of 1 g of liver is required and it should be stored and transported to the laboratory frozen.

REMOVAL AND EXAMINATION OF THE ALIMENTARY CANAL, SPLEEN AND LIVER

This should be carried out by cutting the lower oesophagus and incising the skin around the vent. The cloaca and the attached bursa of Fabricius should be removed intact and care should be taken not to contaminate the rest of the carcass. The spleen should be attached to the underside of the caudal end of the proventriculus (anatomically the dorsal side) and lying behind the gizzard.

The spleen

The spleen is globular in most species but may be triangular in ducks and geese and is usually about one-quarter to one-third the size of the heart. Never ignore an enlarged or angular-shaped spleen or one that may have ruptured. It may indicate *Chlamydia* infection. However an enlarged spleen is not always present with *Chlamydia* infection. If other signs are present and the clinician is suspicious of the presence of *Chlamydia*, the spleen should be checked by using an impression smear stained with the modified Zeil–Neelson technique. If this is positive it is wiser to proceed no further. The spleen may be slightly enlarged and hyperaemic due to a septicaemic infection or, as in the case of the liver, mottled with the foci of a neoplasia. The signs of tuberculosis, *Pasteurella*, *E. coli* septicaemia and aspergillosis are similar to those seen on the liver.

The lower alimentary canal

Before dissecting out the gut, examine the pancreas enclosed within the duodenal loop which can usually be seen before the alimentary canal is removed from the abdomen. The pancreas should be examined for evidence of atrophy or neoplasia, neither of which is common in birds. If paramyxovirus is suspected (particularly in neophema parakeets) specimens of pancreas and also brain and lung should be placed in separate pots, cooled to 4°C and dispatched to a laboratory for histopathology.

The accompanying duodenum may look congested or distended with gas which often occurs if the bird has been dead some time before post-mortem. Take a sterile sample of the contents, in the same way as harvesting a sterile sample of heart blood. *Clostridia* sp. may be cultured.

If the ingesta are too viscid, dilute by injecting a little sterile saline. Examine the sample for *Coccidia*, by Gram stain and culture. The Gram stain will enable assessment of the relative numbers of Gram-positive and Gram-negative organisms. The latter should not be predominant in most healthy birds. Look for signs of intestinal haemorrhage, which could be generalised or patchy throughout the intestine. If this is accompanied by pathological signs in other parts of the body it may be an indication of Newcastle disease. However, the pathological signs of Newcastle disease vary greatly among different species and lesions may not be present in any of the viscera. Always look at the pattern of pathological change in the intestine together with other changes in the rest of the viscera. A single intestinal haemorrhage may not be due to a bacterial enteritis but rather caused by terminal venous congestion brought on by right heart failure as a result of toxaemia. A condition of stress enteropathy has been described by J.R. Baker (personal communication) when a seepage of large quantities of blood takes place into the lumen of the intestine resulting in rapid death. The stress can have occurred hours or days previously and the condition has often been noted by the author.

Fiennes (1969) has pointed out that sporadic haemorrhage occurring anywhere in the body, both internally and externally and unassociated with any other signs may be due to vitamin K deficiency. Vitamin K is partially synthesised by normal gut flora. This may have been disrupted by disease of the bowels or indiscriminate use of antibiotics. Haemorrhage may be due to warfarin poisoning as mentioned previously when discussing examination of the pectoralis muscle.

Examine the caeca; these vary considerably in shape and size in different species (see Fig. 1.8). They are large and obvious in poultry, in passerines they are small and in pigeons and parrots they are rudimentary. They have lobate ends in the barn owl. In turkeys, chickens and game birds the lesions of blackhead may be seen. The caeca are swollen, the mucosa extensively ulcerated and the lumen contains a lot of necrotic material. In *Salmonella* infection, the caecal wall may have a white, glistening appearance.

After an external examination of the bowel the whole alimentary canal should be opened to expose the lumen. The interior may be filled only with a green fluid without any ingesta indicating anorexia. The lower intestine may contain grit or undigested seed from the gizzard indicating increased peristalsis. The mucosa of the bowel may be congested and swollen or flaccid and dilated. If the lumen is filled with catarrhal exudate this could be caused by a parasitic infection. The contents of the bowel and scrapings of the mucosa should be examined for *Coccidia* or *Capillaria* (up to 1 cm long) or helminth eggs or even *Cryptosporidia*. The scraping should be stained with Giemsa to confirm diagnosis when numerous minute spherical organisms will be seen adherent to the mucous membrane. For parasites the specimen is best stained with Lugol's iodine. The gut may contain ascarid worms which may be so numerous as to cause impaction and rupture of the bowel.

In the case of *Salmonella* infection the mucosa may show signs of desquamation or show small nodules of necrosis. Even if the gut looks normal it is always wiser to take a swab for *Salmonella*.

Foreign bodies such as fish hooks and small nails are sometimes found in the lumen of the gut and occasionally penetrate the bowel wall.

The proventriculus and ventriculus (or gizzard) should be examined for evidence of the cheesy exudate of Trichomoniasis which is more commonly found higher up in the alimentary canal. Also examine for signs of ulceration sometimes caused by megabacteria particularly in budgerigars (*Melopsittacus undulatus*) but also in other small psittacines.

The proventriculus may be enlarged and filled with grit and undigested food. This is an indication of psittacine neuropathic gastric dilatation (originally known as macaw wasting disease) and occurs in all species of psittacines. The mucosa of the proventriculus should be scraped and stained with Gram stain to show the large Gram-positive filaments of the megabacterial organism.

Signs of *Aspergillus* infection are occasionally found in the lumen of the bowel.

Striations seen in the muscle of the wall of the gizzard may be due to vitamin E deficiency. The koilin layer of the gizzard of granivorous and herbivorous birds may be stained with bile. If staining is intense or extends into the proventriculus this may indicate antiperistasis.

Lastly the cloaca together with the bursa of Fabricius should be examined. The latter should be small and involuted in the adult bird. It is only easily recognisable in the young growing bird when it looks like a large lymph node. A prominent bursa of Fabricius indicates persistent B-cell production to boost humoral antibody as a response to chronic anti-gen stimulation from chronic infection such as paramyxo virus or psit-tacine beak and feather disease. The cloaca may be impacted with urate crystals forming a crumbling calculus or it may be filled with blood clot as the result of damage during artificial insemination. The mucosa of the cloaca can show signs of inflammation or neoplastic change (papillo-mata) sometimes seen in New World psittacines such as Amazon parrots and macaws.

EXAMINATION OF THE HEART AND ASSOCIATED MAJOR BLOOD VESSELS

The exterior of the heart together with the pericardium will already have received some attention when the carcass was first opened but must now be examined in greater detail. The normal heart of a bird is roughly triangular in shape; any tendency to a spherical shape is abnormal. The pericardial sac should be examined for any increase in fluid content, the amount of which is normally imperceptible. If the pericardium is unu-sually opaque this may be caused by infiltration with urate crystals. Examine the myocardium, endocardium and coronary blood vessels for any sign of petechial haemorrhages, which may be a sign of septicaemia or alternatively of violent struggling just before death.

Occasionally the right atrium may be found to be ruptured as a con-sequence of massive dilation during circulatory failure brought on by an overwhelming disease.

The major blood vessels leaving the heart should be examined. At the same time look for any signs of air sacculitis in the cervical and inter-clavicular air sacs. If this is present, it may be productive to cut through the head of the humerus and take a swab from the medullary cavity since this is connected to the anterior air sacs.

When examining the brachiocephalic trunk and the carotid arteries leading away from it, the crop must not be damaged. The interior of the major blood vessels, as well as those of the abdominal aorta and renal arteries, may show atheromatous plaques and these may be so extensive as to apparently occlude the lumen of the vessel. They may also make the blood vessels less flexible.

These lesions are not uncommon in anseriformes, falciformes and ostriches. They are occasionally found in many other species such as psittacines. Young turkeys commonly suffer from dissecting aneurysms of the arteries, which can lead to sudden death.

After the crop has been carefully dissected to one side, in order to examine the carotid arteries, the thyroids and parathyroids should be examined (Fig. 4.1).

Examination of the thyroid and parathyroid glands

Enlargement of the thyroid is not uncommon in budgerigars and is usually caused by iodine deficiency (see pp. 29 and 39). Neoplasia of the thyroid is not common in birds but a number of clinicians have reported seeing occasional cases when the signs exhibited before death are similar to those of thyroid dysplasia. Secondary hyperparathyroidism occurs in birds that have been fed almost entirely on seed that contains very little calcium but excess phosphorous (p. 85). If these birds have been deprived of soluble grit metabolic osteodystrophy or secondary nutritional hyperparathyroidism may follow. In these cases the parathyroid glands (Fig. 4.1) are somewhat enlarged and white in colour. In the normal bird they are often difficult to find.

Examination of the crop

Normally the crop wall is quite thin – in small birds as delicate as tissue paper. However, where there is infection, as with *Candida* or *Trichomonas*, the mucosa of the crop can become hypertrophied and noticeably thick. If the white, caseous exudate of *Candida* is scraped from the mucosa, the surface will look rather like velvet.

Physiological regurgitation of seed is normal in the budgerigar when feeding nestlings but there is no accompanying hypertrophy of the crop (Baker, J.R., 1984, personal communication). Occasionally a crop will become impacted, a condition affecting all species. The trapped food will ferment with superimposed bacterial infection and inflammation of the crop. The layman's term of 'sour crop' can cover any of the above conditions. Brooks (1982) reports necrosis of the crop wall in a sparrow-

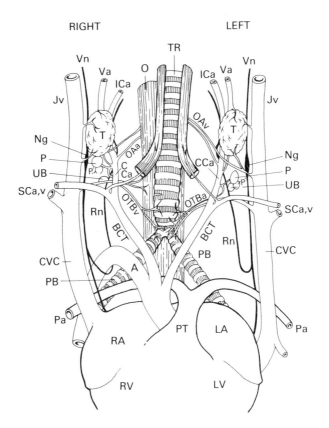

Fig. 4.1 Ventral view of the blood vessels, nerves and glands at the thoracic inlet of the domestic fowl. The carotid bodies are on the medial surfaces of the parathyroid glands. A, aorta; BCT, brachiocephalic trunk; CCa, common carotid artery; CVC, cranial vena cava; ICa, internal carotid artery; Jv, jugular vein; LA, left atrium; LV, left ventricle; Ng, nodose (distal vagal) ganglion; O, oesophagus; OAa, ascending oesophageal artery; OAv, ascending oesophageal vein; OTBa, oesophagotracheobronchial artery; OTBv, oesophagotracheobronchial vein; P, cranial parathryoid gland; P', caudal parathyroid gland; Pa, pulmonary artery; PB, primary bronchus; PT, pulmonary trunk; RA, right atrium; Rn, recurrent nerve; RV, right ventricle; SCa, subclavian artery; SCv, subclavian vein; T, thyroid gland; TR, trachea; UB, ultimobranchial body or gland; Va, vertebral artery; Vn, vagus nerve. After Abdel-Magied & King (1978), with kind permission of the editor of the *Journal of Anatomy*.

hawk leading to a fistula probably caused by a penetrating spicule of bone. Fistulas may also result from external wounds or from scalding in hand reared psittacines. In cases of unexplained death examine the crop contents for signs of poisonous plant material.

The oesophagus and oropharynx

The whole of the oesophagus should be opened by making a parallel cut with scissors along each side. If a pair of strong scissors or a pair of bone forceps (in large birds) are inserted with one blade in the mouth, the quadrate bone can be cut and the lower jaw disarticulated. The whole of the upper alimentary tract can now be examined. A caseous exudate could indicate trichomaniasis, *Candida* or there may be signs of *Aspergillus*. The signs of all these infections can be confused and diagnosis should be confirmed by laboratory examination. Trichomonads are sometimes difficult to find under the microscope. In a newly dead bird the mucosal scrapings should be examined using a hanging drop method after mixing with a little normal saline. Use a × 20 objective and rack the condenser down. However, if the exudate is incubated overnight in a trichomanad culture medium, there is no difficulty (Wallis, A.S., 1984; personal communication).

The clinician should be aware that signs of Trichomoniasis may be superimposed on an underlying *Chlamydia* infection (de Gruchy, 1983) or indeed on other infections such as avipox together with hypovitaminosis A.

Excessive mucus in this region may be indicative of *Capillaria* infection and the worms are sometimes easily seen in the mucus by naked eye although microscopical examination may be necessary.

Abscesses in the mouth of birds, particularly parrots, are not uncommon and may be due to an underlying vitamin A deficiency. However, the small white specks sometimes seen on the roof of the mouth in pigeons (Wallis, A.S., 1984; personal communication) are not considered to be of any clinical significance. The lesions of avipox are much larger.

Haemorrhage into the choanal space or into the oral cavity may be noticed when the mouth is first opened. This may be as a result of trauma. Both wild and pet birds will fly into window panes. Sparrow-hawks in their enthusiastic pursuit of prey may collide with the same window pane as their prey and both be found dead together.

THE RESPIRATORY SYSTEM

The palatine choanal opening

Mites may sometimes be found inhabiting this area. Look for any sign of infection in this region. The upper beak should be cut across just in front of the cere and the sinuses examined. They may contain catarrhal or caseous exudate or there may be a blood clot.

The glottis and trachea

There may be signs of inflammatory change along the edges. Open the trachea by making two parallel cuts. The mucosa may be congested or there may be signs of fungal infection. In those birds that feed on invertebrates, and this includes a wide range of species, the nematode *Syngamus trachea* is commonly found particularly in young birds. Occasionally a foreign body is found such as a seed obstructing the trachea. Caseous plaques are not uncommon in the region of the syrinx and may partially occlude the airway. These lesions should be crushed on a slide and stained with lactophenol cotton blue (methylene blue stain also works reasonably well). Look for signs of mycotic infection.

The lungs

The air sac system has already received attention when first opening the carcass. The lungs should be examined *in situ* and then carefully eased away from the adjoining ribs using the handle of a scalpel. Look for any evidence of abscessation (sometimes only found on the dorsal surface of the lung) or look for haemorrhage. If this is present examine the adjacent rib. There may be signs of a recent or old fracture. Lungs that are dark in colour and exude moisture when compressed are oedematous. This can be due to the inhalation of toxic fumes such as carbon monoxide from a faulty gas heater, polytetra fluroethylene (Teflon) from a chip pan fire or from the fumes of an industrial waste plant upwind from an aviary. This industrial effluent mix may be intermittently discharged. Section the lung and look for smoke particles.

Haemorrhage into the lung substance may be agonal (unorganised clot) and occur as the result of right heart failure. It may also be the result of inflammatory change. If the lung looks solid, try and float a piece in water. If there is pneumonic change the piece of lung will sink. Also if the lung is solid sear the surface with a hot blade and take a bacteriological swab through a cut in the sterilised area. Also send samples for histopathology.

THE GONADS, THE ADRENALS AND KIDNEYS

First look at these organs *in situ*. It may then be possible to strip them out in one piece from their 'bed' ventral to the synsacrum. This is attempted by gripping the fascia just cranial to this group of organs, peeling back gently and easing the organs out with closed scissors. However the sacral plexus transverses the kidney and so makes complete removal difficult. In small birds the kidney and the synsacrum may have to be removed in one piece.

Both ovaries and testes vary considerably in size according to the maturity of the bird and the breeding season. In both cases there may be total or partial pigmentation (black or dark green) of the gonads – which is normal in some species (e.g. cockatoos, gulls and others). In the ovary affected with *Salmonella pullorum* disease, the follicles may become mis-shapen and angular instead of being globular. The disease has been diagnosed in many species. Both male and female gonads can undergo neoplastic change. If there are cysts present in the ovary, examine the bones (ribs, vertebrae, sternum, humerus and skull) to see if there is any distortion or increase in solidity. The condition of polystotic hyperostosis is not uncommon in budgerigars and may occasionally be seen in other birds. It is most often first noticed during radiography and is associated with an increased level of oestrogens seen in females with neoplastic change in the ovary and in male birds with sertoli tumours.

The adrenal gland, closely associated with the cranial end of the gonad, is normally a pale pink or orange colour but it may become hyperaemic during the course of an infection or it may look almost white in colour. The adrenals may be enlarged in the chronically stressed bird. The kidney may be hyperaemic together with the rest of the viscera in septicaemia conditions. Alternatively it may be grey in colour, due to cloudy swelling. The kidneys may show any of the signs seen in the liver due to infectious disease mentioned above. The kidney may be pale in colour, the tubules and the ureters may be prominent when impacted with urate crystals. A condition not uncommon in water-fowl. *Small* quantities of urate crystals in the ureters may be normal. Salt poisoning results in marked deposition of urates. This condition is sometimes seen in aquatic birds in time of drought or in pet parrots fed salted peanuts or crisps. Occasionally neo-plasms or aspergillosis granulomas are seen in the avian kidney. These may result in pressure on the sacral plexus. In geese and some other Anseriformes swollen kidneys covered in white patches may be caused by *Eimeria truncata*.

THE NERVOUS SYSTEM

The peripheral nerves

After the kidney, examine the nerves of the sciatic plexus where these leave the spinal cord and emerge beneath the synsacrum. These nerves together with those of the axillae and the intercostal nerves should be examined for signs of irregular thickening typical of Marek's disease, seen in poultry and occasionally in falcons, owls and pigeons, and possibly other species. The thickening of the nerves is caused by lymphocytic infiltration resulting in tumours as in the viscera. Take a length of nerve from either the sciatic or brachial plexus, stretch out on filter paper, leave to dry then fix in 10% formal saline for histopathology.

Neoplasia of the hypophysis or pituitary gland

In any bird but particularly budgerigars exhibiting polydipsia/polyuria and CNS signs antemortem this gland should be examined. It lies in a fossa dorsal to the basisphenoid bone which forms the cranial part of the brain case. The organ is immediately caudal to the optic chiasma. It is roughly a 2 mm globe in the budgerigar.

The brain

During removal of the skin covering the head, evidence of subcutaneous haemorrhage may be seen. This is only significant if there has been a lot of bleeding.

Next find the foramen magnum and in small birds insert the blade of a scalpel; in larger birds a pair of strong scissors or bone forceps will be needed. Cut around the cranium on each side and raise the calvaria to expose the brain.

Signs of haemorrhage within the substance of the bone, sometimes quite extensive, are of no significance and are caused by blood extravasated from blood vessels very soon after death. However, an organized blood clot either over or under the meninges or in the substance of the brain is important. This is so, even if the blood is not clotted and may be evidence of concussion, particularly if there is also a matching bruising of the skin, or haemorrhage into the nasal cavities.

THE SKELETON

Before finishing the post-mortem examine those parts of the skeleton that were not examined when looking for Marek's disease. Open and look particularly at the joints. Greenish discoloration in the muscles around the joints is evidence of bruising. Signs of a septic arthritis of the joints with discharge of exudate may be signs of *Salmonella* infection in pigeons and poultry. The articular cartilage may also show petechiae.

Urate crystals may be seen in the joints of those birds affected with visceral gout as well as subcutaneous tophi. For the muroxide test to confirm the presence of urate crystals see Chapter 2, p. 43.

Cut off the head of the femur and sample the medullary cavity for blood-borne bacteria and examine the blood corpuscles for signs of any cellular disorder.

Chapter 5
Medication and Administration of Drugs

A problem for the busy practitioner in his consulting room is being presented with an obviously sick bird brought in by an anxious and sometimes demanding owner. He is required to reach an instant diagnosis and to initiate appropriate and immediate treatment. Yielding to these pressures, it is all too common among practitioners, to assume that the bird is suffering from a bacterial infection and to dispense a soluble antibiotic. This is usually one of the tetracyclines and the owner is told to put some of this in the drinking water each day.

This routine is not only ineffective, it may in fact decrease the chances of the bird's recovery by disturbing the normal bacterial flora of the alimentary canal. In addition it increases the chances of the emergence of antibiotic resistant strains of bacteria and some of these organisms are pathogenic for man. Also it has been shown (Gerlach, 1994) that tetracyclines can cause a transient rise in corticosteroids and suppress the immune system by inhibiting the activity of the macrophages.

If the practitioner cannot persuade the client to let him hospitalise the bird so that a more accurate diagnosis can be made, it would be more logical to assume the sick bird is vitamin deficient. The metabolic turnover of the B vitamins is rapid, many birds in captivity are maintained on a restricted diet and some are chronically short of vitamin A. These vitamins can be given safely in the drinking water or by injection and will give the practitioner a little more time in which to make a more considered diagnosis aided by taking samples for laboratory investigation.

ASSESSING THE WEIGHT OF A BIRD

To achieve adequate and safe medication an accurate estimate of the bird's weight must be obtained. For small-and medium-sized bids up to 1 kg in weight, a Persola spring balance, as used by bird ringers and distributed by the British Trust for Ornithology can be used. The bird is placed in a cloth or plastic bag suspended from the balance. If this is not available a mail or letter balance can be used for birds weighing from 30 to

500 g. This is not quite so accurate but will give a reading within a few grams of the true weight. This balance is not accurate enough for birds below 30 g; if possible use an electronic laboratory balance. Larger birds, particularly falcons and some parrots, will sit on a perch attached to the weighing pan of a more robust balance. Falconers often weigh their birds regularly to maintain them in flying condition and may be able to tell the weight of the bird. Ducks, geese and similar birds may be put in a sack, with the head out and the sack tied around the bird's neck.

If for some reason it is not practical to weigh the bird then reference may be made to a table of bird weights. Such a table is included in Appendix 10.

However, the clinician should be aware that weights in normal birds can vary at least 25% on either side of the mean weight for the species. In sick or starved birds the deviation from the average weight could be greater.

CALCULATING THE DOSE OF DRUGS

Few medicines are marketed specifically for use in birds. Doses are therefore based on clinical reports or have to be extrapolated from the doses advised by the manufacturer for use in dogs and cats. However, birds have a higher metabolic rate than mammals and the rate increases as the size of the creature decreases. There are also differences in metabolic rate between passerine and non-passerine groups of birds. In addition, other factors such as the density of feather covering are involved. In general the higher the metabolic rate the faster are drugs absorbed, metabolised and cleared from the body. Nevertheless, Bush et al. (1979) have pointed out that there are anomalies to this pattern resulting from the many metabolic and subtle anatomical differences even between closely related species such as the psittacines. The pharmacokinetics of drugs in most species of birds need much more investigation as has recently been highlighted by Donita et al. 1995.

If there is not a recommended or proven dose for a particular circumstance then it is best to calculate the dose from the bird's metabolic/effective weight using a method of allometric scaling. In general this is derived as an exponential of the body weight raised to the power of 0.75. For example, if the recommended dose of a drug for a cat is 2 mg/kg the dose for a budgerigar weighing 40 g will *not* be:

$$\frac{40}{1000} \times 2 = 0.08 \, \text{mg}$$

But will be

$$\left(\frac{40}{1000}\right)^{0.75} \times 2 = (0.040)^{0.75} \times 2 = 0.178$$

which is well over three times as much as the original dose calculated on a weight for weight basis. This of course is the total quantity to be given in 24 hours and will need to be divided into a larger number of fractions to be administered more frequently than is recommended for the cat. *Doses given in this book are those used by other clinicians and the author. They are not necessarily based on the metabolic effective weight and may need to be adjusted in the light of future experience.* Always be aware of any possible toxicity particularly in the case of a rare, valuable or unusual species in which the drug has not been used before.

THE ADMINISTRATION OF DRUGS

As in the case with mammals medicines may be given to birds by a variety of routes, some of which are more effective and more appropriate to certain disease conditions.

Medication of the drinking water

This is a convenient method when large numbers of birds have to be treated, such as those in a zoological collection or at a quarantine station or in a poultry flock. A number of drugs are formulated for use in poultry by this method. The daily dose has been calculated on the mean water intake of an average bird during 24 hours. At a very rough approximation 150 ml of water is consumed per kilogram of avian body-weight daily. However, there may be at least a 50% increase or decrease on either side of this figure. The water consumption of healthy birds varies considerably depending on bodily condition, ambient temperatures, diet and species. Fruit eaters such as mynah birds and toucans get much of their water from their food. Raptors may not drink very much. Birds whose normal habitat is desert are able to rely almost entirely on metabolic water.

In the diseased bird water consumption will vary even more; not only will this depend on the normal function of the alimentary canal and kidneys but also on the health of the upper respiratory tract. The nasal cavities in the bird are important organs of water conservation. Consequently drugs given by this method must have a wide margin of safety. A bird that is polydipsic could take in much greater amounts of medicament. At best, blood levels of the drug are liable to be irregular. Antibiotics given by this method are at least likely to reach minimal inhibitory concentrations within the lumen of the alimentary canal, providing the bird is drinking some water.

Nevertheless birds are creatures of habit and sensitive to changes in their feeding and watering routine. If the medication colours the water or adds a taste to it the bird is quite likely to refuse to drink and its illness is made worse.

There is little doubt that birds have colour vision. The more brightly coloured the plumage of the species the more acute is their perception of colour likely to be.

It was once thought that birds have little sense of taste. Certainly the number of taste buds per unit area is much fewer in birds than in mammals. Work quoted by King and McLelland (1984, pp. 311–312) has shown that, dependent on the species, birds do have a definite sense of taste. Pigeons are apparently more sensitive than the domestic fowl. Bitter- and salt-tasting substances tend to be rejected. Therefore a drug such as levamisole, with a bitter taste, may not be readily taken by a species with a well-developed sense of taste. Sweet substances such as sugars (but not saccharin) produce variable responses in individual birds. Therefore adding these to medicines to make them more palatable will have varying results.

One advantage to medicating the drinking water of a group of birds with an antibiotic is that it reduces the number of bacterial organisms that may have contaminated the water supply and so limits the spread of infection. Another point in favour of the method is that it is much less stressful for the bird than having to be caught for medication. However, many drugs lose their potency when in solution.

If drugs for water medication are to be dispensed on a regular basis, it is more convenient to have ready-weighed small quantities. These can be added daily to a known quantity of water. Drinking containers for cage birds vary in volume so that it is simpler if the quantities dispensed are sufficient to be added to a common household utensil such as a kitchen measuring jug (500 ml). This is used as a stock solution to keep the drinking container filled. The remainder of the stock solution is discarded. The method is wasteful but the quantities of drug dispensed are small and it is simple for the client. Alternatively, smaller weighed amounts can be dispensed, for example, sufficient to be dissolved in 50 ml of water and at the same time a 10-ml syringe is dispensed so that the client can accurately measure this volume of water.

Oral medication

The same drugs used for medicating the drinking water can be given orally. Also there are a number of human paediatric preparations suitable for oral administration in birds. Galenicals such as liquid paraffin and formulations containing kaolin and bismuth may also be used.

Although it is possible to administer liquid preparations using a syringe, or a dropper (not glass for parrots), or even to let the fluid drip into the mouth from the end of a cocktail stick, it is not very satisfactory. There is a danger of inhalation of the medication and it can be wasteful and messy. It is more sensible to give the preparation using an oesophageal or gavage tube. For many species a piece of soft plastic (used 'drip' tubing) or rubber tubing attached to a hypodermic syringe works well. The length of the tube should be measured against the bird's neck so that when the neck is extended the tube will reach well down to the level of the crop or the thoracic inlet. The diameter of the tube and capacity of the syringe will depend on the size of the bird. Birds the size of small finches (zebra) to swans can be dosed by this method. In the swan a canine stomach tube and a 60-ml plastic syringe are suitable.

In some birds, particularly the parrots, it is imperative to use either a gag or speculum of some kind or a rigid metal catheter. The author prefers the latter since the procedure can then sometimes be accomplished by one person.

During this procedure the bird may need to be restrained by gently wrapping in a towel. Protective gloves may be necessary but can often be dispensed with once the head is controlled. While holding the beak open, the neck is extended in a vertical direction to straighten out the typical avian S-shape curve of the cervical vertebrae. Having placed the lubricated (use liquid paraffin), rigid tube in the mouth, it is then advanced beyond the glottis and allowed to slide down the oesophagus under its own weight. No stomach tube should ever be forced down. The avian oesophagus is thin and easily ruptured.

Using this method birds can be accurately dosed and fed if nutrients are added to the medication. Experienced nursing staff and intelligent owners can be instructed to dose birds in this way. However, strict hygiene of the tube, syringe and utensils is necessary. Suitable volumes that can be given by this method are given in Table 5.1.

Table 5.1 Suitable volumes (in ml) for oral medication.

Canary	0.25
Budgerigar	0.5–1.0
Lovebirds	1.0–3.0
Cockatiel	2–4.0
Amazon parrot	5–10
African grey parrot	5–10
Macaw	10–15

When giving medication orally or in the drinking water it always should be noted that the absorption of drugs from the gut can be adversely affected by parasitism, a diseased mucosa and nutritional deficiencies particularly hypovitaminosis A. The absorption of some antibiotics such as penicillin, ampicillin and lincomycin is reduced in the presence of food. Oxytetracycline has a reduced absorption in the presence of calcium and magnesium and so will be affected if a bird is receiving soluble grit in the diet or the antibiotic is given with antacids.

Medicating the food

Seed impregnated with drugs (e.g. Ornimed: canary seed impregnated with oxytetracycline or vitamin B_{12}) is available for small pet birds, up to 100 g (cockatiel size) in body weight. Provided the bird will eat it, it is a convenient method of medication. If the practitioner is dealing with a situation where a large number of birds will need medicating on a regular basis, then it may be possible to get a feed manufacturer to incorporate the desired drug in the pelleted feed. Most psittacines, except the macaws, will accept pelleted food providing it is introduced into the diet gradually over 2–3 days.

Parrots will sometimes eat powdered tablets or the powder contents of capsules if these are spread on sweet biscuits or on bread with peanut butter or honey. It may be possible to inject some drugs into fruits such as grapes. Toucans swallow grapes whole without crushing them. Seeds can be coated with a powdered drug by moistening the seed or adding a little corn oil. If given too much oil, the bird becomes coated in it. However, since most seed is dehusked before being swallowed this method of giving drugs is unreliable.

For the prophylactic administration of chlortetracycline to psittacines exposed to *Chlamydia* infection, Ashton and Smith (1984) recommend the following mash: two parts maize and two parts rice with three parts of water cooked to a soft, but not mushy consistency. The drug is added at the rate of 5 mg/g of cooked feed. The food is prepared daily and a little brown sugar and seed is added for palatability. At a rough approximation most birds eat about one quarter of their weight in food daily.

Intramuscular injection

Undoubtedly this is the most accurate and reasonably safe route for parenteral administration of drugs. Either the pectoralis or the iliotibialis lateralis or biceps femoris muscles of the leg can be used. Both sites have advantages and disadvantages. If injection is made into the pectoralis this must be carried out at the caudal end of the muscles. The veins are better developed at the cranial end of the muscle and there is a much greater chance of accidental intravenous injection. Quite severe inflammatory reaction can occur in the muscle after injection (Cooper, 1983). But this is only likely to be of any consequence with repeated injections at exactly the same site. Some falconers and racing pigeon owners do not like this area since they believe the flight muscles will be damaged. If the injection is made slightly to one side of the carina or keel of the sternum then the needle is unlikely to go beyond the lateral edge of this bone and penetrate the underlying viscera. Take great care in fledglings in which the bone may not have been fully calcified and is still cartilagenous. It is easy to penetrate this soft bone and give the injection directly into the underlying liver.

Injections into the leg muscles have the same disadvantages regarding bruising. In addition the large ischiadic nerve may be damaged where it courses down the posterior aspect of the femur. Also injections into the legs may pass through the renal portal system before entering the systemic circulation. This is particularly important with drugs that are excreted through the kidney in an unmetabolised state. Some part of the dose may be partly lost before it has a chance to reach therapeutic blood levels (Coles, 1984b).

For the administration of very small volumes to birds a microlitre syringe, which holds 0.1 ml when filled to capacity and which is marked in 0.001 divisions, is very useful. However, these syringes are expensive and need to be maintained with care. A 1-ml tuberculin syringe divided into 0.01 amounts is much less costly. Many drugs in aqueous solution can be diluted in this syringe to measure very small quantities. With those drugs that cannot be diluted, a microlitre syringe is the only answer. Plastic microlitre syringes are less costly.

Subcutaneous injection

This method can be used, but only one or two sites are suitable because the avian skin is not very elastic and fluids tend to leak out through the point of needle puncture. If the area covering the pectoralis muscle is used there is little danger of damage to vital structures but the needle must be advanced well under the skin and only a little fluid can be injected at the site. A much better region is the groin. Greater volumes (2 ml into an African grey parrot) can be injected here and, provided the skin is picked up with forceps before making the injection and the needle is not inserted too far, there is little chance of damaging the nerves and blood vessels beneath. Movement of the bird's leg helps disperse the injection. Dispersion can also be aided by adding hyaluronidase (half an ampoule or 750 IU) to the injection. Another useful site is the skin on the dorsal base of the neck. Care must be taken to hold the loose skin of this area away from the underlying vertebrae and muscles and to make the injection in the mid-line.

The administration of volumes of liquid suitable for fluid therapy in birds is quite practical using these sites.

Intravenous injection

This is most easily given into the brachial vein (Fig. 3.1) but the tarsal vein on the medial surface of the leg can be used in some birds as can the right jugular vein. The medial tarsal vein is particularly useful for blood sampling or injecting conscious swans. The jugular is useful in small birds. Both the right jugular and the brachial vein can be used in the ostrich. Intravenous injection is not always easy not only because of the small diameter of the vein but also because of the fragility of the vein wall. Haematoma formation after intravenous injection is a common occurrence. However, intravenous injection is an effective and important method of treatment in an emergency where a bird's life is threatened by disease.

Interosseous injection

This route provides a stable access port into the vascular system. The canula (20–22 gauge needle with an indwelling stylet (e.g. a spinal needle) can be left strapped in with 'Vetrap' and used for several days. A dorsal approach is made to the intramedullary cavity of the distal extremity of the ulna with the carpal/metacarpal and carpal/ulna joints held in a flexed position. Also the proximal tibiotarsal bone has been used for this purpose (see Fig. 8.1).

Intraperitoneal injection

This method has been used by some clinicians but is not without the hazard of entering one of the air sacs. A small volume of fluid is probably of no great consequence and in fact the method is suggested by Clubb (1984) as a method of treating disease of the air sacs.

If the injection is only to reach the peritoneal cavity, the skin and underlying muscle must be picked up by forceps to form a 'tent' slightly to the right of the mid-line. The injection is made into this area with the needle directed almost horizontally thus keeping away from the underlying viscera. If a $16\,G \times 0.5\,mm$ needle is used the injection should go into the ventral hepatic peritoneal cavity (see Fig. 7.5 and the accompanying text in Chapter 7). This procedure is carried out most easily in the sedated bird.

Intratracheal injection

This has been used to treat disease of the respiratory system. Amphoteracin B can be administered by this route. In small birds this is most easily carried out by using a mammalian intravenous catheter, cut short and attached to the syringe. The drug is then very slowly introduced into the trachea through the glottis, easily seen on the floor of the oral cavity.

The bird's neck needs to be held vertically and slightly extended and the tongue needs to be gently restrained on the floor of the mouth. The method is not practical in the unanaesthetised parrot unless the bird is deeply sedated. There will be some coughing but this is usually only temporary. Obviously the volume of fluid must be kept to a minimum though up to 1 ml has been given to pigeons and parrots (400–500 g) by this method.

Subconjunctival injections

Very small amounts (0.01–0.05 ml) of drugs can be placed under the conjunctiva of the upper eyelid. These are usually antibiotics and steroids and can be very effective *when a specific diagnosis has been made.* Since the technique requires the bird to be absolutely still, general anaesthesia or deep narcosis is advisable. Long-acting preparations are used for this purpose.

Injections into the infraorbital sinus

This technique is described in the chapter on surgery (Fig. 7.2). The method has been used for many years for treating poultry and is quite applicable to many other types of birds.

Topical applications

The local application of ointments and creams can be used but these should only be applied sparingly using a cotton wool bud. If too much is used the plumage becomes damaged. If larger quantities of ointment have to be used then an Elizabethan collar will be necessary to stop the bird becoming grossly contaminated.

Topical applications which are absorbed or dry quickly such as tinctures are more suitable. Dimethyl sulphoxide (DMSO) is a useful preparation applied to the legs and feet of birds. It is rapidly absorbed and may be used as a carrier for other drugs.

Ophthalmic preparations

Ophthalmic ointments can be used but have the same disadvantages as other ointments. Ophthalmic drops are much better but their effect is very short and their use needs constant handling of the bird which is a disadvantage. Subconjunctival injection of slowly absorbed drugs is more effective and less stressful for the bird. The instillation of ophthalmic drops into the nasal cavities for the treatment of sinusitis can be used but direct injection into the infra-orbital sinus is more effective. Also misting the eye with a fine spray of sterile water with the dissolved drug has been used effectively.

Inhalation therapy

A major problem in the treatment of disease of the respiratory system is infection of the air sacs. These thin-walled extensions of the lungs hold about 80% of the volumetric capacity of the respiratory system. The walls are no more than two cells thick and have no blood vessels. There is therefore a large 'dead' space within the bird filled with warm, moist air that is not very accessible to the bird's cellular and humoral defence mechanisms. This area is subject to infection particularly by *Aspergillus* fungi and coliform bacteria. The lungs, which have a good blood supply, are much less liable to be infected unless challenged by massive infection.

Unfortunately air sacculitis can be present for some time and becomes fairly extensive before outward signs are evident.

Inhalation therapy aims to saturate the air in this dead space and reach the internal surface of the air sacs. To be effective the droplet size of the medication must be below 5 µm in diameter otherwise the droplet does not remain suspended in the air stream long enough to reach the target area. Vaporising the medication does not work because most of the droplets are too big and condense in the upper respiratory tract. To be effective the drug needs to be administered from a nebuliser into a chamber in which the bird is housed during therapy. The drug is mixed with a suitable volume of saline, or better, with a vehicle such as tyloxapol which aids better dispersion of the medicament. Suitable doses are listed in Table 5.2. Some custom-made hospitalisation cages for birds incorporate a nebuliser. Alternatively a nebuliser built for human use such as the Porta-Neb 50 can be used with a small air compressor or the oxygen flow from an anaesthetic machine so long as the flow rate is at least 6 litres/min.

Table 5.2 Suitable doses (in mg) for inhalation therapy, to be diluted in 15 ml of saline and administered over a 30 minute period three or four times a day.

Amphotericin	25–100
Tylosin	150
Chloramphenicol	200
Spectinomycin	200
Gentamicin	50–200
Dexamethasone	3

THE LOGICAL USE OF ANTIBIOTICS

No antibiotic should be used unless the clinician is reasonably certain that the bird is suffering from a bacterial infection. However, there is sometimes a rapid deterioration in the condition of a young or small bird challenged by an overwhelming infection. In these circumstances the practitioner may decide to start antibiotic therapy before the results of laboratory tests to confirm his diagnosis become available.

Selection of antibiotic

If the antibiotic is required for systemic use it must be of low toxicity. It should penetrate all the bird's tissues easily and the minimal inhibitory concentration of the drug should be as low as possible. A swab should be taken from the choanal space, the orophanrynx or the cloaca, stained by the Gram method and examined under the microscope. This will at least indicate if the organisms present are mainly Gram-positive or Gram-negative and show their relative numbers. The autochthonous gut flora of most birds consist mostly of Gram negatives; clinical infection is usually dominated by one organism. This may indicate whether it is safe to use an antibiotic that is principally active against the one or the other group of bacteria. However, in the first instance, until subsequent laboratory tests are completed, a broad-spectrum antibiotic will usually be chosen. Ampicillin, amoxycillin combined with clavulanic acid, trimethoprim combined with a sulphonamide and the quinolones (Baytril) are all reasonable choices. If given by injection the quinolones, amoxycillin and trimethoprim combination are bacteriocidal and the tetracyclines are only bacteriostatic and rely on the host's immune response to be effective. The results of more extensive laboratory investigation such as antibiotic-sensitivity testing from swabs taken before and after starting antibiotic therapy may show that it is necessary to change the antibiotic being used.

Bactericidal antibiotics are probably better in the first instance. These drugs work only on bacteria that are dividing. There is a school of thought that considers intermittent exposure or less frequent dosage to be a more effective way of using the antibiotic. Bacteriostatic antibiotics inhibit bacterial multiplication and give time for the mobilisation of the body's defences. However, the maintenance of a plasma concentration for several days, well above the minimum inhibitory concentration, is essential.

The use of broad-spectrum antibiotics inevitably has some adverse effect on the host's normal bacterial flora, particularly that inhabiting the gut. Because of this, once the pathogenic organism causing the illness is identified, together with its sensitivity to antibiotics, it is wiser to select an antibiotic that has a narrow range of activity.

If the bacterial flora of the gut are disturbed, then the administration of natural yogurt-containing *Lactobacillus acidopilus* may help to restore the balance. This can be given by oesophageal tube at the rate of 2 ml/mg. Better still use a custom-made probiotic such as Avipro which contains *Lactobacillus* strains specific to birds. This is soluble and can be given in the drinking water simultaneously with the administration of antibiotic.

In some cases of chronic infection the rate of maturation of the T-lymphocytes may be depressed and cell-mediated immunity may be impaired. In these cases it has been demonstrated in birds and mammals that levamisole used intermittently, at a lower dose than the normal anthelmintic dose, may have a beneficial and sometimes quite marked effect on the progress of the disease.

THE USE OF DRUGS UNREGISTERED FOR USE IN A SPECIFIC SPECIES OF ANIMAL

Although some drugs are listed here for use in a particular species, genus or class of birds this should *not* be interpreted *per se* that the drug is officially or otherwise approved or licensed for use in a particular species, genus or class of birds, but only that it indicates that to the best of the author's knowledge, the particular drug has been used as described. Under the present day law in the United Kingdom, preparations licensed for use in other species, including humans, may be administered under the responsibility of a qualified veterinary surgeon who has the birds under his/her *direct care* and when no other suitable drug is licensed for use in that particular species, genus or class of birds.

Chapter 6
Anaesthesia

GENERAL CONSIDERATIONS

Before selecting an anaesthetic the practitioner should take into account the reasons for its use.

Hypnosis and restraint

Perhaps the main indication for using an anaesthetic drug is to produce chemical restraint while radiography is carried out or endoscopy or some other non-painful procedure is performed. There are a number of drugs or combinations of injectable agents suitable for the purpose but which have little analgesic effect.

Analgesia

The abolition of painful stimuli may be the prime consideration. If this is to produce analgesia of a limited surface area then local anaesthetics can be used. These have not been very popular with many clinicians in the past, particularly the drugs of the procaine-based group which have a reputation for toxicity. This is most probably because many small birds were grossly overdosed. Local anaesthetics are safe in birds if the dose is carefully calculated.

Some operations on poultry such as the relief of an impacted crop or ovarectomy have in the past been carried out without any anaesthetic and with little apparent distress to the bird. There is little doubt that the level of sensory perception is low in many parts of the avian skin. Cutting the integument seems to provoke much less response than stretching or undermining the skin. However the plucking out of two feathers in a lightly anaesthetised bird may stimulate violent wing flapping. Those parts of the bird's anatomy that are most sensitive are the cere, the comb, the wattles, the cloaca and the surrounding skin, the scaled parts of the legs and the pads of the feet. However, there is some individual and interspecies variation in the tenderness of the feet, particularly in raptors.

Some anaesthetic agents such as isoflurane and medetomidine are better analgesics than others such as halothane and ketamine. Some non-steroidal anti-inflammatory drugs such as carprofen (2 mg/kg i.m.) provide good postoperative analgesia.

Muscle relaxation

This may be required during surgery, particularly orthopaedic surgery when there is often contracture of muscle groups around a fracture site. Some anaesthetic agents, although good hypnotics, do not relax muscle.

The relief of anxiety and fear for the patient

Although placed last on this list, it is by no means the least important consideration. Anxiety and fear by the bird considerably increase stress and reduce the chances of survival after an operation. It is for this reason that an anaesthetic technique may be chosen which goes some way in combining all the above-mentioned requirements of anaesthesia and often this can only be achieved by using a balanced combination of drugs.

ASSESSMENT OF THE AVIAN PATIENT FOR ANAESTHESIA

The clinician should be aware that there is not only an interspecies disparity in the response of birds to a particular anaesthetic agent but there is also some individual variation. This is probably due to differences in liver and plasma enzyme systems and the rate of detoxication and excretion of the anaesthetic. This is more evident than is the case in related mammalian species. The bird that panics when handled or is difficult to catch will have an increased adrenaline outflow which will cause anxiety during anaesthesia. Conversely, the bird that is too easily caught and is just picked off its perch is also a worry. Wild birds are normally frightened or aggressive; if they are not, they are ill. It is better to delay anaesthesia in this group of patients for 48 hours so that they have a chance to feed and reach a better nutritional status.

A falcon in flying condition or a racing pigeon is usually athletically fit. However, many falconers keep their birds hungry to make them keen hunters. If the bird becomes sick it may be very near hypoglycaemia with depleted liver glycogen reserves.

An aged parrot (it is not uncommon to see one that is 35–40 years old) may have spent most of its life in a cage and may be obese or have atheromatous arteries. Small birds kept in aviaries are more likely to be fit than their caged fellows. A bird that is chronically ill or suffering from a low-grade toxaemia will have a depressed rate of detoxication of drugs.

Because of all these factors, always carry out a clinical assessment of the patient before giving the anaesthetic. Take a blood sample and do a microhaematocrit. If the PCV is over 55% the bird needs rehydrating with fluid therapy as described in Chapter 8, p. 202 before anaesthesia is attempted. If the PCV is below 20%, then theoretically, the bird needs blood. If a donor pigeon is available blood from this bird can be given on a once-only basis to any species. Subsequent transfusions will produce a reaction (p. 150). For an indication of the quantity that can be given see p. 45.

If there is any doubt about the health status of the avian patient and time is available it is wiser to take a blood sample and carry out a full clinical profile to include the minimum of AST, bile acids, LDH, urea, uric acid, full haematology and clotting time.

Some physiological considerations

The avian lung compared with that in a mammal of comparable size is small and non-expansible. The evolution of the fixed-volume avian lung has taken place along with the development of a rigid meshwork of blood and air capillaries. The largest diameter of the air capillaries of birds is less than one-third the size of the smallest mammalian alveoli. The very small diameter of the non-collapsible terminal airway, produces a high pressure gradient for the diffusion of blood gases (King and McLelland, 1984, pp. 140–142). The system provides a greatly increased gaseous exchange surface about 10 times that in a mammal of comparable body weight. The blood flow in the lung in relation to the air flow is principally cross-current. In the mammal the blood and gas flows are more linear. This again increases the efficiency of gas exchange in the avian lung.

The air sacs take no part in gaseous exchange and act merely as bellows driving the air in a one way flow through the respiratory tract, as illustrated in Fig. 6.1. The air sacs do however greatly increase the dead space (approximately 34% in the chicken). Because of this unidirectional air flow in the avian lung, approximately 50% of inhaled anaesthetic gases go first to the posterior air sacs before any gas exchange takes place, and are then passed through the lung before being exhaled via the anterior air sacs. The remaining 50% of inhaled gas passes directly through the lung on inspiration but also in the same one-way direction as the other 50%. If apnoea ensues because too much anaesthetic gas has been administered, and artificial respiration has to be started, then further absorbtion of anaesthetic gas will take place as it passes through the lung exchange

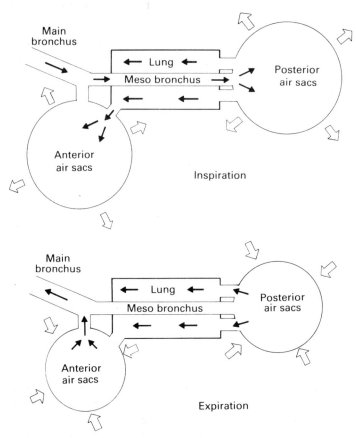

Fig. 6.1 Diagrammatic representation of the function of the avian respiratory system illustrating the uniflow of gas through the exchange surface of the lung. However, see p. 22.

surface from that stored in the posterior air sacs. The net effect of the anatomy and physiology of the avian respiratory system is to make gaseous exchange much more rapid and efficient than in the mammal. Volatile anaesthetics can reach dangerous plasma concentrations very quickly.

Another physiological aspect of the rigid lung is that the chemoreceptors monitoring Pa_{CO_2} are much more important than the mechanoreceptors monitoring pressure changes (Fedde and Kuhlman, 1977). The Pa_{CO_2} of the domestic fowl is normally about 30% lower than in mammals because of the more efficient 'washout' in the avian lung. Birds are thus much more sensitive to hypercapnia.

It is therefore important to maintain high gas flow rates of oxygen during avian anaesthesia. These should be at least three times the normal minute volume. Klide (1973) gives the following normal minute volumes:

(1) domestic fowl weighing 2.5 kg, the minute volume is 770 ml/min;
(2) racing pigeon weighing about 300 g, the minute volume is 250 ml/min;
(3) a small cage bird weighing 30 g, the minute volume is 25 ml/min.

In practice the author uses flow rates of not less than 1.00 l/min for the small birds and 3 l/min for birds the size of domestic fowl. Flow rates higher than this are unnecessary and even wasteful of volatile anaesthetic particularly isoflurane which is expensive. However, see p. 21.

Marley and Payne (1964) demonstrated when using halothane anaesthesia that the Pa_{CO_2} gradually increased during prolonged anaesthesia even in those birds where respiration appeared to be normal. In birds where respiration was depressed the Pa_{CO_2} increased much more rapidly (from 18–27 mmHg to 50–75 mmHg within 10 min). If the Pa_{CO_2} rose to 80 mmHg the bird died. Some volatile anaesthetics may have a depressive effect on the Pa_{CO_2} chemoreceptors.

King and Payne (1964) showed that in the chicken, when the bird was placed in dorsal recumbency the minute volume could be reduced by a factor of 10–60%. This was brought about by the pressure on the air sacs by the viscera. These workers showed that the effect was greater in the female than in the male and was less if the bird was in lateral recumbency.

The effects of hypoxia vary in different groups of birds. Nevertheless the oxygen uptake is higher in all birds than in mammals of comparable size. High-flying birds and diving ducks can withstand the effects of oxygen withdrawal better than surface-feeding ducks and birds that are mainly terrestrial (Dawson, 1975). The gentoo and chinstrap penguin, which remain submerged for long periods, withstand hypoxia better than the Adélie penguin which is a short-term diver.

Many agents used in general anaesthesia are also respiratory depressants. All these factors make the maintenance of an adequate rate of respiration together with relatively high flow rates of oxygen very important, whatever type of anaesthetic technique is being used. Failing this, the Pa_{CO_2} can build up rapidly and without warning. Even if there is a high flow rate of oxygen, the elimination of carbon dioxide may be inefficient. If the bird's respiratory rate is allowed to drop to a level where it is just perceptible it may be irreversible. A condition of respiratory acidosis quickly supervenes, the myocardium is depressed and blood pressure drops. A raised Pa_{CO_2} predisposes to atrial and ventricular fibrillation and to cardiac failure.

Hypothermia, which affects all birds under anaesthesia particularly the small ones, also helps to depress the myocardium. If the core body temperature drops more than 5°C the bird may not recover at all. Use a continually recording cloacal thermometer.

Because of the large internal surface area of the air sacs, there may be a high fluid loss during prolonged anaesthesia. In an already dehydrated bird this could be critical and lead to a reduced circulating blood volume with a fall in cardiac output, reduced tissue perfusion and to anaerobic respiration. This in turn leads to a fall in plasma pH and a condition of metabolic acidosis ensues. Many anaesthetics also depress blood pressure.

Cardiac failure during anaesthesia of birds is most likely to be caused by hypocapnia, but hypoxia, the anaesthetic agent, dehydration, hypothermia and the positioning of the patient are all contributing factors.

SUGGESTED PRECAUTIONARY MEASURES DURING GENERAL ANAESTHESIA OF AVIAN PATIENTS

(1)   Whether employing an injectable or volatile anaesthetic agent always administer oxygen. If possible have an endotracheal tube in place to maintain a clear airway and to enable artificial ventilation, should this prove necessary. If there is a suspicion of food in the crop or distal oesophagus pack the proximal oesophagus with wet cotton wool (see legend to Fig. 1.9 and Table 1.2).

(2)   It is safer to have too high a rate of flow of oxygen than one that is too low.

(3)   Make sure the respiratory rate is not reduced too much and maintain as light a plane of anaesthesia as is possible.

(4)   If possible use lateral or sternal recumbency.

(5)   Use a heat pad (if this is electrical it may take time to warm up). Do not make the bird too wet during pre-operation preparation. Keep the table top dry. Maintain a comfortable high operating room ambient temperature. If there is a forced air ventilation system, reduce any air currents to a minimum.

(6)   Green (1979) suggests leaving a long piece of capillary tubing, with the tip in the oropharynx of a very small bird, to aspirate any excess mucus by capillary action.

(7)   It is useful to have a syringe with an attached piece of catheter ready, in case it is necessary to aspirate any mucus blocking the airway.

(8)   The author has now ceased using atropine for premedication because (a) it has a tendency to increase the viscosity of mucus; (b) it may inhibit the Pa_{CO_2} chemoreceptors; (c) it may lead to respiratory depression.

(9)   Do not stretch the wings out too tightly. There may be damage and stimulation to the nerves of the brachial plexus. In addition if the bird is in light anaesthesia and the anaesthetic agent does not give complete muscle relaxation of the pectoralis muscles, movement of the thorax may be restricted.

(10)   Use fluid therapy if the bird is anaesthetised for any period longer than 20 min. Use 0.1 ml of Ringer lactate intramuscularly for a 30 g budgerigar, every 10 min or 1 ml/kg per hour for larger birds. This is particularly important if the anaesthetic drug is excreted through the kidneys. The addition of glucose to the Ringer lactate solution helps the liver detoxicate drugs. It is much better to give the fluid i.v. or intraosseously, see p. 203 (Nursing and after care).

(11)   For birds weighing more than 1 kg withhold food for 12 hours before anaesthesia. For those between 300 g and 1 kg withhold food for 6 hours, between 100 and 300 g withhold food for 3–4 hours. *For birds below 100 g do not withhold food at all* (see p. 60).

Monitoring anaesthesia

Whenever possible and when practical the anaesthetised bird should be monitored and the operator should not entirely rely on human senses which may not detect subtle changes in the patient's physiological state rapidly enough.

(1)   An *oesophageal stethoscope* is easy to use and is not expensive.
(2)   Recording the *ECG* is better and the silogic EC-60 is a relatively small, easy to use instrument, which many companion animal practitioners may already possess. This model will also simultaneously record the respiratory rate. It incorporates optional audio bleep and alarm on both heart and respiratory rate.
(3)   An *Imp respiratory monitor* (IMP Electronics (Fig. 6.2) or an apALERT apnoea monitor and alarm (MBM Enterprises, Australia) may provide a warning of apnoea.
(4)   An *oximeter* can be used to indicate the arterial oxygen saturation level which should be well above 85%. Below 80% can be dangerous. Some of these instruments also indicate the pulse.
(5)   An electronic continuously recording *cloacal thermometer* is also a useful piece of equipment. The temperature of a small bird can drop alarmingly during prolonged surgery even if it is on a heat pad.
(6)   *Capnography.* The measurement and continuous recording of the regularly varying wave form (either on a video display unit or on a paper trace) of the level of end tidal CO_2 in birds was initially investigated by J.I. Cruz and the author in 1995. Cruz has since continued to research this subject. Since the level of Pa_{CO_2} is one of the most important factors controlling avian respiration and the level of end expired CO_2 is probably very similar to Pa_{CO_2} this method of monitoring avian anaesthesia is likely to become important. The main disadvantage at present is the capital cost of the equipment. However, capnography can provide simultaneous information on

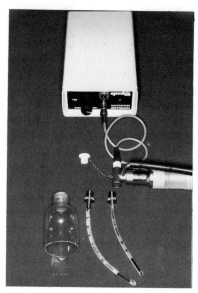

Fig. 6.2 The Imp respiratory monitor, which can be used with all species of birds to weight above 100 g. Also bethume T-piece and portex tubes.

the respiratory rate and the state of the bird's respiratory system including the efficiency of the blood gas exchange barrier. It can also give information on the level of oxygenation and the effectiveness of the anaesthetic circuit. Also capnography can give early warning of a failing heart and of a developing cardiovascular hypotension.

LOCAL ANAESTHESIA

Lignocaine hydrochloride 2% with adrenaline

This is quite safe in all but very small birds which are easily over-dosed. For a 30 g bird 0.3 ml would be fatal. It is always safer to dilute the 2% solution to produce a 0.5% solution and the injection should always include adrenaline to limit the rate of absorbtion. In birds over 2 kg, 1–3 ml can safely be used and in a pigeon-sized bird (400 g) up to 1 ml can be used. Lignocaine ointment may be useful around the vent after a cloacal prolapse.

Procaine hydrochloride 2%

This has been used in the larger birds (e.g. swans and flamingoes) without difficulty but care needs to be exercised with the dosage because of the drug's narrow safety margin. Again the 2% preparation is best diluted to produce a 0.2% solution when 1–2 ml/kg can safely be used.

GENERAL ANAESTHESIA

Pre-anaesthetic medication and tranquillisation

Some of the injectable anaesthetic agents mentioned below, which are not in themselves entirely satisfactory anaesthetics, make very good hypnotic or induction anaesthetics. These can then be supplemented with volatile anaesthetics so that the desired depth of anaesthesia can be achieved.

Assessment of the depth of general anaesthesia

This can be difficult and although it is convenient to classify general anaesthesia into light, medium and deep planes, the response of the individual bird to the stimulation of various reflexes shows considerable variation. Sometimes a bird that is apparently deeply asleep will be awoken suddenly by the stimulation of a particularly sensitive area. The skilful clinician relies on his experience and knowledge of a particular anaesthetic technique and the response of the species on which it is being used. He will primarily observe the depth, rate and pattern of respiration, noting any sudden changes. The aim should be to maintain the patient in light-to medium-depth anaesthesia in which the response to stimulation of the cere, the wattles, the comb and the cloaca together with the surrounding skin is *just* abolished or is sluggish. Pinching the interdigital web of the foot or the undersurface of the foot produces a variable and unreliable response, particularly in raptors. The eyelids may be closed but the corneal reflex, indicated by the nictitating membrane sliding obliquely across the eye, should be sluggish but never entirely lost. If there is no corneal reflex the bird is too deep. Obviously if righting reflexes are not completely abolished the plane of anaesthesia is too light. Respiration should be regular, not too slow (not much less than half the normal resting respiratory rate) and deep. A rapid, shallow or intermittent respiration indicates the depth of anaesthesia is too great.

Injectable general anaesthetics

When using any injectable anaesthetic agent it is mandatory that the bird must first be weighed accurately to enable precise computation of the dose.

Alphaxalone–Alphadolone

This drug has been used widely both by intravenous and intramuscular injection – also intraperitoneally. When given intravenously induction is rapid and anaesthesia lasts for about 10 min, with good muscle relaxation. When first given there is a fall in blood pressure and there is some respiratory depression. The drug is safe for most raptors when given at the rate of 10 mg/kg i.v. (Cooper, 1978) and has been used in dosages as high as 36 mg/kg i.v. (Harcourt-Brown, 1978). However, Cooper and Redig (1975) experienced cardiac irregularities and deaths when using it on red-tailed hawks and Cribb and Haigh (1977) demonstrated serious cardiac irregularities in red-tailed hawks and waterfowl. Haigh (1980) also showed that there was a temporary apnoea lasting approximately 46 seconds after intravenous injection.

Samour *et al.* (1984) considered it to be the injectable drug of choice for *cranes, flamingoes, storks, touracos, vultures and hornbills.*

With the possible exception of the above species mentioned by Samour, the author considers that this drug has no advantages over ketamine and its various combinations. There is also the increased risk of heart failure if the heart is not healthy.

Pentobarbitone sodium

This has been used successfully by a number of workers. At the rate of 30–40 mg/kg i.v. it was used by Graham-Jones (1966) in pigeons and by Hill and Noakes (1964) in fowls. Delius (1966) used it in gulls intramuscularly at the rate of 80 mg/kg. Sykes (1964) gave 0.3–0.5 ml by rapid intravenous injection to fowls weighing between 2 and 4 kg and followed this by 0.5–1 ml given more slowly until required depth of anaesthesia was reached. Pentobarbitone is in current use for the anaesthesia of ostriches in the Jordan Valley, Israel. It is administered i.v. into the right jugular vein at the base of the neck after xylazine has been given i.m. (Ashash *et al.* 1995, personal communication).

Thiopentone sodium

The author has used this successfully intravenously in swans at the rate of 30 mg/kg. Sykes (1964) used it in chickens at the rate of 50 mg/kg.

The margin of safety with both pentobarbitone sodium and thiopentone sodium is narrow and for most birds the use of these anaesthetics is best avoided.

Propofol

Use of this injectable anaesthetic has been investigated by Fitzgerald and Cooper (1990). It is non-irritant to tissue but is so rapidly metabolised its use in birds even as an induction agent is not very practical. Also it has a narrow safety margin.

Metomidate

Use of this drug has been documented by Jones (1977), Cooper (1970, 1974), Camburn and Stead (1966–1967) and by the author in the first edition of this book. However as much better anaesthetics are now available its use has been discontinued.

Xylazine (an alpha₂-adrenoceptor stimulant)

When used by itself in doses of 10 mg/kg i.m. it produces narcosis but not true anaesthesia. However, it is not a very satisfactory anaesthetic or hypnotic agent. Not only is recovery time prolonged but there is nearly always excitement and even severe convulsions during induction in some species. It can cause bradycardia and partial atrioventricular heart block, and there is decreased respiration and often muscle tremors. Although the fatal dose is approximately ten times the therapeutic dose it is not a particularly safe drug to use by itself.

It is not satisfactory at all in the domestic fowl even in doses as high as 100 mg/kg (Green and Simpkin, 1984).

Ketamine (a cyclohexamine)

This dissociative anaesthetic produces a cataleptic state and has been widely used in birds both by itself and in combination with synergistic drugs. It has no analgesic effect. It is both a cardiac and respiratory depressant.

In almost all species when given intramuscularly it produces anaesthesia in approximately 3–5 min. Inco-ordination, opisthotony and relaxation are evident within 1–3 min of the injection and anaesthesia lasts about 35 min. The eyes may or may not remain open. A palpebral reflex is present and muscle relaxation is not very good. There may be some excitement during recovery. The blood pressure and heart rate are slightly lowered and there is some respiratory depression.

Mandelker (1972, 1973) used it in budgerigars and other birds at doses ranging from 50 to 100 mg/kg. The author has used it in the budgerigar at a dose of 50 mg/kg for anaesthesia on three consecutive days without ill effect. Green (1979) uses it at 15 mg/kg for induction of anaesthesia which he maintains on 0.5–1.0% halothane in 50% nitrous oxide.

Altman (1980) suggested it has an adverse effect on the thermoregulatory centre in some species.

For raptors it has been used in doses ranging from 2.5 to 170 mg/kg.

Ketamine is broken down by the liver and excreted by the kidney so that it is important that fluid therapy is used if there is any doubt about the bird being dehydrated or having a hepatopathy or nephropathy. It is now rarely used as the sole anaesthetic agent.

Ketamine and acepromazine

Both Stunkard and Miller (1974) and Steiner and Davis (1981) have used this drug combination stating that there is a smoother recovery with less wing flapping than with ketamine alone. These workers use 1 ml of acepromazine containing 10 mg* added to a 10 ml vial of ketamine containing 100 mg/ml. The dose of ketamine is then calculated at 25–50 mg/kg without taking into account the acepromazine in the vial. The bird is therefore receiving a dose of acepromazine of 0.5–1.0 mg/kg. However like ketamine) acepromazine induces bradycardia.

Ketamine and diazepam (or midazolam the aqueous equivalent)

Redig and Duke (1976) used 20–40 mg/kg of ketamine together with 1.0–2 mg/kg of diazepam. Forbes (1984) and Lawton (1984) also report using this combination at the same dose rate given intramuscularly. The combined drugs have been used on psittacines, Galliformes, Anseriformes, Passeriformes and raptors and the results were generally good with deep sedation or anaesthesia and good muscle relaxation. However Forbes reported that recovery was prolonged in raptors. Both drugs have some depressant effect on respiration. This combination of drugs has been used in the ostrich ketamine (2–5 mg/kg i.v.) + diazepam (0.2–0.3 mg/kg i.v.).

Ketamine and xylazine

This combination produces relatively safe hypnosis or anaesthesia in a wide range of species. Muscle relaxation is fairly good and respiration is only slightly depressed. The eyes are sometimes closed and the palpebral reflex is sluggish or absent. The depth, the duration and the length of the recovery time to some degree depend on the dose of ketamine used. The combination has been used in various ratios of the two drugs. Increasing the amount of xylazine in relation to the ketamine has very little beneficial effect since the main effect of the xylazine appears to be to reduce the rate of breakdown of the ketamine. Redig (1983) has two routines when using this combination of raptors.

(1) Three-quarters of the computed dose is given rapidly intravenously; 1 min is allowed to assess the effect; then the rest of the dose is given slowly.

---

* Acepromazine maleate BPC contains 10 mg/ml for large animals and 2 mg/ml for small animals.

(2)   Alternatively, three-quarters of the dose may be given intramuscularly then if necessary the rest of the dose intravenously but to effect.
If this does not produce sufficient relaxation and there is still some
wing flapping a further one-half the original computed dose is given.

Redig (1983) and also Haigh (1980) found that when this drug combination was given intravenously there were some cardiac irregularities
and disturbance of the respiratory pattern. This does not happen if the
combination is used intramuscularly. Haigh at first used a dose intravenously of 30–40 mg/kg of ketamine together with 0.5–1.0 mg/kg of
xylazine. This worker now uses a dose of 2.5–5.0 mg/kg for the ketamine
and 0.25–0.5 mg/kg for the xylazine and finds there is no adverse effect on
the heart. Anaesthesia lasts 4–15 min and the bird is perching in about 30–
40 min.

There is some individual species response to this drug combination and
Redig (1983) has worked out the optimum dose for a number of species of
raptors. In general a sliding scale of doses which is approximately
equivalent to 30 mg/kg of the ketamine for birds in the 100–150 g range,
20 mg/kg for those near to 400 g in weight and 10 mg/kg for larger birds
weighing 1 kg or slightly more. In eagles weighing 4–5 kg Redig uses
4.5 mg/kg. Haigh considers, and it is also the author's experience, that the
nocturnal raptors metabolise the drugs more rapidly than diurnal raptors.
The author has also recorded (Coles, 1984a) that the genus *Buteo* seems
unusually sensitive to this drug combination when used intramuscularly
– going into deep anaesthesia, sometimes with apnoea – and that recovery
times were prolonged. Redig (1983) also found that the goshawk and
Coopers hawk needed higher doses and that recovery time was
prolonged. Steiner and Davis gave 50 mg/kg of ketamine together with
10 mg/kg xylazine intramuscularly in the budgerigar. These workers
consider that induction and recovery are somewhat rough.

The author has used this drug combination on a wide range of species
and found it to be safe and effective. The dose used is 20 mg/kg of
ketamine and 4 mg/kg of xylazine given intramuscularly. The bird is
weighed accurately and the dose of ketamine computed. An equal
volume of xylazine is then added. Signs of sedation occur within a few
minutes and induction is complete in 5–7 min. Using this dose anaesthesia lasts 10–20 min and birds are usually standing and able to perch in
1–2 hours. There is inco-ordination and sometimes a little excitement
during recovery so that it is best to loosely roll the bird in a sheet of paper
towel.

The combination is not satisfactory or safe in the pigeons or doves and
several authors, Forbes (1984), Green and Simpkin (1984), Samour *et al.*
(1984) and Coles (1984a), have all recorded that it is not satisfactory in the
Galinules. Also *it is unsafe in the long-legged birds* which are liable to
damage themselves during recovery. In penguins there is a prolonged

recovery period. It is also not safe in some pheasants, touracos, vultures and the large owls.

Medetomidine (and ketamine)

Like xylazine this is also another alpha$_2$-adrenoceptor stimulant but is more potent. Both cause a dose dependent reduction in the release and turnover of noradrenaline at the synapses in the central nervous system. In this way it results in sedation, muscle relaxation, analgesia, brady-cardia and peripheral vasoconstriction which in turn results in some rise in blood pressure. However, it has a wide margin of safety. Like xylazine it is best used in combination with ketamine and is given intramuscularly. The author has found this combination particularly useful in swans and other waterfowl. Its use has also been reported in a variety of species of birds by Jalanka (1991), Reither (1993), Scrollavezza *et al.* (1995) and Lawton (1996). Because of its potency the dosages of medetomidine are much less than for xylazine. A range of doses have been used but for practical purposes the author suggests the doses shown in Table 6.1.

Table 6.1 Doses of medetomidine and ketamine.

	Medetomidine	Ketamine
Diurnal raptors	100 µg/kg, i.m.	5 mg/kg, i.m.
Owls	150–100 µg/kg, i.m.	10 mg/kg, i.m.
Geese, swans and other waterfowl	200 µg/kg, i.m.	10 mg/kg, i.m.
Psittacines (because the health status of many captive psittacines is often suspect, minimum doses are best used)	75 µg/kg, i.m.	5 mg/kg, i.m.

After induction of anaesthesia with this combination (which takes approximately 2–3 min), anaesthesia can be maintained with very low doses ($\frac{1}{2}$–1%) of halothane, or preferably isoflurane.

Atipamezole

This is a selective alpha$_2$-adrenergic receptor antagonist which reverses all the sedative, analgesic, cardiovascular and respiratory effects of medetomidine and xylazine. It should be given at the same dose as the previously administered medetomidine. If given too soon after induction with the medetomidine and ketamine combination (i.e. within 10–15 min) and the full effect of the ketamine has not yet had time to be reduced by metabolism, some violent wing flapping may occur. Also atipamezole is metabolised more rapidly than medetomidine so re-sedation can occur and for this reason higher doses of atipamezole than medetomidine are sometimes used.

Neuroleptanalgesia (i.e. deep sedation together with analgesia)

Etorphine, an opiod at least 1000 times more potent than morphine used in combination with acetyl promazine has produced this type of anaesthesia in the ostrich. The commercial preparation, Large Animal Immobilon contains 2.45 mg/ml etorphine hydrochloride and 10 mg/ml aceproma-zine maleate and the same dose as used in the horse (i.e. 0.01 ml/kg) was used in the ostrich (Lyon and Walker, 1996).

General anaesthesia using volatile anaesthetics

Administration and anaesthetic circuits

Volatile anaesthetics have in the past been given by using an open drop technique but nowadays by using an anaesthetic chamber or more usually administered from an anaesthetic machine.

A custom-made glass box is best used as an anaesthetic chamber for small birds. The volatile anaesthetic in oxygen can be fed into the chamber via a small bore tube from the anaesthetic machine. However adequate monitoring of the patient when using this method is difficult. The gas mixture may be delivered directly from an anaesthetic machine and into a mask. Whichever method is used for induction, the bird is maintained on the volatile anaesthetic preferably by connecting it to the anaesthetic machine using an endotracheal tube in all birds above about 300 g in body weight; in smaller birds a mask usually has to be used. It is safer to use some form of semi-open circuit such as an Ayre's T-piece or better a mini-Bane since in only the very large birds is the tidal volume sufficient to move anaesthetic gas through a closed circuit. The author has used a Waters' to-and-fro system in the adult swan. Using the mini-Bane co-axial circuit helps to warm the inhaled anaesthetic gas mixture which may be particularly important if cylinders of oxygen are stored outside in the cold with the gas piped to the operating theatre. Also if possible the oxygen should be humidified since the air sacs are regions of high water loss. The Rees' modification of the Ayre's T-piece, using an open-ended rebreath-ing bag attached to the exhaust limb of the T-piece enables intermittent positive pressure ventilation to be applied if necessary. The Bane circuit can also be fitted with an open-ended bag. The most useful T-piece is the Bethune 'T' which has minimum dead space and can be connected to a respiratory monitor.

Endotracheal tubes and face masks

Plastic endotracheal tubes oral/nasal size 2.5 mm and 3.0 mm suitable for birds down to the size of a pigeon are manufactured by Portex and Cook (Fig. 6.3). Rubber, uncuffed endotracheal tubes sizes 3 or 4 can be used for slightly larger birds such as some Amazon parrots or macaws. A canine urinary catheter can be adapted by cutting the end obliquely and smoothing the end in a flame. These catheters can be fitted to an 8-mm endotracheal tube adaptor using a cut off nozzle end of a 2-ml plastic syringe. The length of all tubes should be reduced as far as is practical to reduce the dead space. The tube should loosely fit in the glottis to allow the escape of gas around it so that there is no danger of over inflating the air sacs or trauma to the trachea which in birds has complete rings of cartilage. If the bird is in light anaesthesia, particularly when using ketamine, there may be some temporary apnoea after the tube is passed. The glottis can be seen just behind the root of the tongue. In some birds (e.g. cockerel and heron) the glottis is further back in the oropharynx and in the parrots the bulbous tongue hides the glottis. In all cases intubation of the trachea is made easier if the tongue is pulled forward. The tube should be lubricated and good spot lighting is advantageous.

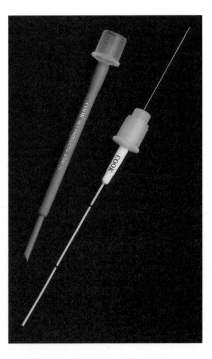

Fig. 6.3 Endotracheal tube and stylet (Cook Ltd). Can be reduced in length if necessary by cutting the proximal end.

The use of a mask may be the only practical way of maintaining small birds on volatile anaesthesia. Suitable masks can be made by cutting the base off a small plastic bottle (Fig. 6.4) or by adapting various sizes (10–60 ml) of plastic syringe cases. Tall plastic bottles or plastic drinking cups can be used to make masks for birds with long beaks (e.g. sandpipers, herons and toucans). If the plastic is transparent then the bird's eye can be seen during anaesthesia. To make a better fit the open end of the face mask can be covered with a latex surgical glove held in place by an elastic band and this can then be pierced for insertion of the bird's head.

A number of gaseous anaesthetics have been successfully used in birds.

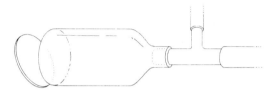

Fig. 6.4 Method of constructing a small anaesthetic face mask from a plastic bottle with the base removed.

Ether

This agent is highly soluble in the plasma and used as the sole anaesthetic for both induction and maintenance, the induction and recovery from anaesthesia is prolonged. The speed of induction and the rate of recovery from volatile anaesthetics is inversely proportional to the solubility of the anaesthetic in the plasma.

The use of ether was described by Sykes (1964) who administered it in air to chickens for up to 60 min. The author has used ether and had no problems but its use has now been superseded by much better agents. Its main disadvantage is that it is highly inflammable and explosive, and as a T-piece system is being used, the room soon becomes filled with the pungent vapour.

Halothane

This anaesthetic has been used by many workers among whom are Marley and Payne (1964), Jones (1966), Graham-Jones 1966). The author has been using this agent on birds for the last 25 years, often as the sole anaesthetic. Many of these anaesthetic sessions have lasted over an hour and Marley and Payne used it for up to 3 hours. Jones (1977) considered that there was a great risk of overdosage. However, in the author's opinion, once the clinician understands the physiology of the avian respiratory system and administers the drug accordingly, it is relatively safe. Halothane is not very soluble in plasma so that induction and recovery of anaesthesia is fairly rapid. Although some workers like to induce anaesthesia with 3–4% halothane in an oxygen flow of 0.5–2.0 litres, the author prefers to introduce the anaesthetic slowly, gradually increasing the concentration from 0.5–1% and raising this to 2.5–3% until the desired level of anaesthesia is reached. It is seldom necessary to go above 3%. Induction by this method takes longer but if the bird is struggling there is less chance of having the posterior air sacs filled with concentrated anaesthetic, should apnoea occur. Halothane is a direct myocardial depressant and cardiac and respiratory arrest are simultaneous.

The practitioner should be aware that if an older type of Fluotec vapouriser is used, before the Mark III, much higher concentrations of anaesthetic are given if the flow rate is low.

Redig (1983) considered the only disadvantage of halothane is that it requires an expensive precision vapouriser for its safe application. However since 20% of halothane is metabolised by the liver it is mildly hepatoxic.

Nitrous oxide

Halothane can be given with 50% nitrous oxide and induction is somewhat smoother. It is unwise to increase the ratio of nitrous oxide above 50% because of the danger of hypoxia. Never use nitrous oxide if there is any suspicion of respiratory disease. Discontinue use of nitrous oxide at least 5–10 min before the end of the operation.

Birds can usually be maintained on 2.0–2.5% halothane if this is the sole anaesthetic agent. If an injectable drug has been used or nitrous oxide is used in the gas mixture lower levels of volatile anaesthetics can be used for maintenance.

Methoxyflurane

This anaesthetic is much more soluble in plasma than halothane so that induction and recovery take longer. Also the plane of anaesthesia takes longer to alter. Redig (1983) found it dangerous in bald eagles, which went into apnoea within 1 min of its use and required mechanical ventilation. As 50% is metabolised in the liver it is more toxic than halothane.

Induction with methoxyflurane can be carried out using 3.5–4% and this takes approximately 8–10 min. The bird can then be maintained on 1.5–2.0%. This anaesthetic can be given without an expensive vapouriser but this is probably more wasteful. Because methoxyflurane has a high boiling point it is difficult to achieve a concentration above 3.5%. The anaesthetic is a good analgesic and analgesia apparently persists after recovery. The drug is absorbed into the fat depots from which it is gradually released and metabolised in the liver. It is not now considered to be a very suitable safe anaesthetic for birds.

Isoflurane

This volatile anaesthetic is a fluorinated ether and it is by far the safest anaesthetic to use in avian practice. Its advantages are:

(1) It is relatively insoluble in plasma so that the induction and recovery from anaesthesia is smooth and rapid so that stress for the bird is reduced to the minimum. The bird is rapidly perching without any apparent hangover effect.

(2) The depth of anaesthesia can be altered quickly by increasing or decreasing the percentage of isoflurane in the gas mixture.

(3) It has much less effect on the myocardium and the decrease in blood pressure is largely due to a reduction in peripheral vascular resistance.

(4) Cardiac arrest does not occur until several minutes after apnoea so that, unlike the case with halothane, the anaesthetist has plenty of time to 'wash out' the respiratory system and so reduce the level of inhaled anaesthetic gas.

(5) Only 0.3% of isoflurane is metabolised by the liver so that it is much less hepatoxic and safer with patients with possible undiagnosed hepatopathy. It is also less toxic to theatre staff.

(6) Because of its safety and the ease with which it can be given it can be administered if necessary two or three times daily for the routine taking of blood samples, the changing of dressings or the administration of parental fluids, etc.

The author has used it for the last 8 years for very many birds (over 3000) of a variety of species with very few anaesthetic fatalities. The method generally used for most birds is to induce with 5% isoflurane in a flow of oxygen of just over 1 litre. When light anaesthesia is achieved (usually 2–3 min) the amount of isoflurane is maintained at $2\frac{1}{2}$–3%. Waterfowl may take longer to induce anaesthesia and the maintenance setting may be somewhat higher. With these species induction with medetomidine and ketamine and then maintenance with isoflurane is easier. The author has used isoflurane as the sole anaesthetic for an adult rhea (*Rhea americana*). A flow rate of 4 litres of oxygen was used containing 5% isoflurane. Induction took approximately 7 min.

The vapour pressure of isoflurane is similar to that of halothane so that it is possible to use the same vaporiser. However, this is not recommended because the vaporiser needs to be thoroughly soaked and flushed out with ether after using halothane to rid it of preservatives in the liquid halothane.

The only real disadvantage for the practitioner when using isoflurane is the initial capital cost of a dedicated vaporiser and the greater cost of isoflurane compared with halothane. However, if used sensibly without using unnecessarily high gas flow rates, which waste a lot of anaesthetic, the significant advantages far outweigh the increased cost.

Desflurane

This is another fluorinated ether with a very low blood solubility and may in time be found to be suitable for avian anaesthesia.

ANAESTHETIC EMERGENCIES

Apnoea

The most likely causes are too much anaesthetic, the toxicity of the anaesthetic and hypercapnoea. Apnoea will also occur after primary cardiac arrest.

Switch off any volatile anaesthetic and nitrous oxide. Increase the flow rate of oxygen and start gentle mechanical ventilation immediately by intermittently occluding the exhaust arm of the Ayer's T-piece with the finger or by using the rebreathing bag. Do not over inflate the bag and the air sacs. Quite satisfactory ventilation can be obtained in all but the larger birds by this method. In small birds even if an endotracheal tube is not in place, providing the oxygen flow rate is relatively high (e.g. 2 l per min and the escape of gas between the bird's head and the mask is prevented by a latex surgical glove, cotton wool or tissue, adequate ventilation can be carried out. Do not over-ventilate – the aim is to get a moderate excursion of the abdominal wall together with slight movement of the thorax. Over-ventilation washes out carbon dioxide and inhibits the chemoreceptors stimulating respiration. If very forceful, it may rupture the air sacs or even damage the air capillaries.

If a volatile anaesthetic is not in use it is still important to have an endotracheal tube in place so that artificial respiration can be carried out. Trying to ventilate a bird artificially by pressure on the sternum is not likely to be very effective and may cause damage to the ribs, liver or other organs. It is a mistake to take the bird off the oxygen immediately at the end of the operative procedure.

If spontaneous respiration does not start within 2–3 min of artificial respiration give doxapram at the rate of 7 mg/kg (0.3 ml/kg). This can be diluted 1:3 and given to a large bird by slow i.v. injection or i.m. injection. In small-or medium-sized birds it can be dropped into the mouth so that it is absorbed through the mucous membrane.

Depression of the respiratory rate during a long period of anaesthesia

Stop the operative procedure. There may be a build up of Pa_{CO_2}. Increase the oxygen flow rate and gently artificially ventilate to wash out anaesthetic from the air sacs.

A blocked endotracheal tube

This may be indicated by more forceful and exaggerated respiratory movement and is more likely to occur with small birds and very fine endotracheal tubes. Clicking, gurgling or high-pitched squeaking sounds that could be mistaken for the bird awakening, all indicate some obstruction to the airway. Cyanosis is not usually seen except perhaps in chickens, and by the time this is recognised it is usually too late to rectify the situation. Immediately insert an air sac catheter as described below and administer oxygen via this route.

Remove the tube, blow it out, or preferably replace it with another tube. If there still appears to be some mucus present aspirate using a syringe and catheter.

Cardiac arrest

This usually occurs sometime after respiratory arrest. Marley and Payne (1964) using halothane anaesthesia in chickens noted there was a lag of about 10 min between respiratory and cardiac arrest. However this is not typical of birds in general in which with halothane cardiac and respiratory arrest are simultaneous. Unless some method of monitoring the heart is in use it will not be appreciated that cardiac arrest has actually occurred. The practitioner can try intermittent digital pressure on the sternum but this is not usually very successful, neither are intracardiac injections of adrenaline or lignocaine. In birds above 350–400 g (e.g. African grey or Amazon parrot) direct cardiac massage using the finger through an abdominal incision or using a moist cotton wool bud may be tried but is not usually successful.

SUGGESTED ANAESTHETIC ROUTINES

Short procedures lasting no more than 10 min where a quick recovery is required

There is little doubt that isofluorane administered in a gas flow of 50% oxygen and 50% nitrous oxide is the best anaesthetic for all species for quick procedures requiring general anaesthesia. However it *must* be administered *carefully* from an accurate dedicated vaporiser. Halothane is a second choice but it needs extra care during administration.

In large birds always consider whether local anaesthesia plus sedation (low dose ketamine + diazepam or xylazine or medetomidine) may be more applicable.

For prolonged anaesthesia where this may be required for a period of up to an hour or more

The following routine is satisfactory for most species.

Anaesthesia is induced with a mixture of ketamine and medetomidine (or diazepam) given intramuscularly and the bird is maintained on 0.5–1% isoflurane (or if this is not available halothane) given in 50% oxygen and 50% nitrous oxide.

If practical, weigh the bird and compute the dose of ketamine and medetomidine or diazepam. If it is not practical to weigh the bird, estimate its weight from the tables given at the back of this book. Give 75% of the computed dose intramuscularly. Wait 5 min, and if narcosis is sufficient proceed with the volatile anaesthetic. If the bird is not sufficiently sedated give a further 50% of the computed dose. Wait a further 5 min before giving any gaseous anaesthetic.

Always use an endotracheal tube wherever possible. Always flush out the anaesthetic circuit with oxygen every 5 min.

Air sac anaesthesia

This method is used after induction of anaesthesia by another method or as an emergency procedure.

A plastic cannula either fashioned from a cut-off endotracheal tube or commercially available from Cook Instrumentation (Fig. 6.5) is inserted into the left side of the bird's abdomen just posterior to the dorsal part of the last rib and above the level of the junction of the vertebral and sternal parts of the rib cage. The purpose is to insert the cannula into the caudal thoracic air sac and not into the abdominal air sac which is deeper in the

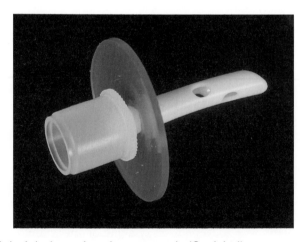

Fig. 6.5 'Coles' design avian air sac cannula (Cook Ltd).

abdomen. In larger birds (above 1 kg) it may be possible to insert the cannula between the last two ribs. After surgical preparation of the selected site the skin is picked up with rat-toothed forceps to form a 'tent'. A snick is made with scissors and their points used to spread and enlarge the hole to reveal the underlying muscle and ribs. The point of a closed pair of straight mosquito forceps or round pointed scissors is quickly thrust through the muscle and into the abdominal cavity. The points of the instrument used are then opened sufficiently to enable insertion of the plastic cannula which can then be sutured in place. The surgeon can check if air is moving freely through the tube by holding a wisp of cotton wool or fine suture material near to the opening and watching for fluctuation during each respiration. The anaesthetic circuit can be connected to the tube and gaseous anaesthesia or just oxygenation maintained via this route. The method is useful for surgery of the head or used as an emergency procedure to relieve partial obstruction of the airway. Although Korbel et al. (1993) has demonstrated in both pigeons and buzzards that Pa_{O_2} and Pa_{CO_2} levels, oxygen saturation and blood pressure are within reasonably normal limits, considerable disruption of the normal pattern of air flow occurs and the percentage of anaesthetic gas often has to be increased to maintain anaesthesia. The altered air flow is necessarily confined to the left side of the respiratory system. The right side will continue to function much as it did before the introduction of the cannula unless the normal main airway (i.e. the trachea) is blocked. This disadvantage can be overcome by inserting the tube into the interclavicular air sac but this is more difficult to carry out and maintain the tube in position together with the added risk of damage to the heart and its major blood vessels.

Total gas flows need to be higher than normal to make sure fresh gas is always entering the caudal thoracic air sac and reaching the exchange barrier in the lung.

There is no completely safe anaesthetic for birds. Always get an anaesthetic consent form signed.

Chapter 7
Surgery

GENERAL CONSIDERATIONS

Selection of avian patients for surgery

Before carrying out any sort of operation on a bird it is wise to carry out a thorough clinical examination and if necessary a complete clinical profile on sampled blood. Obviously, birds which are in a state of shock due to trauma are bad surgical risks. The obese budgerigar which has been confined to its cage throughout life is also a bad risk. However, the author has been surprised on a number of occasions by birds that have been abnormally thin and in poor condition which have survived anaesthesia and surgery. If possible, it is better to try to improve the nutritional state of these patients first. Probably the bird at greatest risk is the one with an obvious respiratory problem. Any bird that is dyspnoeic or one that becomes dyspnoeic with the minimum of handling is a bad surgical risk. A bird that has ascites or a large abdominal space occupying mass is a bad risk.

Positioning of the patient during surgery

Any bird placed in dorsal recumbency will have a reduced air sac volume, so that in birds with space occupying lesions of the abdomen this condition is exacerbated. This problem is discussed in more detail in Chapter 6, p. 129. Although the vast majority of surgical patients can be placed on their backs and are less liable to be moved in this position, it is better to have them in ventral or lateral recumbency. When in lateral recumbency care should be taken not to forcibly fold the wings too far back above the body, as this may restrict respiratory movement.

Essential equipment

A selection of small instruments such as those used in ophthalmic or microsurgery should be used. The following list is the most useful and the minimum that should be available.

(1) 114 mm enucleation or strabismus scissors.
(2) Tissue forceps with 1 × 2 teeth such as Lister's conjunctival forceps.
(3) Straight Halsted mosquito forceps.
(4) Curved Halsted mosquito forceps.
(5) A blunt-ended probe. Sterile cotton wool buds will serve this purpose and will also act as swabs for clearing blood or exudate.
(6) Fine needle holders.
(7) A Spreull needle attached to a sterile 10-ml syringe is useful for suction or irrigation.
(8) Suitable suturing materials, e.g. No. 2 pseudo monofilament polyamide, 3/0 chromic cat gut or polyglactin 910 swaged on to round-bodied, taper cut pointed needles. If absorbable sutures are used in the skin the bird will not need handling again for suture removal.

When using instruments for delicate surgery the hands are under better control if the surgeon is seated and it may be possible to rest the elbows on the table. Also some form of magnification combined with good illumination is advisable. An operating microscope is the ultimate choice but this is costly. Binocular loupes or magnifying spectacles are also useful. The least expensive system is a combined lens and circular fluorescent light. This is marketed by several surgical instrument companies and a number of different designs are used in industry by persons carrying out delicate work. Harrison (1984) suggests mounting the fibreoptic laparoscope (see Chapter 3) on a flexible arm, like that used for some table lamps, and using this for magnification and lighting. This gives excellent lighting and magnification but the field of vision is somewhat restricted.

Electro surgery

Although not essential it is desirable to have the use of an electro surgical (i.e. radio surgical) instrument for both incision and coagulation. Preferably the equipment should have a frequency range up to 5 MHz such as the Ellman Surgitrom. Most equipment of this type operates through a monopolar active electrode using an indifferent plate placed under the bird. Bipolar forceps with both active and indifferent electrodes incorporated into the same hand-held instrument are better since the current does not have to pass through the whole body of the patient.

Haemorrhage

There is little doubt that many avian surgical patients die of blood loss. Systemic blood pressures in birds are high compared with mammals. Blood loss from severed vessels is therefore rapid and the control of bleeding is of paramount importance, particularly in small birds. However, Kovách *et al.* (1968 and 1969) have demonstrated that several species of birds are able to tolerate blood loss better than mammals. Circulating blood volume is usually little more than 10% of body weight (see p. 45), yet Kovách has shown that pigeons can survive blood loss of 8% of body weight during prolonged haemorrhage. Although the blood pressure and heart rate dropped, these returned to normal within 30 min to 4 hours. This effect is apparently due to the greatly increased capillary surface area (3–5 times that found in the domestic cat) that is available for the absorbtion of reserve tissue fluid and to a very pronounced vasoconstriction in the skeletal muscles. From the practical point of view the author has often noticed that birds presented at the surgery because of trauma have suffered considerable blood loss, as shown by their surroundings, and yet they have survived.

The arterial capillaries in the muscles are more influenced by autonomic nervous control than by the level of local metabolites (H^+, CO_2 and lactic acid) than is the case in mammals. Although the resting heart rate of many birds is lower than that in mammals of comparable size, stress or excitement very soon leads to a much more rapid heart rate. Struggling due to an inadequate depth of anaesthesia can result in considerable haemorrhage. Harrison (1984) and the author have used blood transfusions in birds. It has been shown that blood from heterogenous species can safely be used for a first transfusion (p. 127). However, blood for transfusion is unlikely to be readily available and in view of the above mentioned observations of Kovách *et al.* the discrete use of blood volume expanders such as the gelatin artificial colloidal plasma substitutes which also contain electrolytes is all that is necessary. If there is any suspicion of a hepatopathy a pre-operation vitamin K injection should be given.

Cleaning and antisepsis of the operation site

To obtain a clear operating area every feather has to be meticulously plucked. If cut, the feather does not grow until the bird's next moult. Plucking can be tedious and it sometimes is easier using forceps. The shaft of the feather must be firmly gripped and pulled out cleanly so that the germinal layer of the feather papilla is not damaged and the feather will regenerate. Regeneration will occur in most cases within a few weeks of plucking. If the feather is fully grown, it is a dead structure which will not bleed when plucked. If the feather is plucked before growth is completed and the feather has not completely emerged from its sheath haemorrhage is likely to occur. Only the minimum number of feathers consistent with clearing the operation site should be plucked to avoid excessive heat loss, particularly in small birds. For the same reason the surgical site should be cleansed with minimal antiseptic solution. Cleaning and sterilisation can be carried out using a quaternary ammonium solution, chlorhexidine, benzalkonium chloride or one of the tamed iodine antiseptics such as providone iodine.

To limit heat loss the patient should be placed on an electrically heated pad or on a rigid hot water bottle covered in sterile cloths or a water circulating heat pad.

SURGERY OF THE SKIN AND ASSOCIATED STRUCTURES

Overall the skin of birds is much thinner than that of mammals of comparable size. In the feathered area the thickness and strength varies between the feather tracts (pterylae) and the featherless areas between these tracts (apteria). In the apteria the dermis has a stronger mesh of collagen fibres (Stettenheim, 1972).

Surgical incisions are best made in the apteria, parallel and mid-way between the adjacent feather tracts, and the subsequent sutures placed in the apteria.

The subcutis and dermis contain only a few horizontal sheets of elastic fibres so that avian skin is not very elastic. The skin is not firmly attached to the underlying muscle, but in some areas (the skull, the carpus, the digits, the pelvis) the skin is firmly and extensively attached to bone. Avian skin is therefore not very mobile and easily tears, particularly where it is attached to the bone. The skin is best sutured using suture material swaged on to atraumatic needles. There are numerous blood vessels, both capillary and larger vessels, within the skin and haemorrhage can be a problem. When possible, incisions should be made with a radio surgical or ophthalmic diathermy knife. The scalpel should not be used at all for most types of avian surgery or radio surgery. If diathermy is not available an incision can be made by nicking and blunt dissection with scissors after first crushing the skin with artery forceps along the line of the intended incision.

Lacerated wounds

These are sometimes caused by attacks from aviary mates or flying into sharp objects, particularly during stormy and gusty weather. Racing pigeons not uncommonly return home having been blown into telephone or barbed wire. If these wounds involve the anterior sternum, as they often do, there may be damage to the clavicular air sac with resulting subcutaneous emphysema. This usually resolves spontaneously, but if necessary, can be deflated with a hypodermic needle and syringe. Providing the wound is fresh and haemorrhage has been controlled the wound can be treated on a routine basis and usually heals by first intention without secondary infection. If skin has been lost and the wound has started to granulate, debride the wound and then cover with a hydrophilic dressing. Some types of this dressing, e.g. Granuflex, are rigid enough to lightly suture in position and will help epithelialisation of quite large areas.

Subcutaneous abscesses

These are not uncommon around the head, particularly in parrots. They often involve the paranasal sinuses around the eye but also occur in the submandibular region. These abscesses are usually filled with inspissated, caseous pus. The abscess should be opened with a scalpel fitted with a No. 11 blade, by inserting the point first and directing the cutting edge away from the bird. The pus is then scooped out and the cavity curetted. A Volkmann's spoon can be used, but a useful instrument for a small bird is a canine tooth scaler with a rounded spatulate end. When opening a submandibular abscess care should be taken to avoid the large subcutaneous blood vessels in this region. Before suturing the skin, a bacteriological swab should be taken for culture and antibiotic-sensitivity testing. An injection of ampicillin may be given at the time of opening the abscess although this antibiotic may need to be changed later in the light of the results of bacteriological culture. In the case of very small birds of 15–20 g size it may not be practical to suture an abscess after opening. In this case the cavity can be cauterised with a silver nitrate pencil and left to heal by granulation.

Abscesses sometimes occur around and in the ear. The surrounding skin can become thickened and the ear canal filled with exudate. These abscesses need great care because of the risk of haemorrhage and damage to the tympanum which is relatively near the surface. It may be wiser to try and first reduce the swelling with topical steroids combined with antibiotics.

Feather cysts

These are usually seen in the region of the carpus but can occur in other parts of the body. The author has never seen them in the many thousands of wild birds he has examined. They are most often seen in some breeds of canary but do occur in other captive birds. They may be genetic in origin or caused by mechanical damage to the developing feather follicle or excessive preening by the bird. They are usually dry and contain the remains of the undeveloped feather which has been unable to emerge in a normal manner from the follicle. However, some neoplasms may look like feather follicles and bleed profusely when opened. Since the feather follicle persists in maintaining an abnormal direction these cysts will recur if they are merely opened. The whole section of skin including the cyst should be carefully dissected out. Dissection is not easy without damaging the neighbouring follicles and the skin is adherent to the underlying bone in the area of the carpus.

Subcutaneous tumours and cysts

These are seen in all species but are most common in the psittacine birds, particularly the budgerigar. They are not usually invasive but can become ulcerated. They are usually easily dissected free of surrounding tissue by using a closed pair of mosquito haemostats or preferably radio-surgery. Great care should be taken to search out and clamp and coagulate any blood vessels supplying the neoplasm. This is particularly the case with the common lipomatous tumours found over the thorax of the budgerigar which often have a large blood vessel beneath them and which can bleed profusely. Meticulous attention should be given to any haemorrhage into the wound after surgery. For this reason any loose skin left after removing a large tumour should be trimmed and dead space diminished.

Fatty tumours in budgerigars are best reduced before surgery by strict dietary and medical routines. This also improves the general physical condition of the bird. The seed should be rationed to one heaped teaspoonful twice daily. Add soluble vitamins and diluted Lugol's iodine to the drinking water (p. 267).

Tumours of the uropygial or preen gland

These may be benign adenomas or malignant adenocarcinomas that can become adherent to the underlying bone. Haemorrhage is not usually a problem but if the tumour has been allowed to reach an appreciable size some difficulty may be experienced in repair. Removal of the preen gland does not seem to have any adverse effects. It does not seem essential to the maintenance of budgerigar plumage and it may not be essential to other species of birds since it is absent in some species such as many pigeons, parrots, emus, cassowaries and bustards (King and McLelland, 1975). The composition of the secretion varies in different species but usually contains a complex of water repellent waxes, lipids and proteins. It may also contain a precursor of vitamin D (Stettenheim, 1972). The vitamin D precursor may only be important in growing birds.

THE HEAD REGION

Accidental wounds

Apart from the fractures of the beak, dealt with below, other fractures are liable to result in instant death. However, less serious injury may cause damage to the skin including the eyelids. The skin over the whole of the skull in most species is not very elastic and is adherent to the bone. Any wound more than a few days old will have contracted with resultant fibrosis and it will be difficult to suture the skin edges together. If the upper eyelid is damaged at the nasal canthus it may be possible to slide the remaining part of the eyelid forward, by making a lateral canthotomy, as shown in Fig. 7.1. Do not remove a wedge of skin below this incision, as is sometimes done in the mammals for this type of plastic surgery. In the bird this only results in too much tension across the lower eyelid. In birds it is the lower eyelid that carries out most of the movement in covering the eyeball.

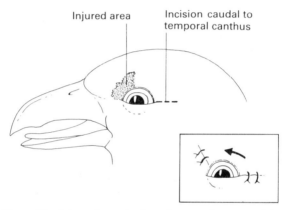

Fig. 7.1 Position of incisions for suturing damage to upper lid.

Corneal ulcers

These can be the result of trauma or a variety of infections including avipox virus and *Chlamydia*. Fluorescein can aid diagnosis. Surgery for indolent ulcers can be achieved using good magnification and standard ophthalmic techniques. If suturing the nictitating membrane over the cornea the direction this travels across the cornea is from the ventral nasal canthus to the dorsal temporal canthus in a somewhat different direction than is the case with mammals.

Enucleation of the eye

Before this is undertaken the following factors should be taken into account. The eye in birds is relatively much larger than in mammals of comparable size, particularly in raptors. In fact, avian eyes are much larger than they appear to the casual observer and occupy more space in the skull than the brain. The extraocular muscles have been greatly reduced in size and the resulting loss of movement in the eyeball is compensated for by an increased movement of the whole head supported by the very flexible neck. Reduction in the eye muscles has resulted in much less space for the surgeon to work between the eyeball and its socket. The globe of the eyeball is much more rigid than in the mammal. Not only is the sclera cartilagenous but there is a ring of bony plates around the circumference near the corneal scleral junction. There is only a thin interorbital septum between the two eyes, which is particularly evident in the owls. In removing one eye the optic nerve of the other eye can easily be damaged. At the back of the eye in some species there is a U-shaped bone in the sclera surrounding the optic nerve. There is a well developed venous plexus near the corneal–scleral junction (see Fig. 3.8).

The simplest method of enucleation is by lateral canthotomy, then an incision of the cornea to remove the aqueous, the lens and the vitreous. The sclera and choroid should then be carefully collapsed into the resulting free space using scissors and forceps. It may be wiser to leave the back of the sclera with the attached tissues intact and to plug the socket with an absorbent fibrin or gelatin sponge. The eyelids are then sutured together after removing the margin of each lid.

Tumours of the nictitating membrane are occasionally seen in birds. Apart from the cosmetic aspect, which worries the owner, the surgeon should always consider whether the removal of this membrane is absolutely necessary. As in mammals, but probably more so in birds, the nictitating membrane has a very important protective function to the eye. Removal of the membrane can lead to a keratitis.

Cataract surgery

Cataracts are not uncommon in birds. If bilateral surgery is justified it should be carried out by an ophthalmic veterinary surgeon using phacoemulsification techniques.

Cannulation of the infra-orbital sinuses

This is a simple procedure that can be carried out in a quiet bird without anaesthetic. It may be required in any species with a chronic sinusitis (see section on clinical examination of the head). The point of entry is illustrated in Fig. 7.2. A 20–22 G hypodermic needle is held almost parallel to the skin surface with the needle pointed to a position halfway between the orbital globe and the external nares. Care must be taken not to pierce the globe of the eye. In bad cases the sinus is well-distended and entry can be made without any difficulty into the area of greatest distension. In the

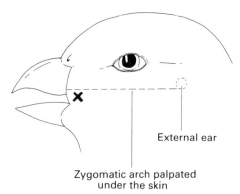

External ear

Zygomatic arch palpated
under the skin

Fig. 7.2 The ×-cross shows the point of entry for cannulation of the infra-orbital sinuses. This is just dorsal to the commisure of the mouth where the distal end of the zygomatic arch can be felt to impinge on the premaxilla (i.e. the skeletal element of the upper beak). (See Figs 1.1 and 3.8.)

budgerigar the hypodermic needle needs only to be advanced horizontally to a depth of approximately 2 mm. A suitable volume of fluid for injection is 0.1–0.3 ml. Excess fluid will exit through the nares and may also flow into the pharynx so care must be taken that none flows down the glottis.

Hyperkeratinization of the cere and nares

In budgerigars a horn-like projection sometimes develops from the cere and occasionally may obstruct the nares (see Fig. 2.2). This is purely excessive keratin that has not desquamated from the basal tissues. It is dry and bloodless and can be cut with scissors or nail clippers, care being taken not to go too close to the sensitive cere.

The larger psittacines may also develop rhinolyths or collections of dry exudate within the nares which can act like a ball valve. They may partially obstruct breathing and cause annoyance. It is a simple matter to scoop these out with a dental scaler. Some underlying infection may be present.

Abscesses in the oral cavity

These can occur anywhere in the mouth. They may be seen around and partly blocking the choanal opening from the nasal cavity or on the tongue, particularly in parrots. They should be opened and thoroughly curretted. It is not practical to suture those over the choanal opening so they should be cauterised.

Beak problems
Deformities and overgrowth

Budgerigars often are seen with overgrown or distorted beaks. There is very little that can be done surgically to correct these defects. Regular clipping with nail clippers is the best routine. Other psittacines also get overgrown beaks sometimes through lack of proper wear or they may become distorted through excessive wear caused by climbing the metal bars of their cage. Other species of birds also occasionally suffer distortion of the beak through trauma to the germinal layer. Metabolic bone disease not only affects the other parts of the skeleton but also affects growth of the premaxilla and mandible so that the overlying beak becomes distorted. The rhamphotheca or heavily cornified covering of the beak is a constantly growing structure. The cornified surface of the tissue obliquely slides towards the tip of the beak (Stettenheim, 1972), the edges and surface of which are continually worn away during use. Falconers regularly 'cope' or cut the upper beaks of their birds to counteract overgrowth.

In all cases the beak can be trimmed to shape (not just cut off square) with nail clippers and then smoothed off with fine sandpaper. An emery board is very suitable. Sometimes the beak can be ground into shape with a modeller's cordless 'hobby' drill fitted with a small carborundum stone. A diamond chip dental cutting disc is also a useful attachment. If bleeding occurs, it can be cauterised with a silver nitrate pencil or solution of ferric chloride after which it is neutralised with sodium chloride. Occasionally a beak is seen that has either developed abnormally from hatching or has been fractured and allowed to heal in an uncorrected position. The lower beak may stick out at an angle to the upper beak. The owner might think this is due to dislocation, but because of the double articulation of the avian lower jaw (Fig 1.1), dislocation is unlikely. There are two joints of the quadrate bone, dorsally with the temporal bone and ventrally with the articular bone, that distribute any disrupting force applied to the mandible.

There may be prehension difficulty with soft food tending to lodge at the side of the beak. There are two methods of dealing with this problem – both of which require osteotomy. First, the difference in the lengths of the two sides is measured carefully. Procedure number one is to remove a section of bone from the longer of the two mandibles and then wire the bone back in position with one or two stainless steel wire sutures. The second technique is to use a sliding osteotomy. This is carried out just anterior to the commissure of the integument covering the upper and lower beaks. In this area the bone is fairly accessible and there are no large blood vessels overlying the bone. The pseudotemporalis muscle closing the beak overlies the posterior part of the section to be made in the bone. The size of this muscle depends on the species and the power of closing

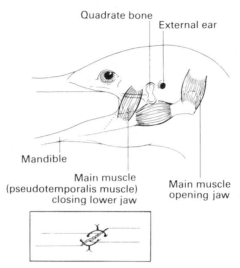

Fig. 7.3 Diagrammatic representation of the articulation of the mandible in a typical bird, showing one method of osteotomy. The dotted line indicates where the bone is sectioned.

the beak, which depends on the bird's feeding habits. Fortunately, most of those birds where the operation is required have weak pseudotemporalis muscles and relatively long, straight mandibles. The part of the muscle which may overlie that part of the bone to be sectioned is partly freed from its insertion onto the bone. Having decided on the direction of the oblique section through the hone a line of fine holes is drilled along this position. The bone is then cut with a saw. The anterior part of the mandible can then be slid cranially in relation to its posterior half and again wired in position with stainless steel wire sutures. If the upper pair of holes drilled for the wire are large enough, they will take a catgut, or better, polyglactin suture as well as the stainless steel suture. This absorbable suture can be used to hold the pseudotemporalis muscles back in place (Fig. 7.3).

In carrying out both these methods, the integument covering the bone needs to be carefully stripped for a little way down on each side of the section through the bone. As far as is practical it is better to try and suture the integument so that the suture line does not lie over the union in the bone but more to one side. For sectioning the bone a sterile junior hacksaw blade can be used. This is sometimes easier if the blade is first snapped in half. The wire sutures should be tight enough only to bring the bone together; overtightening usually results in the wire cutting its way through the fine trabecula structure of the bone. Birds show little discomfort after both these procedures and are surprisingly rough with their beaks. They usually start to feed straight away. Because of this some external support is recommended. A splint made of hexcelite thermoplastic splinting material can be moulded around and form a cradle for the mandible. This can then be wired into position with the wire going through the skin and over the bone. The success of these operations will depend not only on the skill of the surgeon but also on the correct selection of cases. The temperament of the bird is important. Ducks usually make good subjects. Success also depends on the size and shape of the lower beak. One needs a relatively long and straight area on which to operate. One disadvantage of these operations is that the mandibular branch of the fifth cranial nerve runs through a canal in the mandible and is quite likely to be destroyed when the bone is sectioned. When using the second method on a reasonably large bird it may be possible to cut carefully round the circumference of the bone providing the predrilling has not already damaged the nerve. However, the nerve distal to this area is only sensory and the bird is not apparently affected by anaesthesia of this area.

These techniques are not suitable for parrots, in which other techniques can be used.

(1)   In the case of an upper beak which diverges to one side producing a scissors beak, a prosthetic ramp is built up on the lower beak so that as the tip of the upper beak bears on this it tends to be pushed into the correct position. The ramp is fashioned from dental acrylic or Technovite and anchored to the lower beak with a Kirschner–Ehmer (KE) wire and stainless steel mesh, after the surface of the beak has been scarified with a dental burr.

(2)   A KE wire is passed through the frontal bone and hooks formed on each end. A second KE with a hook is passed through the central area on the upper beak. Acrylic or Technovite is used to help hold this in position. Elastic bands (or dental rubber bands) are placed across the hooks to pull the beak into position.

Both methods work best in birds which are not fully grown. For more information on these methods see Martin and Ritchie (1994).

Splints or fractures

If the damage is a simple crack in the bone, particularly if only one side is affected, then a stainless steel wire suture will suffice. If only the cornified integument is damaged it can often simply be glued back in position using an epoxy resin glue or one of the 'super glues' or better still bone cement (cyanomethylmacrylate).

If the beak is more seriously damaged and is hanging by the intact integument, something more robust than simple wire suturing will be needed. Various methods have been used by different workers. These methods nearly always involve the use of Steinmann's pins or Kirschner wires placed in a cruciate pattern. These are further braced with figures-of-eight stainless wire sutures placed around the ends of the pins. The ends of the pins are best protected by an epoxy resin glue or similar substance. Some sort of cradling device as described above, to give external support, is advised.

Partial loss of the beak

This can happen in any species but is commonest in those birds with rather large or long beaks such as the hornbill, the toucan, parrots, ducks and, occasionally, wading birds. In this last group, because of the long, thin beak, the problem is insoluble. In those birds with a wider base to the beak it may be possible to fit a prosthesis. If only the tip of the beak is broken off, particularly if this does not involve the underlying pre-maxillae, the beak can be filed and shaped with sandpaper. Eventually the beak will return to normal (see Fig. 1.1).

If a small part of the premaxilla is missing, the open end needs to be first plugged before shaping. A surgical glue such as a self-curing acrylic is preferable but if this is not available epoxy resin glues such as those used for car body repair kits can be used and do not appear toxic when used externally.

There are few papers in the scientific literature that record the fitting of a prosthesis. Von Becker (1974) reports a problem in two hornbill ravens, damaged in transit, that was repaired by fitting steel plating to cover the ends of the remaining stumps. Most other reports have used a beak moulded from fibreglass or dental acrylic. The material marketed under the name of Technovit 609 is suitable. The author on two occasions has used high density polyethylene for a prosthesis fitted to two parrots and has used polypropamide to replace a duck's partly-missing upper beak. In the last case the polypropamide upper beak was fashioned from the barrel of a 10 ml plastic syringe. Approximately one-third of the cir-cumference of the plastic tube was used and was found to have about the right curvature. This was then overlapped on the remaining proximal half of the beak and kept in position with stainless steel wire sutures. The bird started to feed as soon as it recovered from the anaesthetic (see Plate 2).

In the parrot cases the prostheses were carved from a block of high-density polyethylene, the material used for making human artificial hips. The problem in both cases is the satisfactory and permanent fixation of the prosthesis to the remainder of the beak. A surgical glue can be used, or wire sutures or Kirschner wires used in a cruciate pattern. In all cases the attachment eventually works loose due to the birds' constant rough usage and to pressure erosion of the bone. The bone, in any case, is not very solid in the region of the nares, being composed of a mesh of interlocking trabeculae enclosed in a thin, outer shell. Nature has provided a very strong and light-weight structure admirably adapted to the function of prehension for the particular species but quite useless as a firm anchorage in orthopaedic surgery. The parrots used the prosthesis quite readily to climb both vertically and across the top of the cage. They did not use the beak to crack nuts. This may have been due to the fact that the natural beak has a number of transverse ridges across the internal surface. They are used in lodging a nut with the tongue in order to crack it with the force of the lower beak. The bird has to be maintained on soft foods such as seed, ground down in a food blender and mixed with peanut butter or mashed potato. These birds readily eat a variety of fruit. Oesophagotomy tubes may be required immediately after surgery in some cases.

It is questionable whether the use of a prosthesis is always justified in parrots. Although the device is well tolerated, apart from the improved cosmetic effect, there may be little advantage to the bird. The birds soon learn to climb and to feed quite effectively on soft foods without an upper beak and appear to be quite happy once the original lesion has healed. A Tasmanian green rosella (*Platycereus caledonicus*) is reported to have fed and reared its chicks normally. A prosthesis is, however, essential if the mandible is lost.

Surgery of the neck

Sometimes a foreign body will lodge in the oesophagus. This could be a long bone from the prey of a raptor or a fish hook in a water bird. The oesophagus in most birds is wide and easily dilated, but the muscular wall is thin. It may be possible to extract the object via the oropharynx in the unanaesthetised subject. In other cases an incision will have to be made in the neck. There are no particular problems but it is as well to make the incision on the left side since the jugular vein is better developed on the right side. The external carotid artery does not form until near the base of the skull and the internal carotids are tucked under the cervical vertebrae.

Impaction of the crop

This can occur through a variety of causes, e.g. foreign bodies, infection, the sudden ingestion of food too high in fibrous content. The aetiology of crop stasis in hand-reared nestlings can be similar to impaction in adult birds but is more often caused by food given either too frequently or in too great a quantity or at the wrong temperature. In chicks the condition can usually be relieved by gentle flushing and aspiration with warm saline. Never be tempted to turn the chick upside down.

The impaction can be felt as a plastic mass situated at the thoracic inlet. Providing an incision is made over the area of greatest distension there is little danger of damage to other structures. This is a simple operation and may be done under local anaesthesia. Both crop and skin should be sutured separately. However, see p. 14.

Fistula of the crop

This is also seen in hand-reared nestlings and results from scalding by food given at too high a temperature. Surgical repair is feasible but defer surgery as long as possible so that the chick reaches maximum weight and the edges of the wound are easily defined. Have a crop tube in place during suturing to facilitate visual differentiation of the crop mucosa and skin. If there has been extensive loss of skin it may be possible to mobilise skin from higher up the neck. The most dangerous situation is food trapped between the skin and the crop resulting in subcutaneous necrosis.

Use of a pharyngostomy tube

This is sometimes useful after neck or crop surgery and is simple to insert. Incision is made through the skin of the right side of the neck just caudal to the mandible. If possible place a finger in the oesophagus and dissect down onto this.

SURGERY OF THE RESPIRATORY SYSTEM

Devoicing birds

This has been carried out on the domestic cockerel or a peacock. It is also recorded as having been performed on some raptors. It is questionable whether this is an ethical procedure for a veterinarian to perform in the light of the opinion on animal welfare in the United Kingdom and United States of America. Some consider this an unjustifiable mutilation and in any case the long-term end result is often not satisfactory. Description of the surgical technique has for these reasons been omitted from this edition.

Acute respiratory obstruction

In parrots, and occasionally in other birds, respiratory obstruction is not uncommonly encountered. There is usually pronounced dyspnoea accompanied by abnormal expiratory sounds. This condition is distinct from the more slowly developing syndrome seen in the budgerigar due to hypertrophy of the thyroid gland. In other birds it is usually due to inspissated pus and occasionally seed husks or chewed carpet material. In parrots often there is a history of respiratory disease. In desperate cases insertion of an air sac auxiliary airway is essential (see p. 146) after which diagnosis can be confirmed by endoscopy. The obstruction can be removed by aspiration using a modified canine urinary catheter (e.g. 6 Fr, 2 mm diameter) attached to a 60 ml syringe. This combination, if the plunger is rapidly withdrawn, produces a good negative pressure.

Sometimes two or three attempts are required. Culture the aspirate. If necessary repeat on two or three subsequent days. Always follow with endoscopic examination (see p. 83).

ABDOMINAL SURGERY

The clinical indications for entering the avian abdomen are: (1) diagnostic, (2) the removal of foreign bodies from the proventriculus or gizzard, (3) the relief of an impacted gizzard or ventriculum, (4) the removal of tumours, (5) the relief of an impacted oviduct, (6) colopexy and (7) salpingo hysterectomy.

The approach to the abdomen is usually through a mid-line ventral incision but if a neoplasm of the gonads or adrenal gland is definitely diagnosed, a flank incision gives better access to these organs and their associated blood supply. The ventral incision is best made slightly to the (surgeon's) left of the mid-line.

The abdominal muscles are the same as those in the mammal but the extent of the linea alba and the thickness of the muscles varies according to the species of bird. It is best developed in strong flying birds since the body wall is the site of the elastic and active movement governing the bellows action of the air sacs driving air through the avian respiratory system. Harrison (1984) suggests extending the mid-line incision by incisions at right angles, parallel to the posterior edge of the sternum, so as to form two flaps. This produces better exposure but if these para-sternal incisions are extended more than a third of the distance from the mid-line to the ribs in some species, the intestinal peritoneal cavity will be entered, which may not be necessary. Just below these outer areas lie the left and right posterior thoracic air sacs. Also depending on the species, the mid-line incision, if extended too far posteriorly, will enter the intestinal peritoneal cavity. This cavity contains the two abdominal air sacs. Taking the above anatomical facts into consideration it is not desirable to incise and deflate all four posterior air sacs (see Fig. 7.4).

If a careful incision is made through the linea alba, with blunt-pointed scissors, while picking it up with rat-toothed forceps to hold it away from the underlying viscera, entry is made into the right ventral hepatic cavity. This initial incision is preferably carried out with a radio-surgical instrument. On the floor of this cavity (anatomically the dorsal aspect of the cavity) is a membrane (right posthepatic septum) that resembles an air sac but is one of the peritoneal membranes. Contained within this first cavity are the organs shown in Fig. 7.5. The gizzard is attached by the central mesentery to the abdominal wall at the mid-line. Distal to the ventral mesentery lies the left ventral hepatic cavity containing the left lobe of the liver. The ventral hepatic cavities contain no air sacs. The thickness and translucency of the posthepatic septal membranes vary

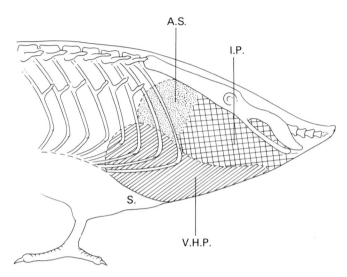

Fig. 7.4 Diagram showing the relative positions of the coelomic cavities. A.S., left and right caudal thoracic air sacs; I.P., left and right intestinal peritoneal cavities. The two cavities are divided by the dorsal mesentery in which is suspended the intestine and reproductive tract. Intimately connected with the intestine are the left and right abdominal air sacs; V.H.P., left and right ventral hepatic cavities. These are divided by the ventral mesentery. The cavities only contain the two lobes of the liver; S., sternum. After Dunker (1978).

with the size of the bird (also if there is any degree of airacculitis or peritonitis causing adhesions). In small birds the posthepatic septum acts as a fat depot, obscuring the intestine beneath. The air sacs are mostly adherent and supported by the surrounding tissues and so will not collapse if punctured. Providing entry into and destruction of the integrity of the air sacs is not extensive, it has no more effect on the respiratory system than tracheotomy does in mammals.

Gastrotomy/proventriculotomy/ventriculotomy

Access to these organs may be required for the removal of foreign bodies. The muscular stomach or ventriculus is easily accessible through the initial abdominal incision. Its muscular wall varies in thickness; in the gizzard of some granivorous birds it is very thick. In these species haemorrhage from the muscle can be a problem if a radio-surgical knife is not used.

The glandular part of the stomach or proventriculus is not quite so accessible but gentle traction on the ventriculus will bring the posterior part of this organ into view (Fig. 7.6). In the ostrich proventriculotomy for the relief of impaction may be required and the surgical approach is somewhat different (Fig. 7.7).

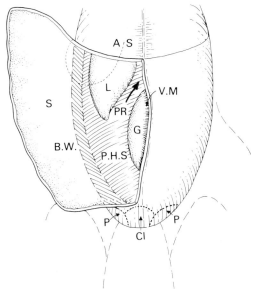

Fig. 7.5 Incision through the linea alba into the right ventral hepatic cavity.
A.S., Dotted line shows the position of the right caudal thoracic air sac below
the level of the ventral hepatic cavity containing the liver; L., right lobe of liver;
P.R., the approach to the proventriculus; G., gizzard attached to linea alba by
the ventral mesentery; P.H.S. right post hepatic septum distal to which lies the
duodenum and pancreas in the intestinal peritoneal cavity and which is
surrounded by the abdominal air sac; C.L., cloaca. An incision in this area will
enter the intestinal peritoneal cavity; P., pubis; B.W., body wall; S., skin flap;
V.M., ventral mesentery.

Surgical access to the rest of the alimentary canal

If it is necessary, an approach can be made via the route used by Durant
(1926 and 1930) and Schlotthauer *et al.* (1933) for ablation of the caeca. This
is to make an incision medial and parallel to the left pubis. There is a large
artery in this area that must be avoided. This approach gives access not
only to the caeca but also the rectum and the distal part of the ileum, the
duodenum, the proventriculus, the ventriculus and the gonads (Fig. 7.8).
    The duodenum and pancreas are best approached via a ventral
abdominal incision. This is made through the mid-line into the right
ventral hepatic cavity and then through the right posthepatic septum
(described above), on the floor of this coelomic cavity, when the duodenum is found directly underneath. This surgical approach also gives
access to the supraduodenal loop of the ileum and some other parts of the
small intestine. However, the intestine in birds is not as mobile as in
mammals, being not only suspended in the mesentery attached both

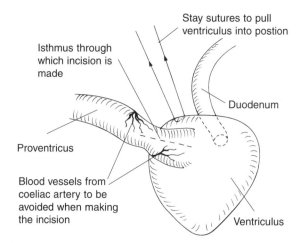

Fig. 7.6 Surgical approach to the proventricus.

dorsally and ventrally, but this mesentery is intimately surrounded by the abdominal air sacs. Any traction on the intestine is liable to lead to a tearing of these membranes and possible rupture of the associated blood vessels together with traction on and stimulation of the nerve of Remak containing the autonomic nerves. Greenwood and Storm (1994) reported the successful reduction of intestinal intussusception in two red-tailed hawks (*Buteo jamaicensis*) and give a useful discussion on possible aetiology in this species.

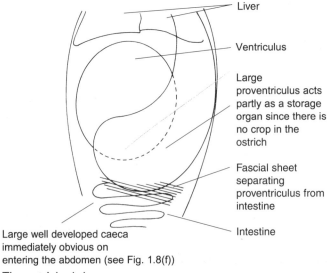

Fig. 7.7 The ostrich abdomen.

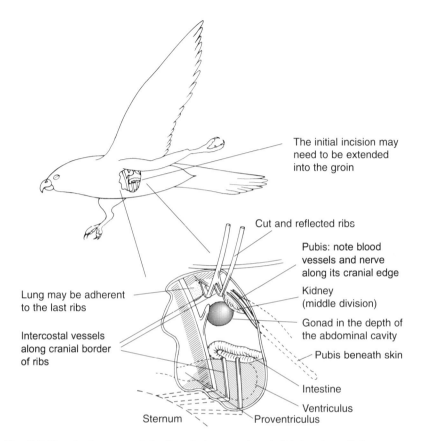

Fig. 7.8 Surgical approach to the abdomen via a left lateral coeliotomy.

The reproductive tract

Egg retention and egg peritonitis

Any lesion causing enlargement of the reproductive tract is likely to displace the stomach towards the right. An incision in the mid-line is therefore quite likely to pierce the ventral mesentery, by which the ventriculum is attached to the ventral abdominal wall, and to enter the left ventral hepatic cavity. On the floor of this and probably displaced upwards by the enlarged oviduct, will be the left posthepatic septum. Incision of this will expose the oviduct. If an egg is to be removed by hysterotomy it is best to put in one or two preplaced sutures before making the incision in the oviduct (Fig. 7.9). Once this is opened the wall of the oviduct contracts and, being very thin, is difficult to suture.

If there is any fluid in the abdomen, as in egg peritonitis, Harrison (1984) suggests draining with a Penrose drain and flushing with

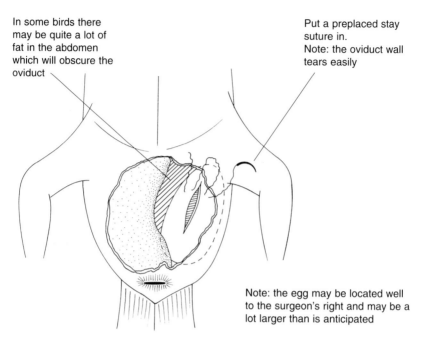

In some birds there may be quite a lot of fat in the abdomen which will obscure the oviduct

Put a preplaced stay suture in.
Note: the oviduct wall tears easily

Note: the egg may be located well to the surgeon's right and may be a lot larger than is anticipated

Fig. 7.9 Hysterotomy to remove an impacted egg.

antibiotics. This is carried out 2–3 days before hysterotomy in the case of an egg impacted in the oviduct. Instead of carrying out a laparotomy, Rosskopf and Woerpel (1982) describe paracentesis of the egg contents by using a hypodermic needle pushed through the abdominal wall and through the egg shell. However the point of the needle easily slides off the surface of the shell unless thrust in with controlled force. When yolk and albumen have been aspirated, the egg shell collapses and the bird is given an injection of oxytocin and calcium. The remains of the egg are then expelled within 2 days.

If part of the impacted egg can be seen through the cloacal opening, the needle can be inserted into the egg through this exposed section of shell. Alternatively an episiotomy type of incision can be employed to extract the egg (Fig. 7.10).

An impacted egg sometimes leads to prolapse of the oviduct through the cloaca. If this is not dealt with quickly the tissues become congested, they can dry and eventually become necrotic. It is essential to moisten the prolapsed parts with normal saline. Use a lubricant such as petroleum jelly or liquid paraffin and moist heat (i.e. just above body heat) to relax the cloacal sphincter to ease the egg out through the opening in the prolapsed oviduct. The blunt end of a sterile thermometer is very useful for this purpose, being slowly rotated around the circumference between the egg and the wall of the oviduct.

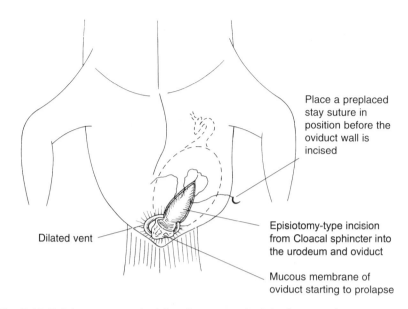

Place a preplaced stay suture in position before the oviduct wall is incised

Dilated vent

Episiotomy-type incision from Cloacal sphincter into the urodeum and oviduct

Mucous membrane of oviduct starting to prolapse

Fig. 7.10 Episiotomy-type incision for removal of the impacted egg.

Cloacal prolapse

After the egg has been removed the cloaca may remain prolapsed. This may also occur after normal egg laying in a weakened oviduct. Rosskopf *et al.* (1983) described the use of No. 0 stainless steel wire sutures around the vent to retain the cloaca in a greater sulphur-crested cockatoo. These authors also describe cloacoplexy by suturing the abdominal wall to the cloaca. Push this into position using a cotton bud. The cloaca is readily accessible through the mid-line incision between the two pubic bones. It should be noted that there is a danger that the prolapse may contain intestine (see previous page), oviduct, or ureter and may lead to obstruction of these organs. Also persistent cloacal prolapse may be due to a tumour (see viral papillomas) or to a cloacitis (see p. 314).

As a short-term measure a purse-string suture around the vent will suffice, but be very careful that this is placed exactly at the cutaneous–mucosal junction, otherwise the ureters may be trapped and the nerve supply permanently damaged. Alternatively use two mattress sutures on either side of the vent. Another solution is to remove a wedge of vent to reduce its circumference but carry this out in the male bird in the dorsal aspect (Lukeij and Westerhof, personal communication). (See p. 25.)

Salpingohysterectomy

Removal of the oviduct but not the ovary may be required to stop persistent egg laying, particularly in cockatiels. The procedure is hazardous and is best carried out using radio surgery, but can be accomplished without this aid if the surgeon is careful and has good anaesthesia (see Fig. 7.11). Greenwood (1992) reported salpingectomy in a 4-year-old hybrid flamingo using two small laparoscopy incisions and the use of a 2.7 mm diameter endoscope and Shae's aural forceps.

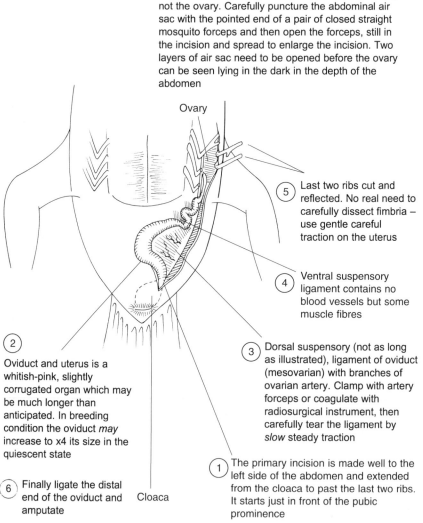

Note: only the uterus (i.e. oviduct) is to be removed, not the ovary. Carefully puncture the abdominal air sac with the pointed end of a pair of closed straight mosquito forceps and then open the forceps, still in the incision and spread to enlarge the incision. Two layers of air sac need to be opened before the ovary can be seen lying in the dark in the depth of the abdomen

Ovary

5 Last two ribs cut and reflected. No real need to carefully dissect fimbria – use gentle careful traction on the uterus

4 Ventral suspensory ligament contains no blood vessels but some muscle fibres

2 Oviduct and uterus is a whitish-pink, slightly corrugated organ which may be much longer than anticipated. In breeding condition the oviduct *may* increase to x4 its size in the quiescent state

3 Dorsal suspensory (not as long as illustrated), ligament of oviduct (mesovarian) with branches of ovarian artery. Clamp with artery forceps or coagulate with radiosurgical instrument, then carefully tear the ligament by *slow* steady traction

1 The primary incision is made well to the left side of the abdomen and extended from the cloaca to past the last two ribs. It starts just in front of the pubic prominence

6 Finally ligate the distal end of the oviduct and amputate   Cloaca

Fig. 7.11 Salpingo-hysterectomy. Although the vasculature is better developed when the bird is in the egg laying condition and some surgeons may decide to delay the operation because of this, the organ is much more easily identified in this state.

Neoplasia of the abdomen

Access to the ovary or adrenal gland, necessary because of a neoplasm, may be made via a flank incision. Arañez and Sanguin (1955) give an excellent description of this approach for poulardisation (removal of the ovary) in the domestic fowl. The incision is made over the last two left-hand ribs (sixth and seventh). The skin is first incised, the sartorius muscle is pushed posteriorly and the incision deepened between the two ribs. The aim is to keep close to the anterior border of the seventh rib to avoid the intercostal artery. The ribs are kept apart with a retractor. Below the ribs the left abdominal air sac is penetrated revealing the intestines, which are pushed aside with a blunt probe. The ovary and adrenal gland should then be visible. In the normal immature organ the base can then be grasped with forceps and twisted off. The same technique can be applied to the testes (see Figs 3.5 and 7.8).

In a bird smaller than the domestic fowl or one where the gonad is enlarged and neoplastic the situation can be more difficult. The same approach as is used for a salpingohysterectomy can be used. Unfortunately by the time many of these cases are finally correctly diagnosed they are too large for successful surgery.

The blood vessels supplying the gonads are short and not extensible, unlike the case in the dog or cat. They are close to the dorsal aorta and vena cava, which can easily be damaged. Very good illumination, magnification and meticulous surgical technique are required for success.

Retained yolk sac in neonates

If the yolk sac is not absorbed during the normal post-hatching period (see p. 222) it is liable to become infected. It is possible to remove this surgically. Indications for removal are abdominal distension, anorexia, inability to stand and inflamed umbilicus. An encircling incision is made around the umbilicus and this is extended by two incisions transversely or longitudinally. Then, carefully rolling the chick over, the yolk sac is encouraged to fall out of the abdomen. The stalk to the intestine must be ligated. Delicate surgery is required. Do not attempt to aspirate the yolk or inject antibiotics into the yolk sac.

The penis

An occasional problem seen in male ducks is prolapse of the enlarged penis. This can be 5–7 cm long and drags on the ground. It can become dry and excoriated and necrotic. The cause is usually due to injury brought about by bullying from another drake. However if several cases occur simultaneously and the ducks look rather ill, then this may be due to duck virus enteritis. In the duck the penis is an extension of the mucous membrane lining the cloaca. There is no vascular corpus spongiosum as in the mammal. The only solution to the traumatic problem is amputation, which seems to have little deleterious clinical effect, except to make the duck ineffective for breeding purposes. In vasa parrots (*Coracopsis* spp.) there is a normal intromittent phallus which may remain protuberant for some time after copulation (see p. 25).

Repair of the ruptured abdominal wall

This is a difficult problem which is more common in the obese female budgerigar. The muscle is weakened by egg laying and infiltration of fat. Gradually the whole abdominal musculature is stretched apart along the line of the linea alba. The weight of the abdominal viscera causes marked enlargement and descent of all the structures so that the swelling becomes pendulant. The results are potentially serious with impaired respiratory and cardiac function. The liver may be enlarged and infiltrated with fat. These cases are bad surgical risks. Since quite large haematomas and lipomas can occur in the same region diagnosis should be confirmed with radiography or possibly ultrasound.

If successful anaesthesia can be achieved, with the bird in dorsal recumbency, it is best not to completely incise the body wall since in these cases the underlying air sacs and contained viscera are easily damaged. The body wall should be picked up so that the underlying viscera falls away, then alternative mattress sutures of 3/0 chromic catgut and non-absorbable pseudo monofilament polyamide are placed through skin and the muscle remaining at the edges of the hernia. The object is not to pull the body wall too tightly together but for the catgut to induce some fibrosis. It is hoped this will produce a renewed and stronger linea alba. Providing the suture needle is placed just below the skin it will not damage the underlying viscera, which are protected by the fat.

ORTHOPAEDIC SURGERY

Before attempting any surgery on the bones of birds it is well to take into account some general considerations. During evolution the avian skeleton has undergone structural responses to the engineering problems of support and movement imposed on a flying vertebrate. Although the elemental structure of the bone, which is a lattice of hydroxyapatite crystals intimately associated with a mesh of collagen fibrils, is basically the same as in mammals, the gross anatomy of the bone has changed. The bulk of an avian long bone is concentrated in a thin porcelain like shell which shows little or no organisation into haversian systems. The interior of the bone contains a network of struts or trabeculae, each one of which is orientated to counteract the external forces imposed on the bone at that particular point. The maximum stress on the bone is at the two ends, so that it is here the bone is expanded with the greatest concentration of trabeculae. The thin, outer shell is the most efficient structure to resist the forces of torque imposed on the bone when this is under twisting and torsional loading, which is exactly what is occurring during flight (see Fig. 7.12). In this situation, a thin hollow cylinder is the most efficient. In consequence of all this, avian bones shatter much more easily during surgery. Except perhaps in very large birds the cortex of avian bones does not form a very sound bed for bone screws. Intramedullary pinning, which in the mammal displaced haemopoetic tissue, in the bird destroys part of the integral strength of the bones.

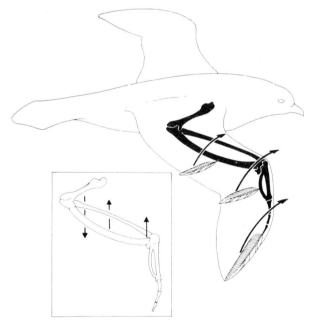

Fig. 7.12 The mechanical forces imposed on the bones of the avian wing during flight. The curved arrows show the torsional stress placed on the bones as the wing descends during flapping flight. The straight arrows illustrate the bending moments applied to the bone at the same time as the torsional stress.

Avian fractures heal in the same manner as those in mammals. This has been demonstrated by Bush *et al.* (1976) who showed that fibrous, followed by cartilagenous callus develops from both the periosteal and endosteal membranes. The rate at which the bone heals is probably a little faster than in mammals. It is most rapid in the smaller birds and one can detect signs of healing on X-ray plates within 8 days. As in mammals, excessive displacement of the fractured ends, movement and infection all retard healing. The so-called very rapid healing of the avian bones reported by a number of workers, may be due to the swift mobilisation of fibroblasts and the formation of collagen fibres binding the bones together, rather than complete resolution of the fracture with the new bone. Under optimum conditions the gap between the fractured ends is filled with fibrous tissue within 5 days and cancellous bone within 9 days. True bony union takes 22 days and complete remodelling takes 6 weeks.

Apart from the healing of bone, there is little doubt that the maintenance of maximum joint mobility is of far more importance in birds than the attainment of perfect bone alignment. This is not denying that perfectly-aligned bones heal more rapidly.

The pectoral limb

The clavicle

Tiemeier (1941) in a survey of 6212 specimens found 3.41% of wild passeriformes had fractures of the clavicle. These are not often diagnosed by veterinarians and when they are, they are best left alone. It is not practical to splint these bones in any way. Note that not all species have a clavicle.

The coracoid

This is a massive bone counteracting the compressive forces of the pectoralis muscle. In a bird of 500 g or more this particular fracture is best dealt with using an intramedullary Steinmann pin. The bone is rather inaccessible, lying deep below the supracoracoideus (superficial pectoral) muscle. The muscle needs to be carefully dissected away from the clavicle or its fibrous equivalent, the edge of which can be felt subcutaneously at the thoracic inlet (Fig. 7.13). If one half of the fractured coracoid has been displaced inwardly, great care must be taken in manipulating the bone back into position, because the great vessels from the heart lie just below this region. In small birds the bone will heal by itself and the bird may be able to fly again, but this could take up to one year. However some of these cases are associated with avulsion of the brachial plexus when surgery would not be justified and the prognosis is guarded.

Luxation of the shoulder

The joint is well-supported by muscle and ligament particularly the coracohumeral ligament. However, the tendon of the supra-coracoideus muscle is sometimes stripped from the muscle belly. Rupture of the tendon leads to upward subluxation of the head of the humerus.

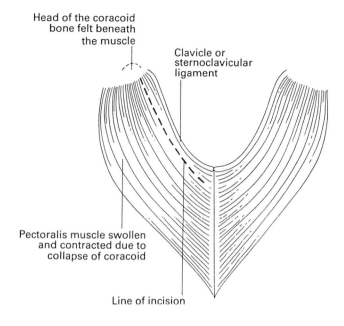

Head of the coracoid
bone felt beneath
the muscle

Clavicle or
sternoclavicular
ligament

Pectoralis muscle swollen
and contracted due to
collapse of coracoid

Line of incision

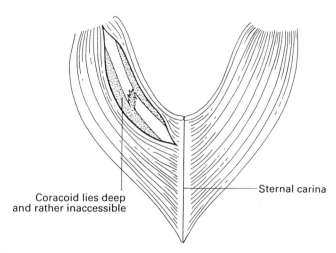

Coracoid lies deep
and rather inaccessible

Sternal carina

Fig. 7.13 The surgical approach to the coracoid bone.

The supracoracoideus muscle and tendon is best developed in birds with a slow flapping flight, in those which hover and in birds which have a rapid jump take off such as pheasants. In fact, rupture of this tendon has been seen only in pigeons and one crow, both of which have fast-forward flight and in gulls which are mainly gliders.

Surgical approach to the shoulder joint is not difficult. The fibres of the overlying dermatensor muscle are split longitudinally in the direction of their fibres and the shoulder joint lies underneath. However, locating and suturing the ruptured tendon back in position is very difficult and an almost impossible task. The retention of complete mobility in the shoulder joint is very important, more so than in any other joint in the wing. All the mechanical forces and differential movements of the wing are concentrated on this joint.

The humerus

The majority of fractures of this bone occur in the middle or at the junction of the middle and lower third of the bone. These are the areas where the bone is least protected by surrounding muscle. In most cases the fractured ends of the bone are well separated and the proximal part is often rotated along its longitudinal axis due to the tension caused by spasm of the contused pectoralis muscle (Fig. 7.14). Although there is an extension of the clavicular air sac into the humerus and damage to this structure can sometimes be seen on X-ray in the region of the pectoralis muscle, it is usually sealed off by blood clot. Emphysema of the tissues is not usually a problem. Since most of the mechanical forces imposed on the wing during flight are transmitted to the humerus it is important to get accurate

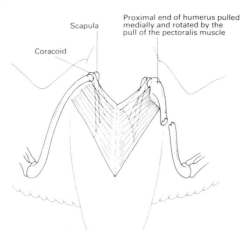

Fig. 7.14 The traction on the proximal end of the fractured humerus by the pectoralis muscle.

alignment and as near perfect resolution of the bone. A slight error in rotational alignment could lead to a change in the angle of attack of the aerofoil surface and aerodynamic properties of the wing (Fig. 7.15). The bird may well learn to adjust to this situation in time but this only increases its problems of rehabilitation. In spite of all this there are a number of recorded instances in wild birds where the humerus has healed in a grossly distorted position and where the bird has been found flying again (Olney, 1958/9; Tiemeier, 1941).

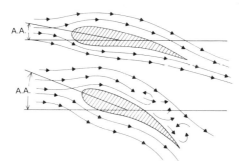

Fig. 7.15 Diagram to illustrate how permanent rotation of the humerus through a badly aligned fracture can affect the angle of attack of the aerofoil section of the wing. The angle of attack (A.A.) affects the airflow across the wing and its lifting qualities.

In a fractured humerus more than 3 days post-trauma, and notwithstanding other considerations such as secondary infection, there is always organisation in the tissue in response to the trauma. This is more rapid, the smaller the bird. If there is extensive dissection to find and free the bone, there is great risk that the nerves and blood vessels traversing the injured area will be damaged. It is difficult to identify the medullary cavity of a long bone of a small bird in a mass of granulating tissue. If the subject is below 100 g in weight (cockatiel size) and a captive bird, it may be wiser to leave the fractured wing alone, except to support it with a bandage for 2–3 days (Fig. 7.16). This only needs to be done if the wing is badly dropped and should not be supported for a longer period, which only leads to excessive fibrosis and stiffening of muscles and joints.

On the other hand if the bird is a falcon and is to fly again, some attempt at perfect resolution will have to be made. The avian humerus is well supplied with blood vessels. This has been studied by Jojié and Popovie (1969) who have shown that there is a separate blood supply to the proximal, middle and distal parts of the humeral shaft. The surgical approach to the bone can be made from either the ventral or dorsal aspect. The latter is probably the easier of the two (Fig. 7.17).

A number of techniques have been devised to repair humeral fractures.

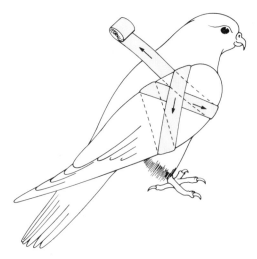

Fig. 7.16 Figure-of-eight bandage using 'vetrap' or similar semi-elastic co-adhesive bandage cut into suitable width strips according to the size of the bird. In some cases it may be necessary to bandage the wing to the body. With the wing bandaged in the flexed position the quills of the primary features act as a strong light-weight splint.

Intramedullary pinning

This can be carried out using the standard Steinmann pin and is the simplest method. In some species such as the goshawk, the humerus is shaped like an extended 'S' so that it is possible for the ends of the pin to emerge from the bone away from the shoulder and elbow joints (Fig. 7.19). This is important because any trauma to soft tissues near an avian joint usually leads to excessive fibrosis and reduction in mobility of the joint. Intramedullary pinning also has the disadvantage that it destroys the trabecular structure of the bone. This will be regenerated when the pin is removed but it does take time. The intramedullary pin does not guard against rotation and, because of the proportionately larger diameter of the avian medullary cavity, a larger and heavier pin has to be used than in a mammal of comparable size. The intramedullary pin does not allow endosteal bone regeneration.

To some extent these disadvantages can be overcome by using one or two smaller diameter pins or Kirschner wires. These may be anchored by a figure-of-eight stainless steel wire through the cortex of the bone above and below the fracture. Place the wire before inserting the pins, after which tighten the wire. A further modification of intramedullary pinning is the modified Harrison-Doyle impaction technique as illustrated in Fig. 7.18. In small birds this method can be applied using suitable hypodermic needles with their plastic hubs notched to receive elastic bands.

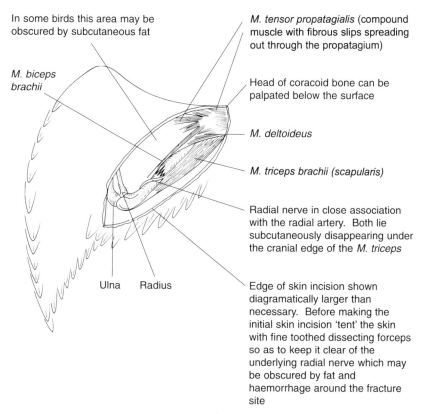

In some birds this area may be obscured by subcutaneous fat

M. biceps brachii

M. tensor propatagialis (compound muscle with fibrous slips spreading out through the propatagium)

Head of coracoid bone can be palpated below the surface

M. deltoideus

M. triceps brachii (scapularis)

Radial nerve in close association with the radial artery. Both lie subcutaneously disappearing under the cranial edge of the M. triceps

Ulna   Radius

Edge of skin incision shown diagramatically larger than necessary. Before making the initial skin incision 'tent' the skin with fine toothed dissecting forceps so as to keep it clear of the underlying radial nerve which may be obscured by fat and haemorrhage around the fracture site

Fig. 7.17 The surgical approach to the humerus from the dorsal aspect after plucking the covert feathers and wetting the area with alcohol. The diagram is not drawn to scale, the humerus being relatively larger for the clarity of the illustration. (After Coles, 1996, *BSAVA Manual of Psittacine Birds*.)

Kirschner splints

This method has been used successfully in large birds by Bush (1981). The pins pass perpendicularly or better at an angle of 45° through the skin and cortex of the bone from one side to the other. Four pins are used – two in the proximal half of the bone and two in the distal half. The four pins traversing the bone are then clamped to a rod running parallel to the longitudinal axis of the bone. This is the so-called half pin method. If the external clamping rod can be placed on the dorsal surface of the wing this causes less discomfort to the bird. If the pins are pushed further through the bone they can be clamped to another pin on the other side of the bone – the full pin technique. In this case the pins must be inserted perpendicularly to the longitudinal axis of the bone. The disadvantage of this effective method is weight. However very light weight Kirschner splints are being developed for finger surgery in humans and may be adaptable

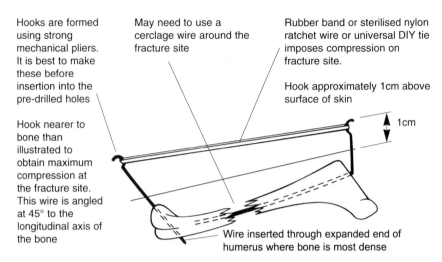

Hooks are formed using strong mechanical pliers. It is best to make these before insertion into the pre-drilled holes

May need to use a cerclage wire around the fracture site

Rubber band or sterilised nylon ratchet wire or universal DIY tie imposes compression on fracture site.

Hook approximately 1cm above surface of skin

Hook nearer to bone than illustrated to obtain maximum compression at the fracture site. This wire is angled at 45° to the longitudinal axis of the bone

1cm

Wire inserted through expanded end of humerus where bone is most dense

Fig. 7.18 The Harrison/Doyle impaction technique using kirschner wires of 0.028–0.062 cm diameter. For accurate placement of the wires holes slightly smaller than the second K-wire are first drilled in the bone. After operation the site is padded and the wing placed in a figure-of-eight bandage. This type of splint is reasonably rigid and prevents rotation at the fracture site. (After Coles, 1996.)

for birds. The technique is relatively rapid and it does allow endosteal regeneration of the bone.

A modification of this method that is applicable to smaller birds (down to 200 g in size) is to use arthrodesis or Kirschner wires and to anchor these to a piece of plastic (not rubber) tubing filled with methyl methacrylate based plastic or an epoxy resin glue or dental acrylic which then sets and holds the pins firmly. The diameter of the plastic tubing can be adapted to the size of the bird. When the pins need to be removed they are cut through and withdrawn. The surgeon must make sure there is enough

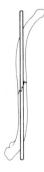

Fig. 7.19 Intramedullary pinning through cortex of curved humerus to avoid the shoulder and elbow joints.

space between the skin and the external bar for this to be carried out. The advantage of this method is that the weight is reduced. When placing the pins in position, the pins farthest apart are first put in position, then joined by the external rod or plastic tube. The bone is aligned and the other pins are placed in position. When using a tube filled with plastic it is sometimes helpful to temporarily anchor the pins to another external pin, parallel to the plastic tube, using wire twisted round the junction. When the whole splint is finished the ends of the pins must be protected, otherwise the bird may be further injured (Fig. 7.20).

Other alternative methods for holding the pins traversing the bone are illustrated in Fig. 7.21.

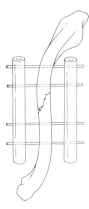

Fig. 7.20 Method of internal splinting a fractured bone using the Kirschner type splint made from Kirschner wire and the barrels of 1 ml hypodermic plastic syringes filled with glue. Leave enough space to enable the pins to be cut when the splint is removed.

Short pin intramedullary devices

The Jonas pin, which is a short pin expanded by a spring when in position, was successfully used by Secord (1958) in repairing fractures on three birds. However, this device is relatively expensive and is unlikely to be readily available in general practice. The author has successfully used short intramedullary pegs made of several materials. These were then held in place by a figure-of-eight stainless wire suture. This method keeps the bone in alignment and helps to put some compression on the fracture site to aid healing (Fig. 7.22). The materials used for the intramedullary pegs have ranged from short lengths of a Steinmann pin, cut-off and smoothed 18 to 4 gauge hypodermic needles, carbon fibre rods and polypropamide rods. The latter were obtained by using the plunger stem of a plastic hypodermic syringe. The stem is cut to approximate size and then cut down and filed to shape during the operation using a sterile file. The material snaps if too long a length is used, but only a short peg is

Note: the brachial artery and vein run approximately below the course of the radial nerve on the dorsal surface

The smallest diameter K.E. wires consistent with the size of the individual bird and rigid stabilisation of the fracture should be used and placed at an angle as far apart as possible

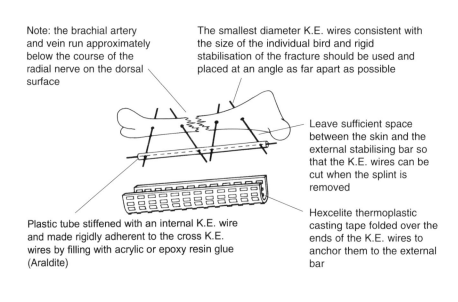

Leave sufficient space between the skin and the external stabilising bar so that the K.E. wires can be cut when the splint is removed

Plastic tube stiffened with an internal K.E. wire and made rigidly adherent to the cross K.E. wires by filling with acrylic or epoxy resin glue (Araldite)

Hexcelite thermoplastic casting tape folded over the ends of the K.E. wires to anchor them to the external bar

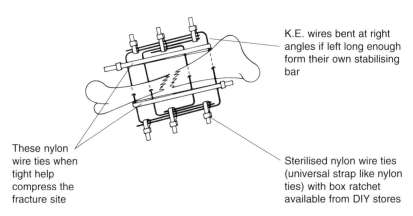

K.E. wires bent at right angles if left long enough form their own stabilising bar

These nylon wire ties when tight help compress the fracture site

Sterilised nylon wire ties (universal strap like nylon ties) with box ratchet available from DIY stores

Fig. 7.21 Alternative methods of stabilising K.E. wires. (After Coles, 1996.)

needed to hold the bone in alignment. If the fracture is more than a few days old the medullary cavity will have to be reamed out of new endosteal bone. The peg is pushed into the longer fragment first and then reversed into the shorter piece of the bone. The reversal is accomplished by pulling on a piece of suture material threaded through a hole drilled at the end of the peg. Holes for the tension band sutures are then drilled with a fine drill bit or a straight triangular needle. This can be held in a mini bone chuck or an instrument maker's chuck and rotated between the fingers. One hole may go through the intramedullary peg but the other hole must be beyond the end of the peg, otherwise the bone cannot be pulled together. Too much tension must not be put on the wire suture; the

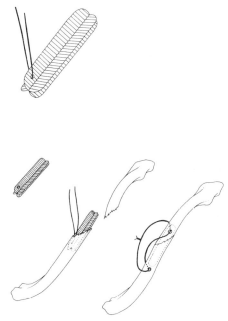

Fig. 7.22 The method of using a peg made of crucate section plastic and a figure-of-eight wire suture to reduce a fractured humerus.

fragments must be carefully brought together to avoid splitting (Fig. 7.22). When passing the wire suture through the drill holes it is sometimes useful to use a hypodermic needle as a wire guide. This method is only really applicable in birds larger than about 600 g in weight.

The method can be tedious but it does allow some endosteal bone formation as the peg has a cruciate cross section. It is also light in weight and the polypropamide is well-tolerated.

Unfortunately many humeral fractures are compound and grossly contaminated. Osteomyelitis does not affect birds systemically so much as mammals but it prevents healing. Bacteriological culture for antibiotic sensitivity should always be carried out. A variety of organisms have been isolated but coliform organisms are common and anaerobes are sometimes cultured.

The whole area should be cleaned and debrided. If the bone is dis-coloured and necrotic it is best removed, even if this means a reduction in the length of the bone. Provided not more than 25% of the length of the bone is lost some birds will learn to adapt and may even fly again (Olney, 1958/9; Scott, 1968).

After operating on the humerus the wing is best strapped in a folded position to the body for 2–3 days. This short period of bandaging should not be extended because the circulation is restricted. Low oxygen tension in traumatised tissue probably predisposes the tissue to excessive fibrosis. A suitable perch should be provided to stop the primary feathers trailing on the floor.

Atrophy of muscle through disuse can be rapid in birds. The white muscle fibres (the glycogen users) as distinct from the red muscle fibres (the fat users) are more susceptible to atrophy when subject to disuse (George and Berger, 1966). There is always a mixture of the two types of fibres in the pectoralis muscle of all birds but the proportion varies with the species. Birds that have a rapid jump take off, such as pheasants, have a higher proportion of white fibres so the chances of disuse atrophy in the pectoralis of these species is higher.

Luxation of the elbow joint

This is not uncommon and can be difficult to resolve. The joint is covered by a weak joint capsule – common to humerus, radius and ulna. There is little surrounding muscle to give protection. Any attempt to stabilise the joint with wire sutures is quite likely to end in fibrosis and even eventual ankylosis. Rodger (J.L. 1981; personal communication) used a hinged splint successfully on a buzzard. Martin *et al.* (1993) devised a method of stabilising the joint and this has subsequently been modified by Forbes 1995 (personal communication) as shown in Fig. 7.23. When attempting to relocate the displaced bones, the covert feathers should be plucked and the whole are wetted so that the anatomy of the parts can be seen.

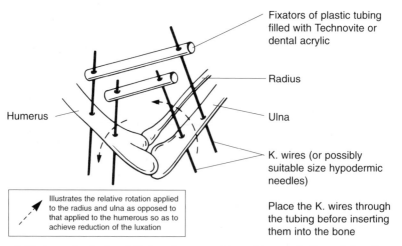

Fig. 7.23 A method of stabilising the repositioned luxated elbow joint. To get the parts into apposition it may be found easiest to *slightly* flex and at the same time rotate the radius and ulna as indicated, then press firmly on a flat surface. (After Coles, 1996.)

Fractures of the radius and ulna

In about 50% of cases either the radius or the ulna is fractured, but not both. When only one bone is fractured it is wiser to leave the fractured bone alone. The normal one will help to splint it. Even if there is not perfect alignment of the healed fractured bone this does not matter, the bird will manage quite adequately and fly again. Strapping of the wing for 2–3 days only is required (see earlier note on pages 178 and 183). If both radius and ulna are fractured some method of splinting will be required.

Occasionally when both radius and ulna have been fractured, during healing a synostosis is formed and both bones become locked in the same callus. For the wing to function normally these two bones should be able to slide longitudinally in relation to each other. The synostosis can be overcome if an ostectomy is carried out on part of the radius or ulna (Rupiper, 1993; Tanzella, 1993).

External splinting

This is more applicable to the smaller birds where the bones may not be thick enough to support some method of internal fixation. One type of external splint is to suture a piece of lightweight plastic material such as a length of Hexcelite or Vetcast casting tape padded with polyurethane foam over the fracture site. The sutures pass through the mesh of the splinting material through the skin and between the shafts of the secondary feathers (Fig. 7.24). It is best to remove most of the covert feathers

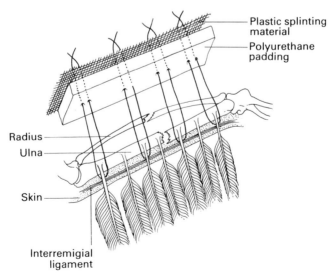

Figure 7.24 Method of external splinting of the fractured ulna using a mesh of plastic splinting material.

and to wet the area so that the anatomy of the parts can be distinguished through the semitransparent skin. The sutures should be placed well behind the ulna so that the main blood vessels are avoided. However, if possible, the posterior sutures should be placed in front of the inter-remigial ligament. All the sutures should be preplaced before being tied so that they can be accurately positioned (Fig. 7.24). This splint is light in weight, is comfortable, and, providing it is properly positioned, does allow some movement of the joints during healing. A similar type but simpler splint, using X-ray film, is applicable to birds the size of a canary (20 g) and is described under fractures of the carpus.

Internal splinting
The Kirschner splint as described for use in fractures of the humerus is quite applicable to fractures of radius and ulna.

The author also once used the barrel of a 1 ml plastic tuberculin syringe cut to size and smoothed off at the ends. This was used as a sleeve to push over the outside of the fractured ulna of a barn owl. A cut was made along the posterior side of this cylinder so that it would slide past the shafts of the adjacent secondary feathers, which are directly attached to the bone. This prosthetic sleeve was sufficiently firm when in position so that no further anchorage was necessary. This provided excellent alignment and the bird was able to fly perfectly with the sleeve permanently in position. The author has also used a rush pin made from a suitable KE wire bent into shape. This needs to be very carefully inserted into the ulna (Fig. 7.25).

Fractures of the carpus, metacarpus and digits

In very large birds it is possible to use a Kirschner–Emmer splint, but in birds below 200 g in weight the metacarpal bone is so thin the method is

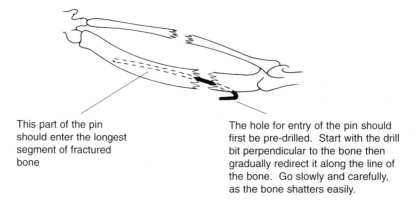

This part of the pin should enter the longest segment of fractured bone

The hole for entry of the pin should first be pre-drilled. Start with the drill bit perpendicular to the bone then gradually redirect it along the line of the bone. Go slowly and carefully, as the bone shatters easily.

Fig. 7.25 Rush pinning of the fractured ulna using a suitable K.E. wire bent into shape. (After Coles, 1996.)

not practical. A method of external splinting that the author has found to work quite well is to use a piece of disused X-ray film or clear acetate sheet. This is bent over the leading edge of the wing and held in position by sutures. The sutures pass through the skin covering the primary feathers. Just posterior to the carpus and metacarpus is the ulnocarporemigial aponeurosis (King and McLelland, 1984, p. 64). This triangular aponeurotic sheet gives very good anchorage for the sutures (Fig. 7.26). This splint is light in weight and allows some movement of the carpal joint. Many medium sized birds (200 g–1 kg) on which this splint has been used have been able to fly again.

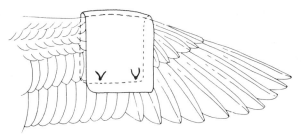

Fig. 7.26 Method of external splinting of the carpus and metacarpus using acetate film.

In very small birds suturing the shafts of the adjacent primary feathers together on each side of the fracture may work – as the shafts are directly attached to the bone.

Pinioning and wing feather cutting for the prevention of flight

The practitioner is sometimes asked to carry out these procedures on free ranging birds to stop them flying. Amputation of the tip of the wing may be required in those birds that sometimes suffer from a so-called 'slipped wing' or 'angel wing' (see Chapter 2, p. 42). Resolution of this condition may be possible in large birds by osteotomy and intramedullary pinning of the large metacarpal bone. A bandage is applied for 4–6 weeks (Yeisey, 1993). Simple cutting short of the primary and most of the secondary feathers will also prevent flight. A sharp pair of strong scissors is sufficient for the operation, and providing the shaft is cut while the feather is not growing (i.e. not in their 'pins'), it does not bleed. It is best to leave the outer one or two primaries which will cover the defect in the wing when it is folded and lead to a better cosmetic appearance. Only one wing is treated since the principle is to unbalance the bird's flight. If both wings are operated on, many birds are able to achieve short distance flight, certainly over an enclosure fence (see p. 230). Some parrot owners like to walk round with the bird perched on their shoulder. It is wise to warn owners of pet parrots that even after clipping the wings the bird may still be able to get over the garden fence or high into the nearest tree.

Amputation of the wing tip for pinioning is usually carried out in fledglings through the third and fourth metacarpal bones, just distal to the carpus. The blood supply to this area, particularly when the feathers are growing, can be well developed. It is therefore wise to place a tourniquet around the carpal area just proximal to the attachment of the second metacarpal or alula digit (attachment of bastard wing) before making any incision. If the covert feathers are well plucked from the area and the operation site is wet, the underlying structures can more easily be seen. An encircling incision is made through the skin at least half way along the length of the third and fourth metacarpal bones, so that there is plenty of skin left to cover the ends of the bone. The skin, tendons and any muscle are then dissected back to the proximal end of the third and fourth metacarpal bones. These are cut at this level with bone forceps or strong scissors (Fig. 7.27). If the temporary ligature is effective, bleeding is minimal, otherwise there can be a lot of haemorrhage which is difficult to control. The skin and other soft tissue is then sutured so that the remaining muscle will cover the ends of the bone.

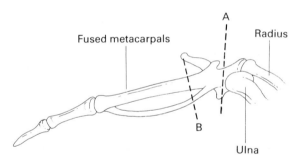

Fig. 7.27 Pinioning of the wing. A, Position of tourniquet; B, Position of amputation.

Patagiectomy

This operation, devised by Mangilgi (1971) and later used by Robinson (1975) is to render large birds flightless. It can also be used in some cases where a wing is so badly injured that amputation is considered necessary. The end result is not only cosmetically more acceptable than amputation but may well enable the bird to maintain better balance. The technique is illustrated in Fig. 7.28.

Tendonectomy of the extensor tendons on the cranial edge of the metacarpal bone has been used to deflight birds. About 8–10 mm of tendon needs to be removed. Also wiring the metacarpus and ulna together in permanent flexion using two or three wire sutures is effective.

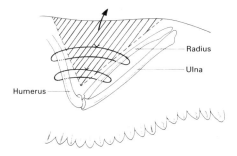

Fig. 7.28 Patagiectomy. The shaded area of the prepatagium is removed after each side is clamped with artery forceps and the area is closed by sutures placed around the humerus and radius. The edges of the skin on the dorsal and ventral surfaces are sutured.

The pelvic limb

Fractures of the femur and the tibiotarsal bone

These can all be dealt with by one of the methods described for internal fixation of the fractured humerus. Harcourt-Brown (1996) has described a tension band technique for proximal fractures of the femur. The surgical approach to the femur is from the lateral aspect and is not difficult so long as the muscles are carefully dissected apart and split in the direction of their muscle fibres. The major blood vessels and nerves lie towards the caudal aspect. The tibiotarsal bone is best approached from the craniomedial aspect to avoid the nerves and blood vessels in this part of the leg.

In the case of the tibiotarsal bone with a transverse midshaft fracture there is a definite tendency for the distal end of the bone to rotate outwardly. While this is often not a problem to the bird, which often manages quite well, it is usually not acceptable to the owner. The rotation is probably caused by the tension of the digital flexor muscles involved in the perching mechanism. This is one reason why intramedullary pinning of the tibiotarsal bone by itself is often not entirely satisfactory without the support of an exterior splint.

Because of the conical shape of the muscles surrounding the tibiotarsal bone, external splinting by itself is not well adapted to this area. However a combination of intramedullary pinning and external splinting often works reasonably well, providing the fracture site is well clear (proximal) to the distal part of the bone and the intertarsal joint. Otherwise developing callus may entrap the free movement of the tendons of the cranial tibial muscle and the m. extensor digitorum longus. To overcome these problems Harcourt-Brown (1996) suggests using a cross pinning technique with two KE wires or pins passed through the lateral surfaces of the epicondyles of the tibiotarsal bone to enter the medullary cavity and then 'bounced off' the opposing cortex to cross each other approximately mid-shaft. The distal ends of the pins are hooked around the epicondyles.

Fractures of the bones below the hock joint

Except in the case of the larger birds, where Kirschner–Emmer-splinting is very suitable or the Harrison–Doyle impaction technique (Fig. 7.18) can be employed for fractures of the tarsometatarsus, external splinting often produces good results. In birds over 100 g (cockatiel) in weight a plastic splinting material such as Hexcelite or Vetcast tape, padded with a 5–6 mm thick piece of expanded polyurethane, works very well. The polyurethane pad is cut generously so that it overlaps the area to be splinted. When the softened Hexcelite is placed in position it is moulded to the part by binding snugly with an elastic bandage such as Vetrap. The excess polyurethane padding and any sharp projections of Hexcelite can be trimmed with scissors.

In small birds like budgerigars and canaries – up to cockatiel size, the use of a splint made of a strip of sticking plaster has been described by a number of authors and is very effective. Any tape material that sticks to itself is effective, but zinc oxide plaster is probably the best. The application of the splint is illustrated in Fig. 7.29 and it can be reinforced by incorporating matchsticks, cocktail sticks, nylon catheter tubing, etc., within the layers of the splint. When applying these external splints, they can always be placed much more effectively if the bird is under light anaesthesia. This allows muscle relaxation and better alignment. Trying to fit a splint on a struggling, conscious bird may result in further trauma. At the proximal end of the splint, if this does not adhere very well because of feathering, two sutures through the tape will overcome this problem.

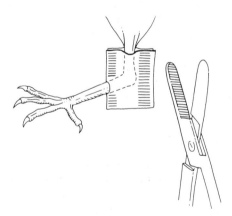

Fig. 7.29 Splint for small birds using adhesive tape crimped together with artery forceps.

A few birds will not tolerate the splint and will remove it in a few days. Even if the splint is only in place for about 4 days it has often been found to be sufficient time in these very small birds.

When the time comes for removal of the splint, soaking the zinc oxide splint in ether or other suitable solvent (Zoff, available from pharmacists) will dissolve the adhesive. Again it is safer to carry this out if the bird is under light anaesthesia.

Valgus deformity

This can be seen as bending of any of the long bones as a result of a calcium:phosphorus imbalance or vitamin D_3 deficiency during the critical period of ossification of the bones in the growing bird. Some of these deformities can be corrected, when growth has ceased and the diet has been corrected, using a wedge or dome osteotomy technique and subsequently stabilising the area with a KE splint. The condition is common in hand-reared parrots and raptors.

The removal of rings around the tarsometatarsal bone

In budgerigars, particularly, but also in other birds it is often necessary to remove a metal identification ring. The ring may have excoriated the underlying scales, or worse, the underlying tissue may have begun to swell, so that the ring acts as a ligature causing swelling of the whole foot. If this is not promptly relieved the blood supply can be cut off and the foot becomes gangrenous. Very often the ring has become buried in the inflamed and swollen tissues by the time veterinary advice is sought. It is most important to have the bird held firmly on a table by another person. General anaesthesia may be necessary. The surgeon can then hold the ring firmly with artery forceps while the ring is cut with the points of a pair of nail clippers. There is a risk that the ring will slip out of the grip of the artery forceps and rotate while being cut. Great care must be taken to avoid this otherwise the tibiotarsus may be fractured. Specially designed cutters are available for this purpose. Also fine hairs from bedding and nest materials can become embedded round the ring and good lighting and magnification is needed to find them.

Luxation of the hip joint

This usually results in a fracture of the femoral head because of the strong round ligament. After this injury the leg becomes fixed in extension and the only solution is a femoral head arthrotomy. Most birds accept this surgery with little disablement. A cranial approach to the joint is made and after excision a slip of iliofibularis muscle (i.e. a large muscle originating on the caudal lateral aspect of the pelvis) is transposed cranially over the proximal end of the femur (i.e. the trochanter) and anchored in through the acetabulum and under the ischiatic nerve.

Luxation of the tendon of the m. hallucis longus (Achilles) the long flexor of the foot

This tendon tends to slip medially away from the trochlea of the tarsometatarsal bone in cases of perosis (see p. 42) causing marked angular deformity of the leg and severe disablement. Before surgery the diet must be corrected.

On examination the joint is noticeably swollen and sometimes the tendon can be pushed back into position. One or both legs may be affected and not all chicks in a clutch are necessarily affected. The author's method to resolve this condition is to make a caudolateral skin incision over the joint and then by careful blunt dissection define the tendon and trochlea. The tendon is then held in position using a suture of polydioxanone through half the tendon thickness through a tunnel made in the lateral epicondyl of the trochlea with a hypodermic needle (used as a guide for the suture).

BUMBLEFOOT

This is a septic condition of the foot leading to abscessation. It has been recognised in poultry for years and is not uncommon among falconers' birds. It is also seen in water birds and occasionally in psittacine birds. It is a serious condition and can ruin a bird for falconry. It is rarely, if ever, seen in wild birds. The infection penetrates the foot from the plantar surface because the integrity of the integument has been impaired. This can take place in water birds if the feet become excessively dry or the skin is abraded. Falcons and heavy, inactive birds, constantly standing on the same diameter perches so that their feet get little exercise are predisposed to bumblefoot. Cooper (1978) discusses the subject thoroughly in his book and points out that puncture of the metatarsal pad or sole by an overgrown claw of the first or hind digit may cause this condition in some falcons.

The feet of birds are covered with scales which are modified areas of the epidermis. The scales are formed by areas of hyperkeratinisation. Between them are sulci or clefts. Some areas of the foot are raised in papillae which increases the grip of the foot. There is constant growth and shedding of the skin surface through normal wear. Sometimes the scales are shed during the moult of the feathers. Anything that interferes with this normal pattern of skin change, such as excessive abrasion, will allow micro-organisms to reach the subdermal tissues. Any bird kept in dirty, unhygienic conditions is subject to bumblefoot. The skin is tight and in places adherent to the underlying bone. Any swelling in this region due to an inflammatory response is restricted and tends to tract along tendon sheaths and other planes of least resistance. Within a few days of the initial infection, fibroplasia sets in – possibly exacerbated by a low oxygen tension through swelling of the tissues and inactivity of the sessile, tethered falcon. The increased fibrous tissue retards any penetration of antibodies to the focus of infection. The whole process is a vicious circle. The abscess may be filled with caseous or serosanguinous pus and may contain a variety of micro-organisms. These commonly include *Staphlococcus aureus*, *Escherichia coli* and *Proteus* species. The infection may track as far as the intertarsal or hock joint. When first presented for veterinary examination the lesion may be 3–4 months old or even older. The obvious swelling is usually covered by a scab caused by hyperkeratinisation. The foot should be X-rayed in the lateral and ventro-dorsal positions because osteoarthritis is a common sequel to a long-standing infection. The scab should be removed and a bacteriological culture taken for antibiotic sensitivity. Swelling of the tendon sheaths and tenosinovitis can sometimes be detected because even when the digits are moved under general anaesthesia small ratchet-like projections on the inside of the tendon sheaths catch with those on the tendons, making the movement feel jerky. This ratchet mechanism is normally brought into play when the bird is perching and there is tension on the flexor tendons. In the relaxed anaesthetised bird there should be no tension on these tendons and the digits can be moved freely.

If the swelling on the foot is very small and there is no sign of the infection tracking, it may be treated with the appropriate systemic and local antibiotics. The local antibiotics may be mixed with dimethyl sulphoxide to help penetration of the drugs. Vitamin A given systematically may help improve the health of the integument.

In the vast majority of cases surgery will be necessary. This consists of opening the abscess and carefully removing all caseous and necrotic material, taking care to avoid nerves, tendons and blood vessels. All sinuses should be investigated with a blunt probe and the whole area should be vigorously irrigated, preferably with chymotrypsin solution. Before starting it is a wise precaution to place a tourniquet around the lower part of the tibiotarsal bone because the granulating tissue within the swelling can bleed profusely. The tourniquet should be released periodically. After thorough curettage the skin is accurately sutured with mattress sutures using non-absorbable suture material, preferably placed across the line of flexion of the skin. The foot is bandaged and the bandage may be left in place 2–3 weeks until healing is completed. A non-adhesive dressing such as fucidin intertulle should be placed under the bandage. As suggested by Remple (1993) better results can be achieved by using a foot cast. After the foot has been covered with a thin sheet of polyurethane foam (obtainable from DIY upholsterers) a cast is made of Hexcelite, dental acrylic, Plastic Padding or Technovite and while this is still plastic it is moulded to the plantar surface of the food and kept in position with strips of Vetrap self-adhesive elastic bandage. When the cast is set hard the bandage is unwound and the cast is removed. A large hole is cut in the centre of the cast and the edges smoothed off so that when re-applied the pressure is taken off the central metatarsal pad and the surgical incision. The same principle can be applied by using human orthopaedic felt pads or the foam-covered material used for the flexible insoles of shoes. Obviously these materials are not so rigid or robust. The surgeon or the owner must regularly inspect the foot to ensure it does not become swollen and the surgical wound can be inspected every 2–3 days without removing the cast. The bird should be allowed on to a perch padded with foam rubber or plastic foam. The patient should be encouraged to use a variety of different sized and shaped perches so that the foot is not constantly held in the same position. The perches may need to be permanently padded and very strict attention to hygiene must be the rule. The owner should be constantly aware of the problem and routinely examine the feet for the early signs of trouble. The use of Astro-turf to cover block perches or in the concrete enclosures of captive waterfowl, also helps to prevent this condition. Use of an apparently unstable but slightly moveable perch (as in the branch of a swaying tree) may encourage the perched bird to constantly shift its weight and help venous return and blood supply to the foot.

Chapter 8
Nursing and After-Care

This chapter is based on a paper by the author published in the *Journal of Small Animal Practice* (1984) **25**, 275–288. Sections of it are reprinted here by permission of the editor and publishers.

Many practices have an appreciable small animal clientele and are already well-equipped with trained nursing staff and facilities for hospitalising cats and dogs and also increasingly for the smaller, children's pets. However, few practices routinely hospitalise birds. This is regrettable because, apart from wild bird casualties for which the public expects immediate expert veterinary attention, diagnosis in individually owned birds is difficult. A practice routine for hospitalising more avian patients will give the veterinarian time to observe and evaluate the bird, leading to a more accurate diagnosis and a higher standard of treatment.

Hospitalising birds is also advantageous to nursing staff. The clinical state of avian patients can change hourly, often with little obvious signs. Nurses, developing their ability to recognise these slight changes, enhance their powers of observation of all patients, and because of the delicate nature of many sick birds, proficiency acquired in nursing these creatures leads to a general upgrading of all nursing skills.

The essential attributes that are common in all branches of nursing are (1) a diligent attention to hygiene, (2) a genuine concern for the well-being of the patient, (3) accurate recording of the clinical progress, and (4) a methodical approach to the task in hand.

Many of the techniques and skills used by the veterinary clinician and the animal nurse have been developed and adapted from those used in human nursing. However, there are dangers in the extrapolation of knowledge from one branch of science to another.

Successful avian nursing depends on the realisation that there are fundamental differences in the biology of birds and mammals.

ASPECTS OF BIRD BEHAVIOUR INFLUENCING AVIAN NURSING

Reduction of stress

When hospitalised, birds are generally more liable to psychological stress than mammals. Bird behaviour is largely instinctive. A routine behavioural response is triggered by a specific stimulus or releaser present in the environment. If there are none of the normal releasers in the bird's hospital environment the creature becomes stressed. Similarly, a bird will make certain ritualistic movements that act as greetings, threats, etc. to a member of its own species. If the bird makes these to an unfamiliar handler and there is no response it becomes stressed. Stress is also related to birds' high metabolic rates and to the fact that most birds are creatures of the air and less used to confined surroundings. Stress, caused by fright or frustration of confinement, will vary among species and be influenced by their degree of habituation to man. Even within species there is considerable variation. Some wild barn owls (*Tyto alba*), for example, willingly eat dead hatchery chicks while others have to be persuaded to do so – this being quite unrelated to the severity of their injuries. Most hospitalised parrots will feed readily, but occasionally one will sulk and feed only on one part of its normal diet (e.g. hemp) for which it has a particular liking. Always accept some of the parrot's normal (usual) food if this is offered by the owner.

Aviculturists recognise that some birds will feed out of, for example, a red dish which they are used to, but will not touch a blue dish of exactly the same type. Some kestrels (*Falco tinnunculus*) are more aggressive than others. Apart from individual differences within a species, some types of bird are more easily handled than others. Amongst raptors, buzzards (*Buteo buteo*) are generally much less aggressive and nervous than goshawks (*Accipiter gentilis*) or sparrow hawks (*Accipiter nisus*).

However, there are some aspects of avian behaviour that are common to all birds with relatively few exceptions. With the exclusion of the ground-living species such as fowls (Galliformes) and waterfowl (Anseriformes), most birds spend a great deal of their time above human eye-level – either in flight or perching. Consequently, when hospitalised, birds are less stressed if they are kept at as high a level as is practical in a room. Their cages, if portable, can be kept on a high shelf. In contrast to this, if one is feeding altricial nestlings, these creatures inherently expect a parent bird bringing food to approach from above. If the nurse is to simulate this pattern of behaviour the chick must be approached from above not from a horizontal direction.

Although all birds have good hearing, abnormal sounds, such as a nearby human voice or barking of a hospitalised dog, seem to disturb them much less than the sight of, or quick movement of, other creatures.

This is particularly so with wild birds which are not accustomed to human contact. The nurse must learn to move slowly and deliberately when in the bird's vicinity. Ideally, hospitalised birds are less stressed if kept in a separate room out of sight and sound of creatures other than birds, where the light intensity can be suitably reduced and where higher ambient temperatures can be maintained. However, in most veterinary hospitals this is not practical because of the other patients and a compromise has to be reached. A reduced light level is most easily achieved by putting a blanket or dark cloth over the cage and in some cases providing the bird with a box or nest compartment in which to hide. A blanket across the front of the cage will sometimes stop a bird continually bouncing the bars of its cage and so causing self-inflicted injury. Nevertheless, care must be taken not to restrict the ventilation or indeed, to restrict the nurse's constant vigilance of the patient. If birds are frequently hospitalised, a thin board, covered in easily cleaned plastic laminate, can be made to hang across the front of the cage. This board can also be used when cleaning out the cage so as to confine the bird to one corner without actually handling it. There is less disturbance to the bird if the cage has a removable tray, similar to those provided in the common type of budgerigar or parrot cage.

When hospitalising dogs, or dogs and cats in a mixed animal hospital ward, it is usual not to have the cages facing each other. This reduces barking and the stress of animal patients and nursing staff. With birds it is often better to let the birds see each other, particularly in the case of social species. Birds often live in flocks of the same or allied species. Some birds, such as hospitalised psittacines, may have led a long, solitary caged existence and sometimes seem to derive benefit from seeing or being near another similar bird. In the budgerigar this is particularly noticeable. A bird that was relatively inactive will suddenly become more alert and interested in its environment. Some parrots will sometimes reduce or cease self-plucking of their feathers.

The one type of bird that all species instinctively recognise is the predator. If hospitalised, this type of bird must be kept out of sight of other birds. Even parrots such as Amazon parrots will recognise and fluff up their plumage if they see a peregrine falcon which does not occur in their country of origin. Hospitalised raptors are usually silent so that other birds do not know they are in the same room unless they see them.

Perches

Many of the birds that veterinarians treat use perches. There is little doubt this type of bird, confined to a cage, is much happier and less stressed if it has somewhere to perch. This instinct in some birds is so strong that even those born with feet so deformed that they are unable to grip will still attempt to perch using the sides of their feet. Ideally there should be more than one perch and these should be of varying size and surface texture so that the muscles of the feet are constantly exercised and do not become cramped. The standard perch used by aviculturists is made of a round wooden dowel and, although easy to keep clean, it is not really ideal because of its uniform diameter and smooth surface. Natural twigs or branches are better and can be replaced when dirty and worn. Branches from most deciduous trees (except oak) can be used, but those from rhododendron and yew are best avoided when used for psittaccines – which like to gnaw. For medium to large birds weighing 200 g to 1500 g, a robust, temporary block perch can be utilised from a brick or an earthenware flowerpot turned upside down. This can be covered with a piece of cloth. A block of wood covered with soft leather makes an even better perch. These coverings need replacement or cleaning when dirty but they provide a good grip and protection from abrasion which predisposes to infection of the feet, and to which birds are prone. Falcons and other raptors are best kept tethered on block perches covered with Astro-turf. All perches should be high enough to prevent the plumage of the birds trailing on the floor – where it is liable to become frayed and soiled. In hospitalised birds, tail feathers can be protected from fraying and damage if bound with a water-soluble, gummed paper tape. Wooden perches can be replaced across the corner of the cages since some birds, such as owls, like to lean against the side of the cage when roosting. Perches should be placed so that when the bird defecates the droppings do not contaminate the food or water containers, or fall on another bird beneath it. The faeces of some falcons are ejected horizontally instead of dropping vertically.

Bathing

Most birds bathe more frequently than most mammals, and many raptors, including owls, will bathe if given the opportunity. Many parrots come from natural habitats of tropical rainforests where during most afternoons there is a tropical rainstorm lasting usually no more than a few minutes. The birds will take advantage of this to have a thorough bath. Aviculturists recognise this, and many of them regularly spray their show birds with a fine mist of water from a spray. Aviary birds can be sprayed with a fine jet from a garden hose or the aviary can be fitted with a sprinkler system activated by an automatic timer. When this is done, birds will purposefully fly into the spray, just as aviary birds will deliberately go out into rain. Falconers put their birds out, tethered to a perch, to weather and offer them regular baths. Consequently, whenever it is practical and when not inconsistent with other veterinary treatment, hospitalised birds will benefit if given a bath or sprayed with a fine mist from a household spray. The depth of water in a bird bath should not be more than half an inch for small birds and not more than one inch for a bird the size of a tawny owl (*Strix aluco*), otherwise there is a risk of drowning. Chicks should not be bathed, since in many species the down does not give them sufficient protection.

Because of the desire of most birds to bathe, their drinking water containers should not be too large and should generally be kept above ground level. The temperature of the water used for bathing should be about 40°C. Bathing keeps the plumage clean and also encourages active preening. This is a normal activity of the healthy bird, since the maintenance of the plumage is not only essential for flight but also for the conservation of body temperature. In water-fowl (Anseriformes) and in gulls and waders (Charadriiformes) the skin of the feet needs constant contact with water to remain healthy, otherwise ulceration and infection may develop. In the Anseriformes, putting the bird into the water of a bath may also act as the releaser to encourage it to start preening.

The advantages and disadvantages of constant handling

Tender loving care by the nurse is of particular benefit to nestlings before their eyes open and will also benefit all ages of birds used to human contact. McKeever (1979) suggests that with baby owls, a piece of dark cloth hung over the top of their box, or a soft toy to nestle up to will be beneficial and simulate physical contact with the adult bird or with the young birds' siblings.

Too much handling and attention can be disadvantageous to an adult wild bird because the creature becomes tame and this may be a danger if release is intended. However, if the bird is to be regularly handled for medical treatment then the sooner it gets conditioned to human contact the better.

PHYSIOLOGICAL CONSIDERATIONS WHEN NURSING BIRDS

The implications of a high metabolic rate

Energy requirements

The animal nurse regularly nursing dogs and cats must be aware that birds have a higher basal metabolic rate. This is directly related to the fact that the body surface area to body volume ratio increases with decreasing body weight. All birds tend to look larger than they really are because the depth of plumage, holding insulating static air in contact with the skin, is thicker than the corresponding layer of hair covering most mammals of comparable size. However, Kendeigh (1970) has indicated that there are other factors, such as the weight of feathers per unit of surface area and the microscopic anatomy and physiology of body organs, which influence the rate of metabolism. Also basal metabolic rate is higher in passerines compared with non-passerines (Lasiewski and Dawson, 1967). High rates of metabolism mean rapid heat loss and rapid utilisation of the body's energy reserves of glycogen and fat. This is so marked that birds will regularly and normally lose weight overnight while they are not feeding (Perrins, 1979). This is particularly marked if the ambient temperature is low e.g. −1°C. Consequently, healthy birds of the order of 10 g body-weight, e.g. blue tits (*Parus caeruleus*), kept under optimum conditions of minimal stress, minimal activity and an ambient temperature of 15.5°C probably cannot survive more than 48–72 hours without food. As size increases, survival from inanition will be longer. Food intake in hospitalised small birds needs to be frequent. If the bird is not feeding itself, nourishment needs to be given at least every hour. Feeding two or three times daily as for small hospitalised mammals is just not sufficient. Small healthy birds need of the order of 1 kcal of energy per gram of bodyweight (Perrins, 1979). One gram of fat yields about 9 kcal and 1 g of carbohydrate yields about 4 kcal. A 20 g canary therefore needs to take in about 5 g of utilisable carbohydrate a day or approximately half this quantity of lipids. Perrins (1979) pointed out that great tits (*Parus major*) feed nestlings between 58 and 78 times daily. Very small birds of 20 g and below this weight which have lost condition through illness need the maximum number of daylight hours in which to feed. It is a wise precaution with these small birds to leave the animal room lights on throughout the night, particularly during the winter months. In larger birds, particularly raptors, the feeding requirements are not quite so stringent. It is reasonable to feed these birds once or twice daily and, provided the food intake is regular, they can with advantage go without food one day a week. The work of Kirkwood (1981) has done much to clarify the rate at which weight is lost in raptors during starvation.

Effect of the inflammatory response

The basal metabolic rate of all homoiotherms increases as part of the body's inflammatory response to disease. This leads to even greater energy demands and a more rapid loss of weight mediated by a complex neuron-endocrine response (Richards, 1980). The nurse should be constantly monitoring the condition of a sick bird by palpation of its pectoral muscles and, where practical, by weighing the bird daily using the methods described on p. 113. Variation in weight is one of the most reliable and easily measurable parameters in a bird's daily progress. The nurse will need to use discretion regarding how much stress is caused to the individual bird by weighing and should not carry this out if the bird gets too excited. As a consequence of an increased metabolic rate, tissues probably heal more quickly. Also irreversible pathological changes, such as fibrosis and the formation of scar tissue in traumatised muscle, takes place more rapidly in small birds than in mammals.

Ambient temperature

To maintain a high rate of metabolism, the normal body temperature of all birds is about 40°C and in very small birds, particularly passerines it may reach 41°C. There may be a diurnal variation of 2–3°C. All sick and severely injured birds, which are rapidly depleting their limited energy reserves, will be less stressed if their environmental temperature is raised to at least 26°C. Sometimes this can, with benefit, be increased to 38°C for a period of 24–48 hours, after which it is gradually reduced. In many veterinary practices warmth will be administered using an infrared lamp. It will be better if this is controlled by an ordinary household dimmer switch; alternatively, the lamp can be gradually moved further away. As with animals, it is essential that the lamp is not too close and that the bird is able to get away from the direct beam. A hot water bottle wrapped in newspaper and placed together with the patient in a cardboard box with ventilation holes in the top of the box will provide warmth in an emergency situation.

It should be remembered that oiled birds have lost their normal insulation and need emergency protection from heat loss.

Special bird hospital cages are available commercially in which the temperature of the cage can be controlled thermostatically. Some of these produced in the USA (e.g. by Snyder Mfg Co., Autech Systems and A. Quabrood) are very good and are fitted with means for a supplementary oxygen supply and a nebuliser for the administration of drugs by aerosol. However, the thermostats in the less expensive and simpler units may not be very sensitive. Also, these cages often do not have any means of controlling humidity and, because the volume of the cage is relatively small, they need to be well ventilated without actually creating a draught. Probably the best means to achieve a high degree of control over temperature and humidity is the use of a hospital surplus premature baby incubator but they have the disadvantage of being low in height and are not very suitable for larger birds. These have a facility for enriching the air supply with oxygen and controlling humidity. Alternatively plastic plant propagators sold in many garden centres can be adapted for the purpose. Incubators need to be adequately ventilated to reduce the risk of infective organisms from dried faecal matter and other body excreta being inhaled by the bird. Incubators are a potent source of infection, not only for the hospitalised bird but also for the handler through many zoonoses (e.g. cryptosporidia) and need to be kept scrupulously clean.

The physiological consequences of the avian air sac system

As mentioned on p. 122 the air sacs are prone to infection. This is exacerbated in the resting bird because flying activity and, in particular, the action of the main flight muscles alternatively contracting and relaxing, helps to pump air through the air sacs and at the same time cooling the hard working muscle. The continual forceful flushing of air through the air sac system reduces the chances of pathogenic organisms contained in this warm, moist, internal atmosphere of establishing themselves on the surface of the air sac.

Because of the large internal surface area of the air sacs and high body temperature, small birds have an inherently high water loss from the pulmonary system. Many birds obtain a lot of their water requirements from metabolised food and body fat stores. Therefore all sick or injured birds that have not been feeding can be assumed to be dehydrated even though this may not be obvious. Many birds normally require much less water than mammals to excrete their waste products of the gastro-intestinal and urinary tracts. Consequently anorexic birds with diarrhoea very rapidly become dehydrated.

Dehydration in birds

Dehydrated birds should be given fluid either by mouth, by subcutaneous injection or preferably by intravenous or intraosseous injection (Fig. 8.1). The injection or fluid can be made over the pectoral muscles, in the propatagial skin fold of the wing, inside the thigh, or at the base of the neck. Normal saline can be given at the rate of 20.5 ml/kg body weight four or five times daily. This volume needs to be halved for small birds, and Steiner and Davis (1981) recommend using 0.1 ml of Hartmann's solution, which helps to counteract metabolic acidosis, given every 10–15 min in the budgerigar, using alternate sides of the body. The rate of absorption is increased if hyaluronidase is added to the fluid. All fluids should be given at 39°C.

Extreme care must be taken in giving subcutaneous injections in birds since avian skin is not as elastic as mammalian skin and aqueous injections tend to ooze out through the needle puncture if too much is given at one site.

Given by slow i.v. injection the bolus for the budgerigar is 1.0 ml, for a cockatiel 2.0 ml, for an Amazon parrot 8.0 ml and for a large macaw or large cockatoo 12 ml.

As a consequence of the usual dehydration in sick and injured birds, constipation easily occurs. Johnson (1979) states that the rectum and coprodaeum are areas of active water absorption, and reflux passage of

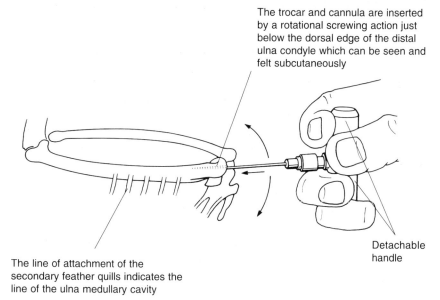

The trocar and cannula are inserted by a rotational screwing action just below the dorsal edge of the distal ulna condyle which can be seen and felt subcutaneously

Detachable handle

The line of attachment of the secondary feather quills indicates the line of the ulna medullary cavity

Fig. 8.1 The dorsal aspect of the carpal joint showing the method of insertion of the author's modification of the Cook Instrumentation intraosseous cannula fitted with a detachable bottle corkscrew type handle. The joint should be flexed and after plucking the covert feathers should be wetted with alcohol or antiseptic to make the anatomy more easily definable.

fluid contents (urine and faeces) occurs from these areas as far as, and into, the caeca. Other considerations apart, dehydration will lead to the cessation of these physiological activities and devitalisation of the associated tissues, resulting in constipation. McKeever (1979) suggests relieving this condition by manual evacuation; the use of a warm saline enema is sometimes useful.

For continuous drip via an intraosseous catheter use a 20–22 G spinal needle with an indwelling stylet. The catheter is inserted into the distal medullary cavity of the ulna or into the proximal tibia. The needle is kept in place with self-adhesive bandage such as Vetrap. An Arnold's pressure drip feed is a useful aid. Instead of a spinal needle Cook Instrumentation make a useful custom-made catheter with a detachable handle for easy insertion (Fig. 8.2).

FEEDING HOSPITALISED BIRDS

There is little problem with birds that are eating. The owner of an exotic cage or aviary bird or the owner of a falcon will be pleased to advise on what to feed, and will often supply suitable food. However, if a falconer's

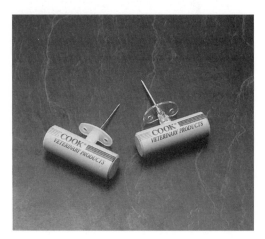

Fig. 8.2 'Coles' modified avian intraosseous cannula (Cook Ltd).

sick bird is received into the hospital, the nurse should be made aware that these birds are sometimes kept short of food by their owners to make them keen hunters, and sick or injured raptors under stress may be near starvation. Wild birds may not have been feeding for some time before being found. The main problems for the nurse arise with the nutrition of the emergency case which cannot, or will not feed readily, or in the case of the wild bird, for which there is none of the normal diet readily to hand. As a rule a 10% solution of glucose or glucose saline given by mouth at the rate of 10 ml/kg body weight will help. However, it needs to be given at least once every half hour for at least 6 hours, but even then it will not meet the daily maintenance requirements of metabolisable energy. Preparations containing amino-acids and essential vitamins are better (e.g Duphalyte) since they provide a more comprehensive range of nutrients. These can be given subcutaneously in quantities similar to those given for fluid therapy.

Artificial feeds made for human infants are useful. They contain fairly high levels of energy-yielding constituents, mainly in the form of carbohydrates with some vegetable fats. The several varieties of Milupa brand baby food contain 422 kcal/100 g and are relatively low in protein. The Milupa fruit salad or tropical fruit varieties are most suitable for parrots, which will often take them voluntarily. The digestibility of their foods is improved if the contents of a Pancrex V capsule is mixed with the food before administration. Vetark Ltd market a 'critical care diet' specifically for sick birds. Also Vetark's probiotic Avipro can be added with advantage to all these foods.

These infant foods can be given in a liquid form with the aid of a stomach or gavage tube (Fig. 8.3) – an easy task, because of the large diameter of the

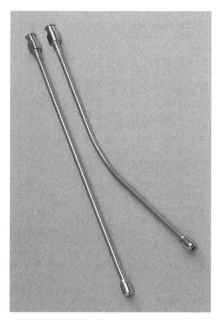

Fig. 8.3 Gavage tubes for the feeding and medication of birds (Cook Ltd).

avian oropharynx and oesophagus (see p. 14). The stomach tube must be placed well down into the oesophagus or crop in most species of birds. Stomach tubes can be devised from suitable diameter pieces of rubber or plastic tubing fitted to the nozzle of a plastic syringe. One can also use a rigid metal stomach catheter if this is well-lubricated and allowed to slip into the oesophagus under its own weight. Custom-made gavage tubes are available (e.g. Cook Instrumentation). When the bird's head and neck are extended in a vertical direction, there is little danger of trauma. However, one must be careful not to force the tube down the oesophagus. When passing a stomach tube the progress of this tube can often be seen particularly in a long necked bird like a swan, as it passes down the dorsal aspect of the neck. It passes under the trachea just before the thoracic inlet.

Other types of preparation that can be used for the general feeding of sick birds are Convalescent Diet or Hill's Prescription Diet 'Canine a/d Feline' which are specially formulated for invalid dogs and cats. These foods are of animal origin and are designed for carnivores. Except for some very specialised feeders such as nectarivorous species (e.g. humming birds and sunbirds), all species of birds are probably capable of digesting this type of food. These foods are soft and can be forced into the barrel of a 2 ml plastic syringe so that when the plunger is depressed the food is extruded from the nozzle as a small worm-like thread which some birds will readily pick at. Another method of administering semi-solid foods is to cut off the nozzle of the 2 ml syringe to enlarge the orifice and then place a plug of the food into the bird's oropharynx. Care must be taken to place the food well beyond the glottis, which in most birds is on the floor of the mouth just behind the root of the tongue. In some birds such as the heron (*Ardea cinerea*) it may be farther back.

A food that is suitable for most species of orphan birds, as well as invalid birds, is mashed, hard boiled, or scrambled eggs mixed with an equal quantity of sweet biscuit meal, or bread crumbs, with a little glucose powder added. This mixture should be slightly moistened and can be given by one of the above methods. If given too dry, the food is not easily swallowed. This mixture can also be offered to small nestlings on the tip of an artist's brush. Some aviculturists feeding parrot nestlings use a small spoon bent up at the tip to form a sort of scoop shaped like the mandible of a parent bird.

A technique for feeding orphaned house martins (*Delichon urbica*), a particularly difficult species to get started, is to offer a drop of water held between tweezers. This is usually readily taken. Follow with moistened Beta puppy pellets which contain a high protein content (Penny Rudd, personal communication).

All these foods require less mechanical work by the bird's alimentary canal and so a more rapid and economical utilisation takes place.

Once the initial emergency period of convalescence has passed, the nurse should consider providing food for the patient which is as near to its normal diet as possible. If one is dealing with a convalescent parrot always enquire what the bird has been fed on in the past. This food may not be what you think is the right diet but nevertheless start with the food the bird is used to and then gradually change to a more suitable diet. Birds will refuse to eat unless they are familiar with the food offered. Start by adding 5% glucose to the bird's normal diet and liquidising this in a food blender – this aids digestion. Birds are very specialised feeders with varied adaptations of their anatomy for this function. The more obvious differences in beak form are also duplicated in the internal anatomy and functions of the oral cavity and alimentary canal. Although many species are quite adaptable, failure to appreciate a bird's normal feeding methods could lead to difficulties in prehension and an inadequate food intake. Parrots, for example, vary considerably in size and need seed which is applicable to their size. Lorikeets, although belonging to the psittacines and looking like small parrots, are adapted to eating fruit and taking nectar.

For most granivorous species the local pet shop can usually supply suitable seed foods and they may also be able to supply more specialised foods such as Sluis Universal which is suitable for feeding insectivorous birds. Granivorous birds also require grit which needs to be the right size for a particular species. A choice of limestone grit, oyster shell and gravel quartz based gravel should be offered. However, there is scientific evidence that some birds may be able to manage without grit.

Most raptorial birds can be maintained for quite long periods on the dead male chicks obtained from hatcheries. If one is constantly dealing with raptors a supply of hatchery chicks can be kept in a deep freeze. However these are low in calcium which could in time result in hypocalceamia. Also they are high in cholesterol contained in the unabsorbed yolk sac. Captive raptors are best maintained on minced hare, rabbit or quail with added vitamin and mineral such as SA 37, Vionate or a probiotic preparation. Some raptors may not readily recognize hatchery chicks as food so it may be necessary to quarter the chick and expose the viscera. It may also be necessary to feed portions of the carcass by hand. If this is done, it is best to discard the head and any sharp parts of the skeleton. A normal healthy bird will deal with these but a weak bird may be injured by them. The pieces of meat can be offered with the fingers or, in the case of the more powerful bird of prey with forceps. The tips of these are best covered with tape to protect the points from damaging the orpharynx, and they must also be kept scrupulously clean. When feeding by mouth, if the sensitive vibrissae at the sides of the mouth, present in some species, are touched the bird will often grab at the food. If the mouth has to be opened by hand the upper beak or premaxilla can easily be raised which has the effect, through the rod like articulations of the palatopterygoid and jugal bones connected to the quadrate bone, of depressing the lower beak or mandible (see Fig. 1.1).

Hatchery chicks can also be used for, and may be taken quite readily by, herons (Ardeidae), cormorants (Phalacrocoracidae), birds of the crow family (Corvidae) and rails. If hatchery chicks are not readily available, small pieces of meat supplemented with vitamins and minerals and mixed with fur and feathers to provide roughage can be given. Always moisten these morsels of food before feeding. Combings of hair from any cat or dog will suffice as roughage in an emergency. As mentioned on pages 15 and 28 all raptors and many other species of birds, regularly produce oral pellets. However, some parts of the skeleton of the prey are digested and are essential, particularly in young, growing raptors if metabolic bone disease is to be avoided. If hospitalised birds of prey do not regularly produce pellets this usually means there is something wrong with the alimentary canal. Nevertheless, if there is insufficient roughage there is no scientific evidence that the production of pellets is essential to the normal function of the alimentary canal. If feeding casualty young chicks, meal worms and maggots are not very suitable. Their chitinous exoskeleton is relatively indigestible. Also if the mealworms have been kept in bran the phytic acid may be harmful.

In the piscivorous species the provision of a fish diet is probably not essential to health. However, these birds will not often feed voluntarily unless the food offered looks like fish, and in some cases unless it is given in water and moves like a fish. Many types of birds only recognise food presented in a familiar form. Once over this difficulty they often thrive on an artificial diet.

Most of the gulls will feed readily on tinned pet food, but forced-feeding of this group of birds is difficult since food is stored in the lower oesophagus and easily regurgitated. Fulmars can eject an evil-smelling oil from the oesophagus a distance of up to a metre; vomiting in other species of birds is usually an indication of upper alimentary disease. When feeding gannets, care should be taken with the sharp edge of their beaks.

Always weigh the bird regularly and do not rely on what it looks like.

PHYSIOTHERAPY

Many injured birds received into a veterinary practice will have trauma to muscle and tendons and to the nerve supply to these tissues. They may also be suffering from concussion. Any fracture present must first be treated; much can be done by intelligent nursing to restore the function of damaged soft tissue.

The nurse must always be aware that hospitalised birds are like human athletes who are out of regular training. The longer they are hospitalised the greater will be the deterioration in the cardiovascular and muscular systems due to disuse atrophy.

Faradism has been used to restore the function in a barn owl's leg (Randall L., 1980; personal communication), but this is unlikely to be available in most veterinary practices. Immersion of an injured limb in hot water at 45.5°C and gentle flexion and extension of the joint as advised by Ratcliffe (J., 1982; personal communication) is simple and can often restore function.

McKeever (1979) recommends the use of a sling and neck brace supports for birds with neurological injuries when the bird cannot support its own weight or the head cannot be held up. The writer has successfully suspended a pigeon in a plastic bag for a total of three weeks whilst both fractured legs were allowed to heal, and has used this support in a Harris's hawk (*Parabuteo unicinctus*) requiring simultaneous operations on both legs.

Once function has been restored to the muscles and other soft tissues these need to be strengthened and built up again. A bird will often do this if it is kept in a large cage or aviary but this can also be encouraged by daily exercising the patient. The bird can at first be held by the legs by hand (gloved if a raptor) and gently raised and lowered to stimulate wing flapping. Later exercise on a leash can be helpful. The leash can be attached to all types of birds by small soft leather straps or jesses as used by falconers, providing of course the legs of the species are stout enough for this purpose.

Chapter 9
Breeding Problems

Increasing demand and monetary value coupled with greater restrictions on supply because of nature conservation will result in more bird owners breeding from stock. The novice will try to replace his losses. The experienced breeder will want to breed for profit and hope to increase his output. Veterinary advice will be sought if these ambitions are to be achieved.

British birds and those from temperate climates breed during a few months of the summer when there is a maximum food supply and favourable weather. Some of the cage birds kept by aviculturists have evolved in tropical conditions but they have been bred in captivity for so long as to be almost domesticated. They are capable of breeding throughout the year and, if kept in outside aviaries, sometimes attempt to breed when the weather is most unsuitable. This can occur in parrots, exotic doves and small finches such as zebra and Bengalese.

Successful bird breeding needs luck, good management and some understanding of the natural history of the species. The breeder should have an empathy with his birds and sense their needs. The zebra finch breeds so easily that the veterinarian may even be asked how to stop them breeding. The solution is either to remove the nest boxes and nesting materials or even to separate the sexes, or in other species to pierce the eggs.

Failure to breed can be due to many causes. These can be catalogued under the following four headings: (1) failure to mate; (2) inability to produce a normal fertile egg; (3) failure of the fertile egg to hatch; (4) failure to rear young.

Some reasons for failure to breed have a single cause but many are multifactorial with varying consequences dependent on the precedence of the different factors.

FAILURE TO MATE

A not uncommon reason is having a pair of monomorphic birds of the same sex. Homosexuality sometimes occurs in birds. Two isolated male lovebirds may copulate and appear to mate normally. The only solution is to sex the birds. The author has seen an instance of four Cloncurry (*Barnardius* sp.) parrots all the same age split into two breeding pairs. When surgically sexed one pair was male and female while the other was two males. The behaviour of both pairs was similar but in one male of the homosexual pair the testicles were much smaller than in the other two males of similar age.

Sexing birds

This can be carried out by several methods. One is direct visual inspection of the cloacal anatomy, as used in poultry, ratites and penguins. This is not usually practical in the smaller species but it is possible for an experienced operator to carry this out on mature specimens of some of the larger parrots. Two other possible methods of sexing birds are to examine either the chromosomal karyotype (from a blood sample) or to compare the relative concentrations of male and female hormones in the faeces (Ivins, 1975; Kock, 1983; Murrell, 1975–76). Both techniques require the help of a specialised laboratory and neither method has been well researched. Some breeders claim to be able to determine sex by measuring the width between the pelvic bones or by noting a slight difference in the lie of the feathering. Both measures are subjective and unreliable.

The most direct method is by surgical sexing. The technique has the added advantage that the conditions of the gonads can also be seen at the same time. The technique is described under laparoscopy in Chapter 3, p. 76. Most parrot species can now be sexed using DNA techniques. (The laboratory carrying out the use of the PCR, DNA probe is Vetgen Europe, PO Box 60, Winchester, Hampshire, UK SO23 9XN. Also University Diagnostics Ltd, South Bank Technopark, 90 London Road, London SE1 6LN, can sex birds on feather samples.)

Stress and aggression

Two birds of opposite sex may not be compatible and dependent on the species, either sex can dominate the other. At worst this can lead to death of the submissive partner or at least infertility due to stress. A female merlin may kill its mate if confined to an aviary at certain times of the breeding season. In *Psittacula* parrots the female is usually dominant to the male except when breeding when their roles are reversed. Sometimes a change of partner, a larger aviary, or more feeding points or nest boxes may solve the problem. The latter is particularly important with falcons, weaver birds and whydahs. Persecution by other species in the same aviary will stop breeding. Some species are incompatible and in some cases, such as the small tropical doves or blue waxbills, will not tolerate another breeding pair of their own kind.

Birds breeding in a colony in an aviary may fight for the highest nest box; consequently these should all be placed at the same height. However aviaries with mixed species may have nest boxes at varying heights to suit different species. The colonial aviary and the mixed aviary should be well established long before the breeding season.

Occasionally a neurotic and aggressive bird will be encountered among a normal breeding group of budgerigars. This one bird can upset the whole flock.

Birds need to be reasonably tame and used to their keeper. Wild birds are reluctant to breed in captivity. It has been demonstrated by Burnham *et al.* (1983) that peregrine falcons taken from the wild breed less rapidly than those bred in captivity. Stress can be induced by excessive noise or any change in the birds' routine management. Observations of shy breeding pairs, such as falcons, can be carried out by a one-way glass window. Prowling predators, such as foxes, domestic cats and rodents around the aviary can disturb birds and prevent mating. Rats, mice, stoats and weasels will get into an aviary and cause havoc. Transportation can cause stress. After capture, foreign species are held by the dealer abroad, then transported by air. They usually undergo a period of quarantine before being sold to their final owners after possibly going through a series of traders. They may take a long time to become adjusted to their ultimate circumstances and then become ready to breed.

The breeder must realise that all birds are individuals in their behaviour, copulation and courtship, and allowances must be made for this Budgerigars and particularly the larger psittacines and also water-fowl tend to form permanent pair bonds so that if one dies it is difficult for the survivor to pair up and accept another partner. It may take 1 or 2 years for a breeding pair to become properly adjusted so that they copulate and produce fertile eggs. It is wise to pair up birds well before a breeding season.

One of a breeding pair may not be sexually mature. Also the two sexes of a pair of parrots may not come into breeding condition at the same time so that there is frustration on the part of the bird ready to breed. Many birds are mature in one year but some of the very large birds of prey may take several years, and macaws take 4 years and the *Psittacula* parakeets, such as the Alexandrine and plum-headed take 3 years to reach maturity. Nevertheless, in most cases if a pair of birds have not bred after 3 years they are unlikely to do so.

Breeding birds should be in good physical condition, good examples of the species and not obviously suffering from any disease. However permanent loss of one leg will not always prevent a male bird from copulating. They should not be obese. This is quite a common problem with captive and disabled raptors which are often overfed and under-exercised. However, the bird must receive food in excess of its metabolic maintenance requirement. The cold weather of a late spring in temperate climates delays breeding in wild birds because they need more food for maintenance (Elkins, 1983). A sudden spell of mild weather stimulates song, courtship and pairing in wild birds and influences captive specimens as well. The increasing number of daylight hours has a major influence on sexual activity providing the above mentioned climatic and nutritional influences are favourable. Increasing the photoperiod in an aviary can help induce breeding. However, the irregular use of artificial lighting can have an adverse effect and therefore it is best to use a time switch.

Many parrot species including budgerigars, cockatiels and lovebirds continue to breed throughout the year, for these species are not natural inhabitants of the European climate. An increase in food supply particularly animal protein may trigger a breeding cycle.

Disease

Only after all the aforementioned factors have been taken into account should the clinician consider disease of the reproductive tracts of one or both breeding partners. General infectious disease is likely to exhibit other signs long before breeding is affected. However, note diseases listed on pp. 280, 298, 314, 318 and 319.

Toxic chemicals

Other remote influences are toxic chemicals, such as chlorinated hydrocarbons used in insecticides and the polychlorinated biphenyls widely used as industrial plasticisers and released when plastic materials are burned. It was thought initially that these compounds only caused thinning of the eggshell but it has been shown that they depress breeding by their influence on oestrogen levels (Peakall, 1970). Wood preserved with chemicals may be detrimental to parrots that chew it. Some parrots become particularly destructive at nesting time and will destroy wooden nesting boxes.

INABILITY TO PRODUCE A NORMAL FERTILE EGG

Feeding

Breeding birds should be chosen from those individuals that will take a wide variety of foods and are not restricted in their feeding habits. In this way a deficiency of an essential element is less likely to occur. Some parrots for instance will eat sunflower seed and nothing else. Where possible home grown foods are better than those harvested abroad. Bird seeds grown in places like Morocco or parts of Australia are more likely to be cultivated on soils deficient in some mineral elements. If the viability of seed is in doubt sow some in a pot and let it sprout. If the green shoot looks normal the seed is probably all right. It is essential to provide increased protein in the diet particularly animal protein with essential amino acids. Also lack of adequate water to drink will stop breeding.

Nesting sites

Birds seen to have mated may not have produced a fertile union because copulation took place on an insecure perch or one or both partners was inexperienced. Birds may not lay eggs in an aviary if there is not a suitably secure or sheltered nesting site or nesting material. Many raptor breeders use enclosed breeding aviaries open only to the sky. It has been shown by Perrins (1979) that great tits and blue tits lay earlier in the season if they have warmer nesting boxes. Nest boxes for aviary birds are warmer if they are as small as practicable. As well as warmth, some hole nesting boxes, such as parrots, need a sufficiently dark box to stimulate the hen to lay. This will not be achieved if there is a crack or warped joint in a wooden nest box. For these birds hollow logs make better nesting sites. Some species need to have a supply of nesting materials such as dried grass (but not hay), leaves, shredded paper, coconut fibre or moss.

Egg laying

In all birds it is normal for the hen to look rather sick and suffer egg lethargy as egg laying becomes imminent. If the bird is disturbed while laying, she may drop the eggs anywhere in the aviary or may crack the shell. Egg eating is a habit formed by some birds which can turn into a vice copied by other birds in the aviary. This can be detected by noticing egg yolk on the bird's face. For budgerigars make a hole in the centre of the nesting concavity in the base of the nest box. The laid egg can then drop through on to sawdust beneath and be hatched under a foster parent.

Infertile eggs are more liable to be laid by an old bird or one which has been allowed to raise too many broods in a season. Nevertheless some macaws will continue to breed at 15 years of age or older.

Candling

If access to the clutch can be gained without disturbing the hen, the eggs should be candled 6 or 7 days after being laid. This enables one to decide if the egg is infertile or 'clear' and to assess the condition of the egg shell, the air cell and the position of the embryo in the fertile egg. Candling can be carried out on thin-shelled eggs, such as those from parrots, using natural light. For others an artificial light source such as a 40 watt bulb can be used. For very thick-shelled eggs such as turkeys, some waterfowl and large raptors, an ultraviolet source is necessary. To avoid harm eggs should not be exposed to the candling light for more than a few seconds.

Artificial insemination

This has for many years been used routinely in poultry, and during the last decade the technique has been successfully developed for breeding raptors. The procedure described by Berry (1972), Grier *et al.* (1972), Temple (1972), Grier (1973), Boyd (1978) and Weaver (1983) has been evolved at a number of centres mainly in the US, but also in Europe (Wilkinson, 1984).

The techniques of collection of semen in poultry and in raptors are essentially the same. They are to massage the lower part of the lumbo-sacral and abdominal regions in a rhythmic manner until a drop of semen is produced at the papilla in the cloaca. The papilla is gently held between thumb and forefinger. There is no technical reason why this technique could not be developed in other species of birds. Samour *et al.* (1986) collected semen samples from budgerigars and Brock (1991) has carried out artificial insemination in parrots.

Boyd and Schwartz (1983) review the technique of semen collection used by a number of workers using a peregrine falcon imprinted on to its handler. An artificial pair bond is slowly formed between the handler and the gradually maturing young bird. This occurs after a long and intensive period of falconry training, including greeting the bird with a vocalisation appropriate to its species and by food transfers. After this long period of socialisation during which time a close physical and psychological relationship has been developed between bird and handler, the tiercel will eventually copulate voluntarily with a specially designed hat worn by the handler. The hat carries a neoprene gutter around the brim which catches the semen. Using this technique semen can be collected several times a day over a period of a number of weeks.

To be successful the handler needs to understand and interpret correctly the courting displays that the bird makes to its 'artificial mate'. The whole process requires a lot of patience and complete dedication from the handler. For an excellent description of the technique the reader is referred to the publication by Boyd and Schwartz (1983).

Once collected the semen can be microscopically examined, or diluted with 50% Ringer's solution before being used for inseminating the female. Avian semen is less liable to temperature shock than mammalian semen.

Also in those species so far examined it is found to be less dense but the spermatozoa should all be the same size and mobile with no abnormalities of the head or tail. Semen should be collected early in the day before the birds are fed and after defaecation. It is then less likely to be contaminated with faeces and urates.

Insemination must be carried out at the correct time in the egg laying cycle. Weaver (1983) states this to be within 6 hours after the last egg was laid and favours insemination after each egg. However, in commercial poultry practice the birds are inseminated at 7–10 day intervals. Gilbert (1979) states that in those birds which have been examined (mainly fowl-like birds and water-fowl), the sperm is stored in the sperm host glands situated at the distal end of the oviduct. Fertilisation, which takes place in the infundibulum at the proximal end of the oviduct, can occur several weeks after a single insemination. Gilbert thinks this is probably the case in all birds.

FAILURE OF THE FERTILE EGG TO HATCH

This is probably the most common problem of all breeders and nearly always caused by a fault during incubation. Only approximately 30% of all raptor eggs laid in private breeding aviaries in the UK hatch and produce surviving young, i.e. for the peregrine, goshawk and merlin.

Development of the egg

During the first few days of incubation the respiratory needs of the developing embryo are supplied by simple diffusion of oxygen and carbon dioxide through the shell and its membranes. As the oxygen demands from the embryo increase, a network of capillary blood vessels forms in the chorio-allantoic membrane. Halfway through incubation this network lies under the whole of the inner shell membrane. Respiration is then taking place across the surface of the shell and oxygen is pumped round by the embryonic heart. Dunker (1977) states that at the end of incubation the embryo absorbs the amniotic fluid and the remainder of the albumen (the so-called breakfast of the chicken). The amniotic cavity becomes aerated and air may penetrate the inner shell membrane. Respiratory movements become regular and serve to ventilate the lungs and air sac system before hatching. Unlike the respiratory system of the mammalian fetus, which undergoes further development after birth, the avian respiratory system is virtually complete and functioning at hatching.

The evolution of this method of development has enabled birds to create a constant-volume lung containing extremely thin-walled air capillaries. The minimum thickness barrier between the twin circulations of air and blood, together with a one-way flow of air, has made the avian lung the most efficient among the vertebrates. This has given birds the ability to reach high activity levels and to be able to fly at altitudes where levels of atmospheric oxygen are low. The developing egg with its delicate embryo and associated blood vessels is a fragile structure. Jerky movements, or vibration caused by nearby machinery, heavy lorries or children at play can all damage incubating eggs, particularly if held in an incubator.

 The two most important environmental factors influencing incubation are temperature and relative humidity.

The influence of temperature

There is a narrow range of optimal temperatures for incubating eggs, which for poultry is 36–38°C and this has been found to be the same for falcons (Heck and Konke, 1983). The experienced bird will maintain the clutch within these limits. Incubating eggs can withstand some cooling, but not rises in temperature, which exceed those of the adult bird. In fact on large commercial ostrich breeding farms eggs are collected twice daily and stored in cooled conditions for up to a week so that they can be incubated in batches and hatching is synchronised. Persistent low temperatures due to cold weather prolong incubation and lead to small, weakly chicks with developmental abnormalities and unretracted yolk sacs. In wild birds, such as swifts and sea birds, where the incubation may have to be left for a period to enable the parent to forage, eggs have adapted to chilling without adverse effect (Elkins, 1983). Chilling of eggs with other birds can occur with a careless or inexperienced hen or from extreme weather with strong winds and rain. Draughty and damp nest boxes can lead to chilling. If birds are being bred inside, the optimum ambient temperature is about 15°C. Overheating of eggs, which could occur if they were in a faulty incubator or if they were exposed to the direct rays of the sun coming through a glass window, is lethal. If the embryo survives it is likely to be deformed.

The influence of humidity

Equally important to the survival of the embryo is the humidity around the egg. Most of the energy needs of embryonic development come from fat stored in the yolk. For every gram of fat metabolised an almost equal quantity of water is generated. If this water is not eliminated the embryonic tissues become waterlogged. Rahn *et al.* (1979) have pointed out that all eggs of whatever species need to lose as water about 15% (some authorities say 12–13%) of their initial weight at lay. This water loss

Plate 1 Goshawk (*Accipiter gentilis*). An apparent insignificant 'cyst' on the upper eyelid was found on histopathology to be a malignant fibrosarcoma.

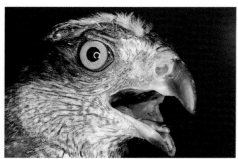

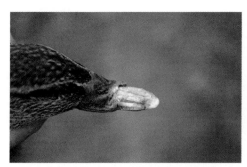

Plate 2 Female teal (*Anas crecca*). Loss of the distal half of the upper beak possibly caused by being ripped off in a struggle with a predator or being amputated by a constricting ligature of fisherman's nylon line. This duck has survived in the wild but will do much better with support feeding.

Plate 3 Little owl (*Athene noctua*). Columboma and hypopyon almost certainly caused by intraspecies aggression to which this species is prone. There were no signs of intraoccular haemorrhage from a traumatised pecten. Providing secondary infection is treated the hypopyon will resolve and although the columboma will remain, vision is not so affected that the bird will not be able to hunt and be rehabilitated into the wild.

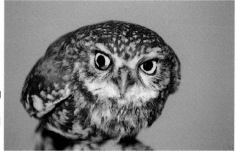

Plate 4 African grey parrot (*Psittacus erithacus*). Bilateral xanthomatosis. This bird lost its upper beak 16 years previously. Use of a prosthesis did not last more than a few months. Subsequently the bird was fed on a semi-solid diet.

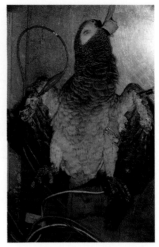

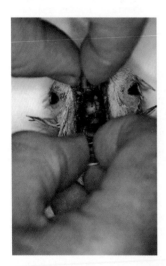

Plate 5 Blue fronted Amazon parrot (*Amazona aestiva*). Choanal abscessation causing occlusion of the single midline lachrimal ducts opening and resulting in bilateral epiphora.

Plate 6 Kestrel (*Falco tinnunculus*). Avipox viral infection.

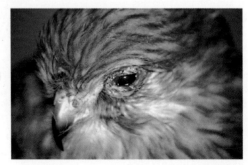

Plate 7 Blue fronted Amazon parrot (*Amazona aestiva*). Viral induced papillomatosis in the choanal area.

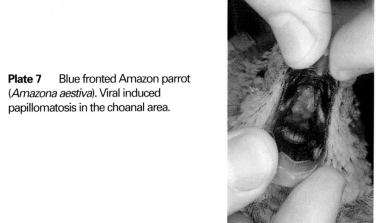

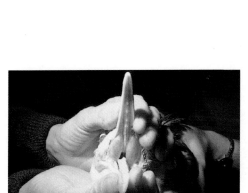

Plate 8 Lesser black backed gull (*Larus fuscus*) with grossly swollen infraorbital sinuses caused by mycoplasmosis.

Plate 9 Tawny owl (*Strix aluco*) with *Capillaria* sp. helminths in the oropharynx.

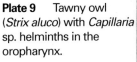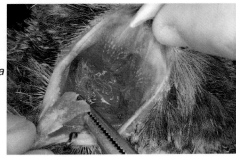

Plate 10 Budgerigar (*Melopsittacus undulatus*). Feather duster syndrome in British show specimen. Probably of genetic origin but may be associated with a herpes virus. (Photograph courtesy of J.R. Baker.)

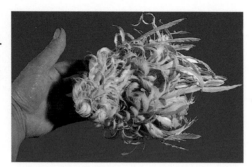

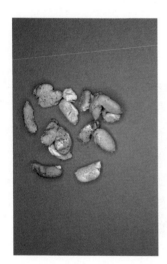

Plate 11 Bulky droppings containing little associated urate content passed by a spelndid parakeet (scarlet-chested parrot, *Neophema splendida*). These droppings had a high undigested starch content due to a pancreatitis secondary to paramyxo virus-3 infection.

Plate 12 Lesser vasa parrot (*Coracopsis nigra*). Dorsum and wings showing marked loss of normal black pigmentation due to psittacine beak and feather viral infection.

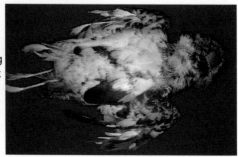

needs to be evenly spread throughout the incubation period and leads to a gradual increase in size of the air cell at the blunt end of the egg. Failure of the egg to lose the correct amount of water leads to a tissue fluid imbalance. Insufficient loss of water vapour molecules through the shell is exactly paralleled by the low exchange rate of oxygen and carbon dioxide. The embryo becomes weak and may develop deformities. If the correct amount of water has been lost from the egg at the end of incubation, the shell is free to rotate around the embryo at hatching. If the egg is water-logged the whole contents are too tight within the shell and this normal process cannot take place. For this reason dead-in-shell chicks are often found to be oedematous. Conversely, if the egg loses too much water the tissue becomes dehydrated and the air-cell is bigger than normal. In all cases of tissue fluid imbalance the chick lacks muscle tone and is unable to force its way out of the shell. In healthy and undisturbed female birds the desire to brood her clutch is very strong and she not only will make considerable efforts to maintain the eggs at both the correct temperature and humidity but will turn them regularly. Most species of birds develop a vascular brood patch over the breast, which transfers heat from the parent to the egg (King and McLelland, 1975). Frith (1959) has demonstrated that the incubator birds, the Megapodiidae are able to use the beak as a thermometer.

In an attempt to increase the humidity, some breeders will provide the nesting birds with damp nesting material. Fortunately this usually dries out before the eggs are laid so has little effect. Rotten wood provided as a nesting material for parrots may contain fungal spores. Also some breeders will spray the eggs of a sitting hen with water to increase humidity. This is of doubtful benefit and may be harmful. The bird is best left to control the situation instinctively. Rahn *et al.* (1979) has shown that the relative humidity of the nest of most wild birds is kept at about 45%, which is about right for the eggs to lose the requisite amount of water.

Incubators

If eggs are incubated artificially correct hatching conditions will have to be duplicated. Management of the incubator, even to the room in which it is kept will have to be meticulous. Temperature and relative humidity must be strictly controlled. Incubators are best kept in a room at a temperature of 21–27°C and the relative humidity should be kept low – no more than 50%. If kept in such a room the conditions within the incubator are less liable to fluctuate. Incubator temperatures for most species are 37.2°C. For safety, incubators should be controlled by double thermostats and any draughts or hot spots within the incubator should be identified. Forced air incubators are better than still air incubators since temperature control is more accurate. The eggs will need to be rotated eight times a day through 45° in alternate directions. Hygiene must be faultless and fumigation using a mixture of potassium permanganate (0.4 g) and formalin (0.8 ml of 37.5%) must be carried out at the end of the hatching season. The eggs must be weighed regularly to make sure the weight loss is correct. The weight can be checked against a graph indicating predicted weight loss. Considering that so few breeders follow these guide-lines it is surprising that any normal chicks are ever hatched.

Influence of the egg shell

Apart from the relative humidity of the microclimate around the egg, the most important factor controlling water loss is the egg shell. The exchange of water vapour, oxygen and carbon dioxide takes place through well-defined shell pores. The pattern and complexity of these channels varies with species. They are more complex in the larger species with thicker shells. Ar and Rahn (1977) have shown that in eggs that are of comparable weight and egg shell thickness the pore size is inversely proportional to the incubation period. Any factor that affects shell quality and shell thickness will have an effect on porosity of the shell. This will affect gaseous exchange and egg weight loss during incubation. In a commercial ostrich hatchery in Israel the eggs are sorted into batches according to the texture of the egg shell which can vary from rough to smooth. This is because farmed ostriches originate from a variety of sub-species. Abnormal shell may be caused by a variety of factors. There may be disease of the oviduct due to micro-organisms such as *Escherichia coli* and *Mycoplasma*. A salpingitis can result in soft-shelled eggs. Some water-fowl and some Galliformes can get trematode infestations of the oviduct. The reasons may be genetic or due to the age of the hen. A dietary calcium/phosphorous imbalance (which should be calcium 1–5 parts to phosphorus 1 part) may result in soft-shelled eggs but is much more liable to result in cessation of egg laying. Soluble grit always must be available for herbivorous birds. There may be a deficiency of zinc, manganese or vitamin D_3. Unlike mammals, birds are unable to metabolise vitamin D_2. One breeder improved egg production in macaws by feeding chicken carcasses and also using a good mixed diet of fruit and vegetables. Use of sulphonamides and excessive use of antibiotics can affect shell quality. The chlorinated hydrocarbon DDT, its metabolyte DDE and dieldrin, as well as the polychlorinated biphenyls have been a notorious cause of thin-shelled eggs, not only in wild raptors but in many other birds such as pelicans and cormorants at the top of the food chain (Peakall, 1970). This cause is unlikely in captive birds unless insecticides have been used in an aviary to control insects, but this must always be taken into account. Shell quality can also be affected if the bird is stressed while the shell is being formed in the shell gland. Some birds such as parrots normally lay thin-shelled eggs which may be related to the more humid environment of a hole-nesting bird. Some parrots can damage the thin shelled egg with overgrown claws. Thin-shelled eggs tend to be laid in very hot weather. Hyperventilation by the bird to overcome hyperthermia leads to respiratory alkalosis. This results in a lowering of the partial pressure of carbon dioxide in the blood with the result that fewer calcium ions are available to the cells of the shell gland. The cause of 50% of dead-in-shell embryos takes place in the last few days of incubation and is due to adverse temperature and humidity during incubation.

Persistent laying of soft shelled eggs may be an indication of hormonal imbalance, i.e. the rate of passage of the egg along the oviduct, or may be due to disease of the shell gland.

Cracked or damaged shells will obviously affect water loss and can sometimes be repaired using clear nail varnish.

Hatching

At the end of incubation, which varies with species, the egg hatches. Incubation times are given in Appendix 11. A few hours (36–48) prior to hatching, the embryo, using its egg tooth (a small projection on the upper beak), pierces the internal shell membrane and starts to inhale from the enlarged air cell – a process known as internal pipping and chicks may start calling to each other at this time. Next a small crack indicating external pipping appears in the shell. The area around the crack starts to break up and eventually a flap with a sizeable hole develops. In ostrich chicks pipping is carried out using the powerful complexus muscle running from the base of the skull along the back of the neck. The chick arches the neck and heaves a crack in the thick shell.

The whole process is gradual, leading to the progressive functioning of the chick's respiratory and cardiovascular systems. Simultaneously, the yolk sac starts to retract into the chick and the blood vessels of the chorio-allantois begin shutting down. From the start of external pipping to the emergence of the chick may take up to 24 hours. A weak chick will take longer. If the chick is taking too long to hatch there is a great temptation on the part of the anxious breeder to help it out of the shell – this is a mistake. There is a grave danger that the respiratory system may not be ready, the yolk sac may not be retracted and the chorio-allantoic vessels may not be completely shut down. These vessels easily tear and a fatal haemorrhage can result. It is better to leave the chick at least 48 hours from the first sign of pipping or hearing the chick chirp and only then, if necessary, carefully extract it. Using blunt ended forceps very carefully prise away bits of shell. Bluntly dissect the shell membranes and tear rather than cut, to reduce haemorrhage. The yolk sac may require ligating. Once the shell is open, fluid is lost more rapidly and prolonged hatching may lead to a dehydrated chick which will benefit from a little subcutaneous sterile saline.

Infection of the egg

The chick embryo has long been the laboratory tool of the microbiologist. The avian embryo has no effective immunological defence mechanism, although passive immunity is acquired from the hen via the yolk. However, the antibodies probably do not pass into the embryonic circulation until about half-way through incubation. Before this, the egg is at greatest risk. Approximately 25% of dead-in-shell chicks die in the early stages of incubation due to infection. Infertile eggs can become infected and act as a focus for pathogenic organisms. Some breeders are in the habit of leaving unhatched eggs in the nest to give support to the chicks. It should not be forgotten that in some species such as parrots, owls and other raptors the eggs do not hatch out on the same day. There may be several days age between each chick. In passerines and many other birds, although the eggs do not hatch simultaneously there is very little interval between hatching. The egg can become infected any time from the start of its formation in the oviduct. However, the most common cause of infection is from dirty nest boxes or unhygienic incubators or from excessive handling and contamination by the owner who can transfer staphylococci to the egg shell. The hands should be washed in antiseptic and disposable surgical gloves worn. All dead-in-shell eggs should be cultured for bacteria and fungi (p. 67). Cultures should be taken from the yolk sac, the albumen and the embryo's liver. The results of these cultures and a postmortem examination on the embryo may give some indication as to how and when the egg was infected. The dead chick should be examined for any developmental abnormalities and its age should be estimated from the size relative to the egg. If pathogenic organisms are isolated, then an assessment of the whole nesting area or incubator together with bacteriological sampling needs to be made.

In summary the veterinarian investigating the failure of the eggs to hatch needs to differentiate between the following common problems: eggs that are infertile, those that are waterlogged or dehydrated and those that are infected or affected by toxins. The investigation will also need to take into account other less common causes such as the age, nutrition and disease status of the female and if the eggs have been handled and stored carelessly before incubation.

For more information the reader is referred to standard text books such as *Poultry Diseases* edited by R.F. Gordon.

FAILURE TO REAR THE YOUNG

As well as deserting eggs, birds will sometimes abandon the chicks and cease to feed them at any stage of brooding. This may be caused by stress or it may be genetic or neurotic in origin. If a bird rears one year but not the next then stress as described in pp. 210–211 is the most likely cause. Similar to the situation in mammals, some birds will attack the chicks as will happen with over defensive cockatoos or goshawks, both species of which can be quite dangerous to humans when breeding.

Fostering

If the survivors are rescued they will have to be reared artificially or by foster parents. These can readily be found from among such birds as zebra or Bengalese finches, redrump parrots, budgerigars, or, in the case of raptors, other falcons. Perrins (1979) found that wild blue tits will feed the young of blackbirds or treecreepers and wrens will feed coal tits. Cross fostering (e.g. Galah, *Eolophus roseicapillus* with Leadbeater's or Major Mitchell's cockatoo, *Cacuta leadbeateri*) has been successfully carried out by breeders. Fostering may result in the young bird becoming imprinted on to the species of the foster parents and may result in pairing difficulties when the birds reach sexual maturity and come to breed. This has not been demonstrated in wild birds. There is an increasing tendency for aviculturists to take the first clutch of eggs in an effort to encourage further laying by the hen. The first group of eggs is then incubated artificially. This may increase productivity but it is not a practice to be encouraged unless performed by trained biologists.

The needs of birds feeding young

All breeding birds should have access to a shallow pan of water. This enables them not only to bathe but to take water, held in the breast feathers, to the chicks or eggs if necessary. Also, birds feeding young may have increased fluid requirements. Pigeons produce crop milk during the early part of brooding and there is increased flow of saliva in parrots rearing young. Smith (1982) suggests that this may have an effect on the activity of plant enzymes when the seed is held for some hours in the crop of the adult bird. This may increase the nutritive value of the food. Smith has shown that such regurgitated seed has a higher nutritive value than that fed to the adult bird. This worker also observes that the primitive bird, the hoatzin, may carry out fermentation in its crop similar to that taking place in the rumen of a cow. Baker (J.R., 1981; personal communication) notes that protozoa are normal inhabitants of the crop in the budgerigar. Birds feeding young need a good quality protein diet. Merlins rearing young and fed a diet of hatchery chicks failed. The fledglings were pale and weak. If the diet was changed to dead (trapped) sparrows the chicks thrived.

Most of the seed-eating birds need to feed their young on animal protein, such as caterpillars and larvae of other insects. Live insects should be provided by the aviculturist during this period, although the use of mealworms is contentious because some chicks may not be able to digest thick chitin. If birds such as parrots are fed too much green food or fruit, their droppings become very moist. This can lead to a damp, unhygienic nest with flies and maggots that will attack the chicks. Many wild birds go to considerable trouble to keep the nest clean either carrying away debris or trampling it into the dry material at the bottom of the nest. Passerines remove faecal sacs from the young and often, egg shells and dead chicks are removed from the nest by many species of birds. Young raptors instinctively defecate over the side of the nest or, if ground nesters, wander away from the nest to defecate. If the birds are used to the handler it is sometimes advantageous to clear out nests daily if the birds are 'wet' feeders. Droppings glued around chicks claws can cause necrosis.

The progress of growing chicks

Properly fed young should gain in weight regularly. A competent bird breeder whose birds are adjusted to him should be able to examine and weigh the chicks regularly. Some aviculturists do examine the chicks but few seem to weigh and record the progress of the chicks. If the weather is cold there may be some temporary loss of weight. By far the commonest problem in growing chicks, particularly hand-reared chicks, is metabolic bone disease. This is due to an imbalance of calcium and phosphorous and insufficient vitamin D_3. Occasionally a chick may develop splayed legs, a condition seen in both raptors and psittacines. This usually is due to a chick being on an unsuitable, slippery surface during growth. If left untreated this can rapidly result in permanent damage. The condition can be treated using a figure-of-eight suture round the legs for about a week or better still by splinting the legs in slots (i.e. splits) made in a suitable block of expanded polystyrene foam or by putting the chick in a cup or small bowl which tends to push the legs under the body. Other congenital abnormalities seen in neonate chicks are opisthotonus, various other joint deviations, scoliosis, hydrocephalus and beak abnormalities. Unabsorbed yolk sacs can occasionally be a problem since these become infected. The yolk sac usually disappears within a few days although may persist in the ostrich for up to 8 days (see Chapter 7, p. 171). The handling of parrot and falcon nestlings does not disturb them but if young passerines are handled 3–4 days before the time when they are due to leave the nest they may erupt and fledge prematurely.

During the first 10 days of brooding, the chicks are poikilothermic gradually become homoiothermic (Elkins, 1983). The adult birds will brood them continuously. During this period the feathers of altricial chicks begin to grow. The rate of growth varies among individual chicks and with different species. At the end of this period when the adults begin to spend less time keeping their brood warm, the least-feathered chicks are at greatest risk. The initial feather cover is not a very efficient heat insulator. Many young chicks die of chilling at this time. The chilled youngster becomes torpid, fails to beg for food and dies of starvation. Nest boxes that are too large, poorly insulated, damp or with only one or two chicks can become quite cold. The larger the number of fledglings in a nest, the greater the body mass and the smaller the ratio of surface area to body volume. Even the totally feathered and active precocial chicks of water-fowl sustain considerable losses if there are adverse weather conditions during the first weeks of life.

Artificial rearing

If chicks are reared artificially in a hatcher, the temperature will need to be reduced progressively during the growing period. As the feathers grow the breeder should take note from their behaviour if the chicks are too hot or too cold and adjust the temperature accordingly. A hot chick will lie with wings and legs stretched out and will keep away from other chicks. The chick will pant and the skin will look red. However redness of the skin could indicate infection. Cold chicks huddle together or, if by themselves, wander around their enclosure. In both cases they tend to make a lot of noise. In chicks being hand reared the breeder should try to assess if a chick's crop and stomach are being filled or emptied properly. This may either be felt or seen through the semi-transparent skin of the neck and abdomen. Slow crop emptying may be due to the humidity of the brooder being too low or if the temperature of the food is too low. However food given too hot can cause scalding and crop burns. Be wary of food heated in a microwave in which hot spots may occur. Crops should be full but not over distended which may lead to impaction and the need to flush out. Sour crop may be caused by either fungal or bacterial infection. Aspirate the contents and examine the sample bacteriologically. Nystatin suspension and Avipro paediatric are suitable treatments.

In conclusion it should be stressed that the three most common causes of death in nestlings are hypothermia, starvation and infection. Infanticide is not uncommon and such factors as vitamin and mineral deficiencies and chemical toxins occasionally increase mortality. Also young chicks are very susceptible to many infections such as the viruses of polyoma, psittacine beak and feather disease, avipox, serositis, infectious bronchitis, reovirus, adenoviruses and duck virus hepatitis. Also trichomoniasis, coccidiosis, giardia, toxoplasmosis (canaries) and various bacteria. All of these diseases are dealt with in more detail in the relevant

Appendices. Prophylactic measures should include meticulous hygiene, quarantine for up to 12 weeks of all newly acquired birds, together with diagnostic testing, and avoidance of bird shows and auctions etc. Keep visitors, particularly from other bird collections, away from hatching and rearing areas.

Chapter 10
Release of Casualty Wild Birds

FACTORS THAT AFFECT SURVIVAL

Considerable interest has been shown and much has been written during the last two decades about the rehabilitation of injured wild raptors. This knowledge has been developed particularly in the United States with the foundation of such organisations as the 'Raptor Research and Rehabilitation Program' based at the University of Minnesota. Concern about raptors is important, since this group of birds is at the greatest risk from extinction. Raptors are often in direct conflict with man and being at the top of the food chain they are most liable to the cumulative effects of the toxic agricultural chemicals. However, the veterinarian in practice is often presented with other groups of sick and injured wild birds, some of which he will want to release. The factors that must be taken into account when birds other than raptors are released vary tremendously. Comparatively little has been written about this aspect of the problem and this chapter is an attempt to examine the task as it affects all species of birds.

As will be seen in the following pages, the release of wild birds is something which should not be undertaken lightly. It not only requires skill as an avian clinician but also knowledge of the bird's natural history. Cooper (1979) has pointed out that in the United Kingdom under the Abandonment of Animals Act 1960, 'the indiscriminate release of wild bird casualties without careful consideration of their chances of survival in the wild could amount to an offence.' On the other hand, any person who keeps any wild bird that could be released is guilty of an offence under the Wildlife and Countryside Act 1981.

The factors can be broadly divided into two areas which are to some extent interrelated. First, there is the bird's physical and mental fitness to cope with its environment. Second, the habitat into which it is released. This is constantly changing and unless a bird is to be released where it was found within a few days of injury, there are many aspects that must be considered. A bird that is in the wrong environment and not completely fit will not only be unable to feed itself properly but will soon be spotted by a predator even if that bird looks normal to the casual observer.

THE ASSESSMENT OF PHYSICAL FITNESS

While it is generally true that a bird needs to be anatomically perfect and 100% fit before release, it is not entirely necessary. How much disability a bird can adapt to will depend a great deal on its normal patterns of behaviour.

Skeletal damage

A healed fracture of the humerus or the ulna may not be in perfect alignment and there may have been some shortening of the bone but many birds will still be able to fly. There are a number of recorded instances where birds have been found surviving with malaligned, healed fractures (Olney, 1958; Tiemier, 1941; Hurrel, 1968). The author has seen several cases in raptors where the fracture had not healed perfectly but where the bird had mated and successfully reared young. This indicates that the bird was hunting effectively enough not only to survive but also to catch enough food for its young. Quite obviously these birds had learned to compensate for the disparity between the normal and abnormal wing.

What is much more important for the bird to be able to fly efficiently is movement in its wing joints. Even here some slight loss in the range of movement may be tolerable and a bird may learn to adapt. A short-winged hawk such as a sparrowhawk or goshawk may be able to cope with the loss of 10% range of movement in its carpal joints. These creatures are birds of fast forward flight and a high wing loading and a high tail-surface : wing-surface ratio. Once airborne the momentum of the bird helps to keep it in the air. Steering and braking depend on the tail. Ducks and pigeons are also birds with short, broad wings and fast forward flight (see Fig. 1.5).

On the other hand a bird such as a barn owl or harrier has quite a different mode of flight. The wing loading is lower, particularly in the owl and full mobility of the carpal joints is essential for the birds manoeuvrability. These birds need the maximum lift on their wings to hunt – slowly quartering the ground and in the case of the owl pivoting in the air. A barn owl with an ankylosed elbow joint was seen to be able to ascend and to glide, but once it tried to turn it completely collapsed.

Large, soaring birds of prey need complete mobility in the digital and carpal joints. The muscles of this area are well developed. The large emarginated primary feathers are splayed out and act like slots in an aeroplane wing to reduce turbulence and increase lift. The distance between the slots is constantly being adjusted by the bird. In the soaring gull mobility of the carpal joint is not so important so long as it can extend the wing completely (see Fig. 1.5).

The kestrel, which spends much time hovering to catch its prey, probably needs complete mobility in all the wing joints. Hovering requires more energy than fast forward flight so that it is possible that the kestrel needs to be a more efficient predator than the sparrow-hawk. However if the casualty kestrel cannot hover but can fly it may learn to hunt from a 'pole perch'. Kingfishers normally hunt from a perch but can hover. Terns (*Sterna* sp.) also hover when hunting but do not have the option of a pole perch if partially disabled.

Some colleagues are of the opinion that all raptors which lose a leg should be euthanased. The author would agree with this view in the case of the larger birds which will inevitably develop bumblefoot on the normal side, but in the smaller species (e.g. kestrel, merlin) this is not the case.

Soft tissue damage to the locomotory system

Some muscles may have been so badly damaged as to be permanently atrophied. The propatagial membrane is often injured in collisions and if scar tissue results, extension of the wing may be severely affected. The author has seen cases where the leading edge of the wing is placed more than one inch posteriorly to the body, than that on the normal side. In these cases flight is affected. In a less severely disabled case the bird may be able to fly but lift on the affected side is reduced because of a reduction in effective wing area. The bird may compensate by trimming the normal wing so that both wings are equal in area and also by flying a bit faster (Fig. 10.1). Lift on an aerofoil, be it a bird's wing or an aeroplane, is not only proportional to the effective wing area but is proportional to the square of the relative wind speed. The author has seen a case of damage to the propatagial membrane in a Harris' hawk where the bird was able to fly but constantly veered off to the left. Quite obviously this bird would not have survived in the wild.

Small birds such as wrens, blackbirds and tits which live in dense woodland cover and do not normally fly great distances may survive with wings which are not quite normal. Providing the distance between perching positions is not too great these birds will adapt. However, if they are released in a more open habitat where the distance between trees and bushes is greater they will be at a disadvantage. They are unable to glide properly like the short wing hawk and ducks mentioned earlier – although they have short broad wings, the frontal body surface area in relation to their body mass is high (i.e. the profile drag is high) and they do not have sufficient momentum to carry them forward. Small birds such as the wren, the robin and the starling need to be able to manoeuvre accurately to be able to get into and out of their hole nesting sites. However, small birds do have an advantage over the large birds. They can sustain a proportionately larger amount of permanent damage to their

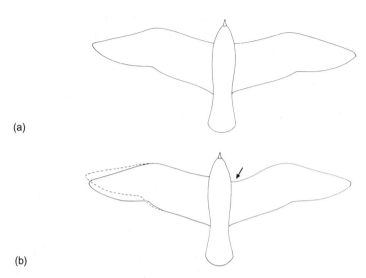

(a)

(b)

Fig. 10.1 (a) This shows the position of the wings in a normal bird.
(b) This shows how the bird trims the wing on the uninjured side by slight
flexion to balance the abnormal wing. The arrow indicates the position of the
scarred and displaced propatagial membrane. To get the same amount of lift,
(b) flies slightly faster than (a).

main flight muscles than can large birds. This is because the power
margin (the energy available from the muscles required to lift the bird
into the air and keep it airborne, beyond the minimum power required for
this activity) is much greater in small birds. In a bird the size of a swan or
large vulture which cannot jump into the air but has to have some distance or a strong head wind to get up relative air speed, the power margin
is low. The bird, in fact, only just makes it. Very little damage needs to
occur to the soft tissue of these large birds and they will not fly again.

No two species of birds have the same flight pattern and probably no
two individual birds fly in exactly the same manner, just as no two people
walk exactly the same.

How a partially disabled bird learns to fly again will depend on the
particular disability and on behaviour pattern of that species. So that a
considered judgement can be made on these matters it is important that
the clinician carries out a thorough physical examination of his patient
before release is considered. This should preferably include the use of X-
rays, the examination of the mobility of all wing joints together with the
extensibility of the wings. This should be carried out systematically even
if no fractures of the wings occurred. This examination can only be done
properly if the bird is relaxed under anaesthesia. One cannot properly
compare the mobility of the joints in each wing in the conscious bird and it
is easy to miss a slightly damaged propatagial membrane.

A bird may look normal when it is alert and perching under observation. Once the observer has disappeared the bird relaxes and both wings may not be held symmetrically.

A bird may feel round and in good condition, its weight may be normal for the species and time of year, but the weight may just be fat. If a bird has been in captivity for some time the ratio of fat to muscle may be too high. Nevertheless some fat must be present as an energy reserve.

Testing flying ability

Having considered all the above factors there is only really one way to assess a bird's flying ability and that is to see it fly. To a limited extent this may be possible in a large aviary. The larger the aviary in relation to the size of the bird the better. Much information can be gained by watching the bird fly in a garage or barn. It may be possible to give the bird daily exercise with these facilities to build up the bird's fitness. Ideally the enclosure needs to be as high and as long as possible. The bird can then practise gaining in height as well as propelling itself forward.

Falconers have developed methods of flying birds on a leash or creance. This is light in weight and the bird is allowed to trail up to 100 m which enables it to be controlled. A large open space is essential although for instance on heather moorland the leash tends to snag on the heather. There should be no obstructions and no distractions for the bird. Obviously the total weight of the leash must not be heavy. If possible it is best to fly the bird uphill and with the wind behind it. This makes flying much harder work and gives a better assessment of how well the bird can fly. This technique is applicable to other types of birds besides raptors. Such birds as pigeons, ducks and gulls, with strong legs are suitable but the method cannot be used in those species with long legs such as herons or waders or any bird with delicate legs.

The method only tests the ability to fly in a straight line, it does not show if the bird can gain height or show how it can manoeuvre. These skills really can be tested only in a large, confined space. If after allowing the bird to fly for a short distance it is dyspnoeic for more than a few seconds it is not fit to release. A normal bird should be able to fly long distances without getting into respiratory distress.

Loss of feathers and damage to the plumage

Before release, the plumage must be in good order. Not only must most of the main flight feathers be present but the thermal, insulating properties of the covert feathers must be effective. Many birds can fly with a few feathers missing – they often do so when moulting but the loss of these flight feathers must not form large gaps in the aerofoil section of the wing. Large birds have an irregular pattern of moulting because they cannot afford to lose too many feathers, to remain airborne. Water-fowl become flightless during moulting. Lorenz (1965) cut off different sections of the remiges in pigeons to see what effect this had on flight. When most of the primary flight feathers had been removed the bird could still fly in level flight but could not ascend. If the secondary flight feathers were progressively removed level flight was affected, although height could be gained.

Falconers use the technique of imping to replace a damaged feather with one that has been moulted or one that has been obtained from a casualty bird. The feather does not have to be from the same species, although the feather must not only be approximately the right size but must be of the same texture. The flight feathers of chickens and pheasants are harder than those of other birds. The shape must be right. In many large birds, particularly the raptors, the outer primaries are emarginated, and the vane on one side of the shaft is very much narrower for part of its length.

The technique of imping is applicable to birds other than raptors. The shaft of the broken feather is cut below the damaged area and the shaft of the new feather is cut so that the upper part replaces the faulty section. The two halves are joined together with a peg made of bamboo, a needle, or the quill of another feather of suitable diameter. Any substance can be used so long as it is the right diameter to be inserted into the ends of the two cut shafts and is strong enough. The whole is held in place with glue.

A new feather can be stimulated to grow by gently pulling out the stump of the old feather. However, growth of the new feather takes time.

The loss of tail feathers is more important in some birds than others. Many can fly without the tail but birds such as sparrow-hawks, hen harriers, magpies, gulls and kites cannot steer properly. The kestrel, the buzzard and the tern cannot hover. The large eagles and the owls can probably manage better than most but the precision of flying will be affected (see also use of tail feathers in climbing, p. 6).

Damage to the legs

The full functioning of both legs is probably not so important as that of the wings. Fishing line can eventually lead to gangrene and loss of part of the leg in birds such as gulls or rails. Some birds lose toes through frost bite. All these birds can and do survive. Some rotation of the tibiotarsus after healing is also quite tolerable. The legs are more important to a raptor but there are reports of these birds hunting and surviving with only one leg functional. Nevertheless the chances of a heavy bird such as a buzzard developing bumblefoot infection are greatly increased if it is constantly standing on one foot. Species such as herons, storks and waders are severely handicapped in their methods of hunting with one leg and should be euthanased.

Damage to the eyes

Fifty per cent of wildlife casualties have intraoccular trauma. The loss of an eye might be thought to be a severe handicap which would affect the judgment of distance but this is not always so. Birds can manage with one eye and are able to judge distance sufficiently accurately to be able to land with precision on a branch. Dr Leslie Brown (an ornithologist in Kenya) in a personal communication (1978) records such a case in a female crowned eagle (*Stephanoaetus coronatus*). This bird survived at least two years with what appeared to be a cataract in one eye. However, Brown notes that the breeding success of this bird was reduced after it developed disease of the eye. It was then probably not a completely efficient predator.

In the peregrine falcon two perfect eyes are thought to be essential. These birds may start their attack on a victim anything from 500 m to 4.5 km away from the target (Brown, 1976). However the author has heard of at least one peregrine which survived in the wild with only one functional eye.

The author has also known of two owls and a buzzard in which loss of an eye occurred and the birds were able to survive.

In the prey species the bird may survive but its chances of eluding a predator would be reduced.

The importance of good hearing

In birds such as owls or harriers which have sustained damage to the head, the clinician should consider if the hearing of the bird is likely to be affected. Both these groups quarter the ground they are hunting with a slow mechanical flight, using their facial discs to pick up the slightest sound. Hearing in these birds is more important than sight. Hearing may be important to some invertebrate feeders. Certainly the thrushes locate earthworms by listening. Also woodpeckers, nuthatches and treecreepers may locate grubs below tree bark by hearing.

MENTAL HEALTH

When considering if a bird's behaviour pattern will enable survival in environment, casualties can be divided into two fundamentally different groups.

First there are those birds that were mature when first caught. These birds have learned to find food for themselves. Provided they still retain their natural fear of man and his domestic animals they pose little problem. Granted if this group are not kept in captivity for more than about 14 days they soon resort to their old habits. If they are released into the exact location where they were found then they know the local geography and where the likely food sources are situated. This group usually survives very well.

If a bird has been captive for several months before it is released it may take a little time to get back to its normal routine. Apart from being out of the habit of continually having to search for food, the bird's food supply will have changed. Summer has changed to autumn or winter. Abundant supplies of insects and vegetable food have changed. Many small birds have migrated and the countryside which yielded a plentiful supply of easily caught young animals for the predator has disappeared. The released casualty will need support feeding from a familiar source while it is learning to adapt to the changed situation.

The group of birds that pose the greatest problem for release are the young which may have been captured at some stage of their development. These birds, which have never lived freely, not only may have to be taught to search for food but may develop undesirable mental attitudes during their nursing period.

The altricial nestings, which include the raptors, are fed by the parents not only during the time they are in the nest but also for a period after they have left the nest. During this post-fledgling period the young bird is not only developing the skills of flying but also, in the case of predators, is learning to hunt and catch prey successfully. Foraging for food in the prey species may also be partly learned by watching parents and also by natural curiosity and investigating a range of potential food items. Jones, (C.S., 1984; personal communication) has noted that the rate at which young tawny owls learn to fly and pounce accurately on a moving prey, varies between individuals. Some birds may never become quite as good as others and may under natural conditions not survive. Mortality in young wild raptors through inefficient hunting is quite high.

Young raptors can be taught to hunt by traditional falconry methods using feeding from the fist, feeding to the lure and 'waiting on' etc. The reader is referred to standard texts on falconry such as Mavrogordato's *A Hawk for the Bush* (1960) and Woodford's *A Manual of Falconry* (1960). A raptor will learn to hunt if it is confined to a barn where there are live mice or rats or if it is in an aviary where small mammals and birds can get through the mesh of the netting but through which the predator cannot escape. To feed live animals to a bird of prey is illegal in the United Kingdom under the Protection of Animals Act 1911–1964.

In the precocial species such as pheasants, plovers and water-fowl, where the young hatch fully feathered, feeding behaviour is almost entirely instinctive but these birds do need to be exposed to their normal habitat during the developing period so that they will learn to investigate all types of potential food items such as invertebrates.

Imprinting

This phenomenon, first demonstrated by Lorenz in geese (1935 and 1937) is seen in all species and has far reaching implications. As the young bird matures its mental awareness of its environment becomes more acute. The bird recognises not only its parents which feed it but also its siblings, nest site and food. These images become fixed in that part of the nervous system controlling behaviour. Alter any of these normal contacts in the developing bird's environment and problems of behaviour occur. The bird fails to recognise or has difficulty in recognising its own species when it reaches maturity. If raptors are not presented with a variety of their normal prey species they may never learn to hunt properly. All birds have great difficulty recognising food items with which they are not familiar although these may be quite suitable as food. Feed a developing raptor entirely on hatchery chicks and it becomes imprinted on them.

Birds often return to the same nest, possibly because the surrounding environment is imprinted on them.

Young fledglings reared and hand fed by humans become imprinted on the handler. They continue to beg for food and can become totally dependent on their human benefactor. These birds may never pair and mate with their own species because they do not recognise them. They may in fact form a sexual pair bond with their human rescuer. When such birds are released they may attack unsuspecting humans in the belief that these persons are a natural food source or that they are a natural mate. McKeever (1979) thought that human imprinted owls released into the wild could be dangerous. In the more rapacious species injury to humans could be severe. Each year newspaper reports appear, usually towards the end of the summer or in the autumn, of a demented owl which has attacked someone. These may be imprinted birds released by well meaning but ignorant do-gooders.

The critical period of socialisation takes place in different groups at different stages of development. In the altricial nesting it is generally later and longer than in the praecocial chick. The rigidity of imprinting probably also varies with the species.

Some authorities believe that imprinting can never be reversed, although there is some evidence that some types of imprinting may be negated. Certainly it is difficult and may take years. For the biologist intent on captive breeding the rare species of raptor this may be practical. For the veterinarian who wants to release a wild bird after treatment, imprinting can produce insuperable problems.

Reversion to juvenile behaviour by an injured bird can sometimes occur (Lack, 1975) and the author has noticed this in an injured parrot which had lost its upper beak. Reverted mature birds open their mouths and at the same time carry out slight fluttering movements of the wings begging for food.

If a young bird is reared, by a well meaning person, in complete isolation in an attempt to stop imprinting on to its human contact, it becomes completely neurotic. It is hypersensitive, frightened of its own shadow and fears all living things – a phenomenon not confined to birds. These birds are excessively aggressive and frightened of their surroundings. The worst effects of imprinting can be avoided by rearing a young bird with its siblings. A good discussion of abnormal and maladaptive behaviour which is important to the releaser of wild birds is given by Jones (1980).

THE ENVIRONMENT WHERE THE BIRD IS TO BE RELEASED

Taking this into account is an equally important part of the problem of releasing wild birds. The summer period in temperate climates is a time of plentiful food supply. Birds that are physically and mentally fit should have no difficulty in finding sufficient food. However, at the beginning of the summer period, there is often intense competition among conspecifics for breeding territory. This biological phenomenon is an attempt on the part of the breeding birds to map out and familiarise themselves with a secure food supply on which to rear their young. An outsider of the same species or even a competitive species released into this territory comes under considerable stress through constant attack and harassment. This is no good for a bird that is trying to rehabilitate itself into the environment.

It would be wiser to pick a release area where the food supply is plentiful and where the number of suitable nesting sites is restricted (Newton, 1979).

As the summer period advances the groundcover in a wood increases and makes it harder for the tawny owl to hunt for its food. But this is an easier time for the prey species including many small birds, as food is abundant and it is easier to hide from the predator. As autumn turns to winter, the groundcover is much less dense giving fewer refuges for the prey and the balance shifts in favour of the owl. These constantly changing circumstances favouring first one group of birds, then another, take place to some extent in all types of habitat. They should always be considered instead of simply releasing the bird. Many birds are migratory, being only in the United Kingdom or other temperate climate regions for a relatively short period during the summer to breed. This is a time of plentiful food supply in such regions. By the time they are fit for release the food supply of insectivores such as swifts, swallows and warblers may have gone.

The short-eared owl and the hen harrier breed on the upland moor during the summer but migrate locally to the estuaries and lowlands during the winter.

Before any bird is released into a habitat it is essential that the releaser makes sure that an adequate food supply is available. The habitat may look right – it does not necessarily mean that the food, for instance the prey species, are present. It is therefore important that to be successful in releasing casualty birds, the veterinarian should either be a competent naturalist or have the cooperation of such a person. The County Naturalists Trusts or the RSPB local groups can be contacted for help. The correct assessment of the complex interactions of the bird and the environment requires a wealth of knowledge of natural history and some practical skill as a field naturalist.

The weather

This is another important and complicated consideration. Prolonged heavy rain can severely restrict the feeding of many species – from the aerial insectivores to the hovering species such as the kestrel. For the barn owl and harrier rain reduces the acuity of hearing. Sea shore waders, and small birds feeding in dense foliage such as the wren, are less affected.

Just after heavy rain there are often many invertebrates, particularly earthworms, near the surface. In dry weather, particularly if prolonged, the invertebrates migrate deeper into the soil. In wetland areas during the drought soil increases in salinity so that fewer invertebrates are available.

Cold weather is important especially if the ground is frozen. Under these conditions the balance between the energy intake of the bird and its energy losses in searching for food and maintaining body temperature may be critical. It is therefore important that the bird has adequate fat reserves before release. Even the barn owl probably only stores sufficient fat reserves to last 3 days. In small birds the energy reserve is much less. Unless the cold weather is very severe the sea shore and estuarine mud is unlikely to freeze as it is periodically warmed by the tide. However, the invertebrates travel deeper in cold weather so that the species feeding near the surface with short beaks are disadvantaged. The wind chill factor with high wind in low temperature can lead to the loss of a lot of body heat. Prolonged frost can have disastrous effects on woodland birds feeding on the pupae and eggs of insects secreted in the bark of trees.

Wind and cold have less effect near the ground and on the leeward side of a wood but are important in the woodland clearings.

High wind churns up large expanses of water including the sea. This stirs up bottom mud making feeding for diving species difficult. A rough sea pounding a rocky shore constantly disturbs the purple sandpiper and the turnstone so that they can spend less time feeding. The subject of weather and bird behaviour is very well covered by Elkins (1983).

Because of all these factors it is wise to consider the weather forecast for the next few days before releasing a bird.

Other factors to be considered before releasing casualty birds

Birds should be released at first light or as early in the day as possible. This gives them the maximum feeding period before darkness and gives them as much time as possible to orientate themselves.

A prey species such as a small tit, a plover or a starling may stand a better chance of survival if it is released near a flock of the same or similar species. Even here there is often a pecking order and the bird will be under some stress until it is accepted.

It is unwise to release birds near a busy main road. Many owls and other species such as crows are attracted to the small vertebrate casualties killed on the road and themselves become injured or killed. Even small birds such as wrens, robins and thrushes tend to fly low over road-ways and become casualties. Some birds of prey such as the buzzard, the little owl and the short-eared owl use telegraph poles or fence posts alongside the road as perches to watch for prey.

When releasing raptors on to farmland or near large estates it is better to have the permission and cooperation of the occupier of the land and his staff.

Releasing a sparrowhawk near an industrial estate or where there is a large complex of buildings would be unwise. These birds often chase prey into a building and then become trapped. The netting of a fruit farm is a similar hazard. Barbed wire fences across open farmland are a particular hazard to barn owls. Swans need a large expanse of water with no overhead wires.

THE TECHNIQUES OF RELEASE

As stated earlier when a bird is building up its strength and initially learning to fly, or convalescing after injury it can be kept in an aviary or other suitable enclosure. If this is situated in a suitable area for release, when the time comes to let the bird go, the netting on top of the aviary can be rolled back quietly. This method has several advantages. The bird has become familiar with the surrounding territory. It can go back to the aviary as a temporary refuge and this can also be a source of support food while the bird learns to forage for itself.

A method that has been used successfully to release falcons is to use a 'hack box'. This is basically the same principle as the aviary method except that it is portable. The box is really a small cage, the size dependent on the species. For falcons it should be about 1.8 m × 1.2 m × 1.2 m. The box is transported to the site chosen for release and left containing the bird on site for 7–10 days. The box needs to be well protected from predators. During this time the bird is fed from behind a screen or using a chute so that the handler cannot be seen. The principle is to try and break the feeding bond and give the bird time to familiarise itself with the surrounding area. At the end of the habituation period the cage is opened but feeding continues for long enough to make sure the bird is foraging for itself. Support feeding may need to be gradually reduced to encourage normal hunting.

Both of the above methods are suitable for most types of birds but may need some modification. Raptors can be released after using standard hacking back techniques. After training they can be tethered to a 'hack board'. This is a wooden platform which acts like an artificial nest site. The bird is tethered for several days, during which time it is fed and gets to know the neighbouring territory, and then is released. Some falconers suggest carrying the bird on the fist around the area surrounding the hack board for several days before release. This helps familiarise the bird with its territory. Regular feeding on the hack board continues and is gradually reduced to encourage hunting.

Survival of all species depends not only on the physical and mental well-being of the bird but also on it having an intimate knowledge of its local environment so that it can find food and shelter.

CONCLUSION

It can be appreciated that the problem of releasing the casualty after treatment is complex. The work can be time consuming and frustrating, because a bird may die at any stage in the rehabilitation process (Appendix 12). However, it is important that veterinary surgeons should be involved in this work and in co-operation with other natural scientists should record their experiences and observations so that others can make use of these records and build on them. The veterinarians' expertise and skill used in this way can help to make some positive contribution to conservation. The techniques worked out on common species can be used on the rarer birds. Today's common bird may become tomorrow's rarity or even become extinct, like the passenger pigeon, which was so numerous in North America during the early part of the 19th century, that during migration flocks containing two billion birds would darken the sky. As HRH Prince Philip has stated, 'It is absolutely inevitable that a very large number of species are going to become extinct in spite of our best efforts'. The Prince warned that in not protecting wildlife our own days will be numbered – 'for we simply cannot survive without the other living species that co-exist with us on this planet'.

Appendices

APPENDIX 1: AN AVIAN FORMULARY

Antibacterial drugs for use in birds

The beta-lactam antibacterials, i.e. the penicillins and the related cephalosporins

These antibacterials are mostly ionised in the plasma and are widely distributed in the body (except for the CNS) because they are not very lipid soluble. They are rapidly excreted unmetabolised primarily through the kidneys although in birds, when compared with mammals, a greater proportion is excreted through the bile. Depot preparations have been developed to prolong their activity in the body. They have a high therapeutic index and consequently are usually relatively safe when used in birds. There are some 74 penicillins licensed for veterinary use, of which only about five are useful for birds. Resistance is developed by those bacteria which produce beta-lactamase; such bacteria are staphylococci, *E. coli*, *Klebsiella*, *Pasteurella*, *Pseudomonas* and *Salmonella*.

Generic and trade names	Formulation	Route of admin.	Dosage	Activity	Comment
Benzylpenicillin or penicillin G, e.g. Crystapen (Malinckrodt Veterinary)	3 g phial of powder for reconstitution	s.c. i.m. i.v.	60 mg/kg body wt q 6–8 h	Bactericidal active against most Gram+ and some Gram–	Safe in birds but rarely used because of the necessity of frequent handling and frequent injection
Procaine penicillin many trade names					*Not safe to use* in many small birds because the procaine fraction is toxic
Ampicillin e.g. Amfipen (Mycofarm) Penbritin (Pfizer)	50 mg & 125 mg tabs.	p.o.	150–200 mg/kg body wt. q 8 h 100 mg/litre drinking water	As above but more broad spectrum active against some Gram–, e.g. *Pasteurella*.	Absorption from the gastrointestinal tract is poor and erratic.
	150 mg/ml injection	i.m. s.c.	15–20 mg/kg i.m. emus and cranes 100 mg/kg body wt q 12h	*Not effective against* haemophilus, *E. coli*, *Klebsiella*, *Proteus*, *Pseudomonas*, *Chlamydia*	These antibacterials should be used for a minimum of 5 days.

Drug	Presentation	Route	Dose	Activity	Comments
Amoxycillin e.g. Clamoxyl (Pfizer) also many other trade names and formulations	150 mg/ml injection	i.m. p.o.	250 mg/kg q 24 h 150–175 mg/kg q 12 h or q 24 h		Amoxicillin is better absorbed from the GI tract than ampilicillin but this is still erratic.
Carbencillin e.g. Pyopen (Link)	1 g & 5 g phials of powder for reconstitution	i.m. s.c.	100–200 mg/kg body wt. q 12 h	Active against some Gram–, particularly *Pseudomonas* and *Proteus*	
Ticarcillin e.g. Ticar (Link)	1 g & 5 g phials of powder for reconstitution	i.m. s.c.	100–200 mg/kg	More active against *Proteus* than carbencillin	Ticarcillin is broken down by beta-latamase produced by some strains of *Pseudomonas*. It has therefore been combined with clavulanic acid, see below
Piperacillin e.g. Pipril (Lederle)	1 g & 2 g phials of powder for reconstitution	i.m. s.c.	75–100 mg/kg q 8–4 h	Less active against most Gram+ than amoxycillin but more active against Gram– organisms and anaerobes	
Amoxycillin and clavulanic acid (co-amoxiclav) e.g. Synulox (Pfizer)	140 mg amoxycillin & 35 mg clavulonic acid/per ml 40 & 100 ml phials	i.m.	100 mg/kg body wt. q 24 h	Effective against resistant staphylococci, some anaerobes and some Gram– including *E. coli, Klebsiella*	Must use a dry syringe and a dry needle otherwise moisture precipitates the preparation and clogs the needle.
	Tablets 40 mg amox & 10 mg Clav acid Drops 40 mg amox & 10 ml Clav acid per ml 15 ml dropper bottle	p.o.	125 mg/kg q 6 h		Clavulanic acid is a beta-lactamase inhibitor but by itself has no direct antimicrobial action.

Generic and trade names	Formulation	Route of admin.	Dosage	Activity	Comment
Ticarcillin and *clavulanic acid* e.g. Timentin (Beecham)	Powder for reconstitution ticarcillin 1.5 g clavulanic acid 100 mg 1.6 g phials	i.m / i.v.	100 mg/kg	Effective against many Gram-, particularly to resistant strains of *Pseudomonas*	

There are at least 13 cephalosporins licensed for veterinary use, but only two of these have been used in birds. Cephalosporins penetrate most tissue including bone and their prophylactic use before orthopaedic surgery is recommended.

Generic and trade names	Formulation	Route of admin.	Dosage	Activity	Comment
Cephalexin e.g. Ceporex (Malinckrodt Veterinary) A first generation cephalosporin	Tablets 50 mg & 250 mg; Oral suspension for reconstitution 100 mg/ml 10 ml phial; Inj. (oily) 180 mg/ml 30 ml & 100 ml phials	p.o. / p.o. / i.m.	35–50 mg/kg q 6 h or q 2–3 h in small species	Some Gram+, some anaerobes and most Gram-, including *E. coli*, *Proteus* and *Pseudomonas*	Cephalosporins have a wide margin of safety in birds and are resistant to beta lactamase enzymes. Well absorbed from G.I. tract. Can be nephrotoxic if given with some diuretics, e.g. frusemide. Can be stored after making up in bulk and used for up to 6 months.
Cephotaxime e.g. Claforan (Rossel) A third generation cephalosporin	Powder for reconstitution 500 mg 1 g & 2 g phials	i.m.	75–100 mg/kg q 8–4 h	Active against a wide range of Gram-, particularly *Pseudomonas*	Penetrates CSF & CNS

The tetracyclines

The most widely used in avian medicine of the antibacterials but far from being the most suitable. They are widely distributed in the body's tissues except the CNS. They are metabolised in the liver and excreted both in the bile and through the kidneys. Injectable preparations often cause irritation and can cause tissue necrosis. They often depress gut flora and cause GI disturbances. Oral absorption is very variable. They are chelated by calcium and magnesium salts (important if administered orally to graminiferous birds which take in calcium and magnesium-containing grit into the ventriculus). If given i.v. they can chelate blood calcium ions with resulting cardiovascular collapse. They can be immunosuppressive and cause photosensitivity. Their toxicity is variable dependent on species, the particular compound and the length of treatment. The major use in avian medicine is in the treatment of *Chlamydia* infection.

Generic and trade names	Formulation	Route of admin.	Dosage	Activity	Comment
Oxytetracycline e.g. Terramycin soluble powder (Pfizer). Many other trade preparations	An oral powder for addition to drinking water or for mixing in food. 225 g & 2 kg packs	p.o.	4–12 mg/litre of drinking water 5 g/kg of food 100 mg/kg body wt by mouth	Only bacteriostatic. Broadspectrum effective against many Gram+ and Gram− (but not *E. coli, Salmonella, Proteus* or *Pseudomonas*. Also active against some protozoa and flagellates.	Oral absorption is erratic and in graminferous birds the dose should be increased to maintain the minimal inhibitory concentration in the plasma. Can precipitate hypocalaemic seizures in African grey parrots which already have nutritional secondary hyperparathyroidism.
e.g. Engemycin (Mycofarm), Oxytetrin (Malinckrodt Veterinary)	As the hydrochloride for injection 5% i.e. 50 mg/ml, 50 ml & 100 ml phials	i.m.	58 mg/kg body wt q 24 hr for birds over 400 g body wt. 100 mg/kg body wt for birds below 400 g body wt		Do not be tempted to use the higher concentrations available for large farm animals (e.g. 100 mg/ml instead of the 50 mg/ml) in an attempt to reduce the bulk of the injection; only results in tissue necrosis.

Generic and trade names	Formulation	Route of admin.	Dosage	Activity	Comment
Doxycycline e.g. Vibravenos (Pfizer)	Long acting depot preparation	i.m.	75–100 mg/kg every 5–7 days cockatiels 0.5 ml budgies 0.25 ml	Antimicrobial activity as for other tetracyclines but because of its pharmacokinetic properties much more effective	Vibravenos is only available for medical use on the continent of Europe but can be obtained by special order from Pfizer. It has a very prolonged half-life. It is more lipid soluble than other tetracyclines and so better penetrates intracellular tissue. However, its half-life is much shorter in Amazon parrots and cockatoos than other species of parrots. Doxycycline has fewer side effects, both hepatic & renal than the other tetracyclines but the side effects of Vibravenos can be: (1) Blood clotting time increased (2) Haemorrhages (3) Possible hepatotoxicity (AST & ALD†) To counteract add vit. K to injection.

e.g. Ronoxan (Rhône-Mérieux)	Tablets 20 mg & 100 mg	p.o.	40–50 mg/kg body wt (for Amazons & cockatoos) i.e. 0.16 tablets per Amazon 25–30 mg/kg i.e. 0.1 tablet per African grey parrot 0.3 tablet per macaw		Is much less affected by cations than other tetracyclines so that absorption from the GI tract is almost 100% & in contrast to the water soluble tetracyclines only 30% is excreted via the kidneys. If regurgitation occurs reduce the dose by 25%. 70% of doxycycline is excreted in the bile and some undergoes enterohepatic recirculation which helps maintain plasma levels. The tablets are really too large except for the larger birds.
Chlortetracycline e.g. Aureomycin sol. powder (Willows Francis) & others	Soluble powder for solution in drinking water or incorporation in food 225 g pack	p.o.	0.25–0.5% in food, i.e. 2.5 g/kg food or 6–12 level teaspoonful/ pound of cooked food or 2.5–5 g/litres, i.e. one level teaspoonful/ 1–2 litres of drinking water (see p. 118)	Mainly of use against *Chlamydia* and *Mycoplasma*. Only bacteriostatic	Needs to be used for at least 45 days continuous treatment against *Chlamydia* since it is only bacteriostatic. Retest birds for infections at the end of this period and continue treatment if necessary. Has a bitter taste therefore food may be refused leading to partial starvation and failure of treatment. Add sugar, etc. to make food more palatable. Using the lower levels of chlortetracycline in the food often leads to an increased palatability and an overall increased intake of the drug.

The aminoglycosides

All these antibacterials have a narrow therapeutic margin and are all relatively toxic. If possible their systemic use in birds is best avoided, *particularly in dehydrated birds or birds with raised uric acid or polyuria/polydipsia*. This group includes streptomycin, dihydrostreptomycin, neomycin, kanamycin, framycetin, gentamicin, apramycin, spectinomycin, tobramycin and amikacin. They are often the most effective antibiotics against many Gram negative bacteria.

They are all *bactericidal*, except spectinomycin, but enteric bacteria rapidly acquire resistance to them. None is absorbed from the GI tract so when used p.o. are relatively safe. They are poorly distributed in the body and toxic to kidney and CNS (ototoxocity). Extrapolating doses for birds from those used for mammals is very hazardous. Only those of real use in birds are listed below.

Generic and trade names	Formulation	Route of admin.	Dosage	Activity	Comment
Spectinomycin e.g. Spectam soluble (Sanofi)	A soluble powder for solution in drinking water. 1 g sachets licensed for use in pigeons	p.o.	1 g/2 litres, 3–5 days 1 g/50 kg dose for pigeons	Bacteriostatic, only active against a wide range of Gram–, including *E. coli* & *Salmonella*, also *Mycoplasma*, also some Gram+ but not streptococci	
Amikacin e.g. Amikin (Bristol-Myers)	Injection as the sulphate 50 mg/ml & 25 mg/ml 2 ml phials	i.m.	15–20 mg/kg body wt q 8 or 12h psittacines In Amazon parrots probably only has a half-life of 1.5 h, less than in some other species of parrots	Very effective against Gram–, particularly *Pseudomonas*	This is the parental aminoglycoside of choice in birds since it is much less toxic than the other antibacterials of this group. However, it is approximately four times less active, but nevertheless when combined with the beta-lactams, it is very effective but this combination may increase its neprotoxicity slightly.

Tobramycin e.g. Nebcin (Lilly)	Sulphate for injection 10 mg/ml 2 ml phial	i.m.	2–5 mg/kg q 8 hr	Similar to Amikacin	Not so nephrotixic.
Apramycin e.g. Apralan (Elanco)	Soluble powder 1 g & 50 g packs	p.o.	25–50 g/100 litre	Primarily of use against *Salmonella*	Licensed for poultry.

Macrolides and lincosamides

This group of antibacterials includes tylosin, tiamulin, erythromycin, tilmicosin, spiramycin, carbomycin, leucomycin, oleoandomycin, clindamycin and lincomycin. They are variably absorbed from the GI tract and well distributed in the body. They are primarily eliminated via metabolism in the liver. Toxicity is low and is confined to the GI tract. However, in some mammals some of these drugs have caused a fatal enterocolitis but this has not been reported in birds in which they are generally considered to be safe antibacterials with a high therapeutic index.

Generic and trade names	Formulation	Route of admin.	Dosage	Activity	Comment
Tylosin e.g. Tylan (Elanco)	Injection 50 mg/ml 50 ml phial	i.m.	10–30 mg q 8 h	All macrolides & lincosamides are only bacteriostatic active against Gram+, *Mycoplasma* and a few Gram– *Campylobacter*	In cranes the i.m. injection is reported to have caused tissue necrosis.
	Oral powder (as the tartrate) 100 g pack	p.o.	500 mg/litre drinking water (dose for pigeons)		Do not add this solution to galvanised drinkers with a zinc coating – toxic effects reported.

Generic and trade names	Formulation	Route of admin.	Dosage	Activity	Comment
Tiamulin fumarate e.g. Tiamutin (Leo)	Oral solution for addition to drinking water 125 mg/ml 20 ml phial	p.o.	1.8 ml of the solution/litre drinking water × 5 days, i.e. 225 mg/litre (dose for pigeons)	Bacteriostatic. Broader spectrum than tylosin. Active against *Haemophilus, Bordetella, Pasteurella, Mycoplasma, Strep.* spp. and *Staph. aureus* and some anaerobes, also some spirochetes & protozoa (e.g. toxoplasma)	
Clindamycin e.g. Antirobe (Upjohn)	Capsules 25 mg & 75 mg	p.o.	10 mg/kg q 8-12h	Particularly useful for Gram+ anaerobes, bacteriocidal to *Streptococcus*	Has been used by the author to treat anaerobes in raptors with no noticeable side effects. A very useful prophylactic for orthopaedic surgery. 2-10 times more active than lincomycin
Dalacin (Upjohn)	Injection 150 mg/ml 2 ml & 4 ml	i.m.			
Lincomycin combined with spectinomycin (an aminoglycoside) see above notes e.g. Linco-Spectin (Upjohn)	Oral powder for addition to drinking water 33.3 g lincomycin 66.7 g spectinomycin in 150 g/120-180 litres (dose for poultry)	p.o.	175 mg/kg q 12h raptors (Forbes, 1995, personal communication)		Licensed for poultry.

Chloramphenicol

This antibacterial is very lipid soluble so it is widely distributed in the body including the CNS and eyes. It is metabolised in the liver and is potentially toxic for several liver functions (neonates are particularly susceptible to toxicity). Also potentially toxic for the bone marrow it is excreted via the kidneys. There is known to be a wide variation in the pharmacokinetics among different species of birds. Oral absorption is erratic. Its use in birds is best avoided.

A small percentage of humans can develop a *non-dose related irreversible aplastic anaemia even with mild cutaneous* contact. Therefore *always* use surgical gloves when handling.

Generic and trade names	Formulation	Route of admin.	Dosage	Activity	Comment
Chloramphenicol e.g. Chloromycetin succinate (Parke-Davis)	Injection, powder for reconstitution 300 mg & 1.2 g	i.m. s.c. Subconjunctival	50–100 mg/kg q 8 h for 10 days	Only bacteriostatic, fairly broad spectrum, active against Gram+ *Chlamydia, Pasteurella, Haemophilus, E. coli & Salmonella* but not *Pseudomonas*	Its use in birds is only justified when penetration of the CNS or eyes is required, or against *Salmonella* where no other antibacterial is suitable. It is antagonistic to the beta-lactams and quinolones. The analogue florphenicol is less hazardous and *may* become useful in avian medicine.

The potentiated sulphonamides

These sulphonamides, when combined synergistically with the dihydrofolate reductase inhibitors baquiloprim and trimethoprim are active against a wide range of bacteria and some protozoa. They are well distributed in the body's tissues. Excretion is primarily via the kidneys but there is also some degree of hepatic metabolism which varies with the species. Usually five parts of sulphonamide are combined with one part of trimethoprim or baquiloprim. They have few toxic side effects but like all sulphonamides will crystalise in the kidney if used in dehydrated birds. *Occasionally* causes irritation and necrosis at the site of injection. To be effective both parts of the combination are at optimal levels in the tissues. Since their pharmacokinetics differ it is essential *not* to use subtherapeutic doses.

The baquiloprim preparations have not yet been used much or assessed in birds but may be more effective since the baquiloprim takes longer to be broken down and inactivated in the body than trimethoprim – so frequency of dosing is likely to be less.

Generic and trade names	Formulation	Route of admin.	Dosage	Activity	Comment
Trimethoprim + sulphonamide e.g. Borgal (Hoechst)	Sulfadoxine 62.5 mg & trimethoprim 2.5 mg & 1 mg lignocaine in 50 ml	i.m. s.c. p.o.	20 mg/kg q 12 h 16–24 mg/kg q 4 h or q 6 h	Broad spectrum, often bactericidal, sometimes only bacteriostatic against many Gram+ and Gram– (not *Pseudomonas*) & *Chlamydia*. Generally not effective against anaerobes or *Mycoplasma*	Do not use if dehydration is suspected. *Occasional* toxic side effects after more than 7 days use: agranulocytosis, haemoloytic anaemia, haemorrhagic diathesis due to avitaminosis K. Sometimes vomiting after administration p.o. therefore best given in small frequent doses in food. Macaws may vomit, often several hours after p.o. administration but not after parenteral administration.
e.g. Cosumix Plus (Ciba) many other preparations	Oral powder sulphachlorpyridazine 100 g, trimethoprim 20 g	p.o.	2.4 mg/kg for addition to drinking water or food		
Duphatrim (Solvay-Duphar)	Sulphadiazine 500 mg/g, trimethoprim 165 mg/g 500 g pack oral granules for addition to drinking water or food	p.o.	30 mg/kg for broiler chickens and turkeys more than 21 days of age		
Scorprin (Willows)	Suspension sulphadiazine 50 mg, trimethroprim 10 mg per dose of 1.1 ml	p.o.	$\frac{1}{2}$ × 1.1 ml dose per pigeon		
Delvoprim (Mycopharm) Duphatrim (Solvay-Duphar	Tablets sulphadiazine 100 mg, trimethoprim 20 mg per tablet	p.o.	$\frac{1}{2}$ tablet per pigeon		

Many other formulations of trimethoprim + a sulphonamide are available, those listed above are the most applicable to avian medicine.

The fluoroquinolones

This group includes norfloxacin, ofloxacin, perfloxacin, enrofloxacin, ciprofloxacin and marbrofloxacin. They are widely distributed in body tissues including intracellular tissue. They undergo some hepatic metabolism excreted via the kidneys. They have low toxicity but can cause occasional GI disturbance due to reduction in GI flora. Can cause occasional anorexia. They have potential neurological side-effects, so do not administer to birds with CNS signs. Known to cause articular defects in the joint cartilage and feather development problems in growing pigeons. Antagonistic to tetracyclines, macrolides and chloramphenicol. They are bactericidal acting by blocking bacterial DNA synthesis.

Generic and trade names	Formulation	Route of admin.	Dosage	Activity	Comment
Enrofloxacin e.g. Baytril (Bayer)	Tablets 15 mg, 50 mg, 150 mg 2.5% or 5% injection 2.5% or 10% oral solution	p.o. i.m. In drinking water	7.5–15 mg/kg q 24 h psittacines × 10 days 5–15 mg/kg q 12 h 1–2 ml of 10% soln. per litre of drinking water	Bacteriocidal broad-spectrum, active against wide range of Gram+, Gram– and *Mycoplasma* (not *Pseudomonas*), *Chlamydia*. Not active against anaerobes	Note: eliminated more rapidly in African grey parrots than Amazons and cockatoos. Injection may cause some irritation and pain.
Ciproxin (the primary metabolite of enrofloxacin)	No veterinary preparation, only human preparations	i.m. p.o.	15 mg/kg q 24 h psittacines × 10 days 380 mg/litre drinking water		Slightly better activity against Gram–, has a bitter taste.
Marbofloxacin ie Marbocyl (Univet)	Tablets 5 mg, 20 mg, 80 mg	p.o.	6 mg/kg q 24 h		Longer half-life period in dogs and cats possibly also in birds.

Anti-mycobacterial drugs

Treatment of tuberculosis in birds is not recommended because of the serious zoonotic hazard and the increasingly frequent resistance of mycobacteria to available drugs. However in the case of a particularly valuable bird or an insistent owner who appreciates the hazards, treatment may be justified but does require skilled management with constant monitoring.

Generic and trade names	Formulation	Route of admin.	Dosage	Activity	Comment
Clofazimine e.g. Lamprene (Geigy)	Capsules 100 mg	p.o.	1.5–4 mg/kg q 24 h	Human drug originally produced for the treatment of leprosy	May produce gastrointestinal side effects
Ethambutol hydrochloride e.g. Myambutol (Lederle)	Tablets 150 mg & 400 mg	p.o.	15–20 mg/kg q 12 h	Human antituberculous drug	Visual side effects in humans non-documented in birds.
Isoniazid	Tablets 300 mg Elixir 50 mg/5 ml Injection 25 mg/ml	p.o. i.m.	15 mg/kg q 12 h 10 mg/kg q 12 h	Human antituberculous drug	May be hepatoxic and may cause vomiting
Rifampicin e.g. Rifadin (Merrel)	Capsules 150–300 mg Syrup 100 mg/5 ml	p.o.	15–20 mg/kg q 12 h	Human antituberculous drug	May be hepatoxic and may cause gastrointestinal disturbance

Antifungal drugs for use in birds

For the treatment of infections caused by aspergillosis, yeasts, *Candida, Cryptococcus*, sporotrichosis, blastomycosis and histoplasmosis.

It is difficult and time-consuming to carry out antifungal sensitivity testing as for antibacterials. Also: (1) many tests are not standardised; (2) they are expensive; (3) they take a long time before results are known; (4) many antifungals look good when tested *in vitro* but turn out to be poor when used *in vivo*. Therefore antifungal drug use is largely empirical. There are hundreds of strains of *Aspergillus* with varying pathogenicity. Many antifungals often work best in combination with other antifungals, e.g. either an 'azole drug combined with amphotericin or flucytosine (this second combination is best if CNS involvement is suspected).

Most of these antifungals are only fungiostatic and fungal infections require much longer periods of treatment than for bacterial infections. Usually several weeks treatment is required. Aspergillosis infections are often systemic but fungal hyphae may be enclosed in locally concentrated granulomas where the ability of the drug to penetrate the lesion is important.

The imidazoles

Those listed here occur in order of their discovery and also in order of decreasing toxicity and increasing effectiveness. Only those of current importance in avian therapeutics are discussed in detail: miconazole, econazole, clotrimazole, ketoconazole, enilconazole, fluconazole, itraconazole. All are absorbed with varying degrees of effectiveness from the GI tract.

Generic and trade names	Formulation	Route of admin.	Dosage	Activity	Comment
Ketoconazole e.g. Nizoral (Janssen)	200 mg tablets soluble in a slightly acid media	p.o.	30 mg/kg body wt q 24 h × 14 days dose for pigeons and cockatoos	Broad-spectrum, active against fungi, yeasts and some Gram+	Some strains of *Aspergillus* (of which there are many hundreds) are resistant, therefore always combine with other antifungals. Readily absorbed p.o. and widely distributed in the body's tissues, but not C.N.S. Eliminated by hepatic metabolism and can cause heptocellular necrosis – jaundice and vomiting, anorexia, therefore usually only used for 2–3 weeks. Also possibly teratogenic. More toxic than later imidazoles. The crushed tablets can be mixed in food or fruit juice or dissolved – one tablet/4 ml (0.8 ml of a one molar HC1 solution diluted with 3.2 ml water). Take care if used with potentially hepatoxic drugs.

Generic and trade names	Formulation	Route of admin.	Dosage	Activity	Comment
Fluconazole e.g. Diflucan (Pfizer)	200 mg tablets	p.o.	Limited studies in birds indicate a dose of 2–5 mg/kg q 24 h	*In vitro* × 100 more potent than ketoconazole. Excellent against yeasts but variable activity against *Aspergillus*	Very soluble, readily absorbed p.o. Widely distributed in the body including CNS. Eliminated via the kidneys. Toxicity low with mild GI upset and CNS signs (but only reported in humans). Since liver enzymes are sometimes elevated it would be wiser to monitor these during treatment. Take care if used with potentially nephrotoxic drugs.
Itraconazole e.g. Sporanoz (Janssen)	100 mg capsules Also oral liquid (peppermint or cherry flavoured)	p.o.	10 mg/kg × 35 days macaws 7 mg/kg × 29 days King penguins 10 mg/kg other penguins: all at q 24 h	5–10 × more potent than ketoconazole	Well absorbed if taken with food. Widely distributed (but not CNS or eye). Degraded in liver, excreted in bile. Can cause hepatitis in mammals. Adverse reactions recorded in some species of birds particularly African grey parrots. Mostly used in birds at 10 mg/kg q 24 h × 30 days +

The polyenke antifungals

Generic and trade names	Formulation	Route of admin.	Dosage	Activity	Comment
Nystatin ie Nystan (Squibb)	Tablets 500,000 IU Suspension 100,000 IU/ml 300 ml phial	p.o. & topically	300,000 IU/kg q 8 or 12h × 5–10 days	Effective against most strains of *Candida* and some other yeasts but not aspergillosis	Not absorbed from GI tract. To be effective must come into direct contact with yeast cell, therefore best not mixed with food or other media. Causes occasionally GI upset with vomiting but generally not toxic and not expensive.
Amphotericin-B e.g. Fungizone (Squibb)	5 mg/ml injection	Slow i.v. Intratracheal nebulisation direct into air sac	1.5 mg/kg q 8h	Broad-spectrum, active against fungi, yeasts, some strains of *Aspergillus* resistant	Not well absorbed p.o., irritant if injected i.m. or s.c., therefore must be given i.v. but *slowly* otherwise cardiac arrythmia occurs and in some species, mild convulsions. Widely distributed in the body. Metabolised and excreted by the liver. Not thought to be nephrotoxic in birds in contrast to mammals, nevertheless monitor kidney function. Turkeys and raptors excrete the drug more rapidly.
		p.o.	0.2 ml per budgerigar q 12h	Active against megacteria	Because the pH of the proventriculus in megabacteriosis changed from a normal of 0.7–2.7 to approximately 7.0, this drug is best administered in a slightly acid solution, i.e. 1 ml of 10% (approx. 1 normal HCl diluted in 30 ml water. Give to the bird 0.5 ml p.o. of this diluted acid solution (Baker, 1995; personal communication).

Generic and trade names	Formulation	Route of admin.	Dosage	Activity	Comment
Flucytosine e.g. Alcobon (Roche)	500 mg tablets	p.o. (gavage) or in feed	50 mg/kg q 12 h × 2–4 weeks for prophylaxis in raptors and waterfowl 65 mg/kg q 24 h in cockatoos 50–250 mg/kg of feed for psittacines and mynahs	Broad spectrum but resistant strains rapidly develop. Effective for yeast but not systemic fungi except in combination with other antifungals	Well absorbed from GI tract and widely distributed in the body's tissues including CNS, excreted almost unchanged. Since may have an adverse effect on the bone marrow, best to monitor haematology. May cause slight GI upset otherwise not thought to be toxic in birds.
Chlorhexidine 20%	Hibitane concentrate solution contains 25% chlorhexidine, marketed as an antiseptic	Drinking water	10 ml/gallon (USA) (3.8 litres) 12 ml/gallon (Imperial) (4.5 litres) 7–14 days		Consult manufacturer before use. Has been used in the USA for flock treatment of candidiasis. Also slows the spread of some viral infections (e.g. psittacine herpes virus). May be viricidal. Not absorbed from the gut (Clubb, 1984). Used by the author in budgerigars and not found to be toxic at 3 × this dose. Can be used as a plumage and skin spray.

Anti-parasitic drugs

A large number of parasites infect birds, nematodes, cestodes, trematodes, protozoa and arthropods. Parasitic infection varies geographically and also depends on the bird's origin, e.g. tapeworms are sometimes seen in imported parrots, but not in parrots bred in the UK because the intermediate is absent. However nematodes, e.g. *Ascaridia* and *Sygamus* are common and found in many specis of birds, particularly those kept in outside aviaries.

Drugs for the treatment of metazoan endoparasites

The benzimidazoles: many are licensed in the UK for veterinary use. These include albendazole, fenbendazole, flubendazole, mebendazole, oxfendazole, oxibendazole and thiabendazole. Only those of relatively safe use are listed below.

Generic and trade names	Formulation	Route of admin.	Dosage	Activity	Comment
Fenbendazole e.g. Panacur (Hoechst)	2.5% 25 mg/ml oral suspension	p.o.	50–100 mg/kg q 24 h once, repeat after 10 days or daily × 3 days, microfilaria daily × 5 days	Broad-spectrum, active against adult and larval nematodes and is ovicidal. Also active against tape worms and some flukes	The suspension has been used for finches in the drinking water at a dose of 10 mg/litre although quite how it remains in suspension has not been stated. Even at this low dose it can be toxic for finches.
	4% oral powder or 40 mg/ml for incorporation in food	p.o.	Trematodes 40 mg/g of dry food – used for grouse, formulated in grit-like pellets		Should not be used when birds are actively growing feathers. Shown to be teratogenic in sheep. Otherwise when used at the recommended dose a relatively safe drug. *Resistant strains of nematodes can develop.* A tasteless and odourless drug.
	Capsules containing 8 mg (licensed for pigeons)	p.o.	One capsule per pigeon over 2 months of age		
e.g. Wormex (Hoechst)	2% 20 mg/ml oral suspension for incorporation in feed. 300 ml pack licensed in UK for game birds	p.o.	7–10 mg/kg body wt q 24 h		

Generic and trade names	Formulation	Route of admin.	Dosage	Activity	Comment
Mebendazole e.g. Mebenvet (Janssen)	Oral powder 1.2% i.e. 12 mg/g 250 g pack, 5% i.e. 50 mg/g 2.4 kg pack	p.o. for addition to food	60 g/tonne of feed for poultry 120 g/tonne of feed for game birds	GI roundworms, gapeworms and tapeworms in poultry and game birds	Contra-indicated in psittacines. Has been **reported to have caused death in pigeons, cormorants, pelicans, raptors and finches.** *Use best restricted to those species for which it is licensed where there are resistant strains of nematodes, i.e. poultry and game birds.*
Flubendazole e.g. Flubenvet (Janssen)	Oral powder 25 mg/g	p.o. for incorporation in food	Turkeys: 20 g tonne of feed geese: 30 g/tonne of feed Game birds: 60 g/ tonne of feed		Use in species other than those for which it is licensed is not documented.
Thiabendazole e.g. Thibenzole (MSD Agvet)	Oral suspension 176 mg/ml	p.o. mixed in food	50 mg/kg body wt in feed for 7–10 days	Roundworms, gapeworm and some flukes	Not a very safe drug for birds, although it has been used in the past. Toxic to ostriches, ducks and cranes.

			Effective against intestinal nematodes, adult and larval forms	
Levamisole e.g. Nilverm (Mallinckrodt Veterinary). Many other trade names	75 mg/ml 7.5% for injection for farm animals 500 ml pack. 75 mg/ml i.e. 7.5% solution for oral admin. 100 ml pack. Note the injectable preparations are all 7.5% but the oral preparations vary 1.5%, 3.2%, 3.0%	All administered p.o.	15–20 mg/kg q 24 h repeat after 2 weeks 100–200 mg/litre × 3 days for finches, dilute 1 in 14	Has a low therapeutic index. Toxicity has occurred when the drug has been injected (i.m or s.c) at doses above 20 mg/kg. Deaths have occurred in budgerigars, lovebirds, pigeons and ibis, caused vomiting, CNS signs, death. Bitter tasting, so reasonably safe when administered in drinking water because tends to be self-regulating. Leave birds without water or fruit for 24 h before dosing. Dose for 6–8 h only
	Tablets of 20 mg for pigeons	p.o.	One tablet of 20 mg per pigeon	Has been used as an immunostimulant at a dose of 2 mg/kg q 24 h i.m. every 14 days × 3 doses. This only works if T-cell function is depressed below normal. It does not elevate normal T-cell functional levels.

Generic and trade names	Formulation	Route of admin.	Dosage	Activity	Comment
Ivermectin e.g. Ivomec (MSD AgVet)	Injection for cattle 10 mg/ml i.e. 1% solution 50 ml, 200 ml and 500 ml phials	Topically drop directly on to skin	200 μg/kg q 24 h repeat once in 10–14 days	Broad-spectrum antiparasitic, effective against invertebrate parasites, intestinal roundworm, gapeworm, microfilaria, knemidocoptes, air sac mite, lice, ecto-parasitic mites. Not ovicidal, not active against tapeworms or flukes. May be effective against *some* coccidia.	Is rapidly absorbed, even percutaneously and spreads throughout the body persisting in the body's tissues for long periods. Therefore, frequent dosing can lead to toxicity, i.e. ataxia, depression, CNS signs. However, generally a safe drug in birds. If the injection is diluted with water tends to settle out unless used immediately – best diluted with propylene glycol. Toxic dose in budgies and some finches may be as low as 0.02 ml. Best used in small birds by dripping directly on to the skin – one drop onto the skin between the scapula on a Gouldian finch is effective against air sac mite.
		p.o.	Dilute 1% solution 1 ml in 3 ml propylene glycol, give 0.1 mg/kg		
		i.m.			
Praziquantel e.g. Droncit (Bayer)	Tablets 50 mg	p.o.	10–20 mg/kg, repeat after 2–4 weeks	Tapeworms. May stop passage of eggs but not get rid of adult tapeworm	A fairly safe drug but can be toxic if the dose is exceeded, particularly by injection and in finches. Tablets are insoluble but can be crushed, mixed in vegetable oil and then mixed in food.
	56.8 mg/ml 10 ml phial	i.m. s.c.	705 mg/kg, repeat after 2.4 weeks (not finches)		

Generic and trade names	Formulation	Route of admin.	Dosage	Activity	Comment
Niclosamide e.g. Yomesan (Bayer)	Tablet containing 0.5 g of niclosamide	p.o. Crop tube In feed	250 mg/kg once	Active against tapeworms	Tablets are not soluble, must be suspended in water or mixed in mash. Death has occurred in pigeons and some Anseriformes at recommended doses.
Piperazine e.g. Biozine (Harkers)	Piperazine dihydrochloride 55% 10 g sachet	p.o.	2.5 g/kg dry food 2.5 g/kg litre drinking water		For use in Galliformes and Anseriformes, but not parrots.

Agents for use against ectoparasites

Generic and trade names	Formulation	Route of admin.	Dosage	Activity	Comment
Piperonyl butoxide e.g. Fleacare (Animalcare)	Powder with piperonyl butoxide 0.8%, pyrethrins 0.113% w/v	External application	Dust on to feathers		Safe and effective. Brush out excess from hand held bird.
Coumaphos i.e. Negasunt (Bayer)	Powder containing 3% w/v coumaphos 2% w/v propoxur 5% w/v sulphanilamide	External application	Dust on to feathers	Active against all external parasites	Contains carbamate propoxur. Useful for fly-blown wounds.
Ivermectin	See above				
Cypermethrin e.g. Dy-sect, Deosan	Dilute to 2%		To treat *premises* infested with *Dermanyssus* spp.		
Fibronyl e.g. Frontline (Rhône-Mérieux)		Spray on skin			Beware – alcohol may dry feathers → brittle

Drugs for the treatment of protozoal endoparasites

Generic and trade names	Formulation	Route of admin.	Dosage	Activity	Comment
Amprolium e.g. Amprol-plus (MSD)	Water miscible solution with 7.68% w/v amprolium hydrochloride BP 0.49% w/v ethopabate BP and aqueous propylene glycol vehicle to 100%	p.o. in drinking water	56.8 ml (2 fl oz) per 18.2 litres (4 Imperial gallons of water) for 5–7 days	*Eimeria* species of coccidia. Resistant strains can develop after repeated use	Licensed for use in poultry and in pigeons. Chemically related to thiamine and competitively inhibits the uptake of thiamine by parasites but may also destroy some autochronous micro-organisms in the GI tract and so produce a thiamine deficiency in the host. Toxic to falcons at 22 mg/kg q 24 h (Forbes, 1995, personal communication).
i.e. Coxoid (Harkers)	Amprolium hydrochloride 38.4 mg/ml 112 ml & 500 ml	p.o. by addition to drinking water	112 ml treatment for 30 pigeons		
Clazuril e.g. Appertex (Harkers)	Tablets 2.5 mg	p.o.	2.5 mg/pigeon 8 mg/kg q 24 h × 3 days, off 2 days and repeat for *Caryospora neofalconis* in merlins (*Falco columbarius*) (Forbes, 1995, personal communication)	Coccidiosis in pigeons	Not very effective in cranes & Galliformes. May cause vomiting in cranes and Galliformes.

Generic and trade names	Formulation	Route of admin.	Dosage	Activity	Comment
Metronidazole e.g. Torgyl (Rhône-Mérieux)	0.5% solution i.e. 5 mg/ml 50 ml phial	i.m. p.o. directly or in drinking water	10 mg/kg or 2 ml/kg q 24h × 2 days 200 mg/litre of drinking water, i.e. 40 ml/litre, 10–30 mg/kg orally q 12h × 7 days	Active against *Trichomonas, Giardia, Hexamita,* clostridia and anaerobes	May be toxic for finches. Injection may cause necrosis at site of injection. Well absorbed orally and penetrates all body's tissues, including CNS. May reduce water intake, and therefore dose taken. A relatively safe drug.
Metronidazole (non-proprietry)	Tablets 200 mg				
Dimetridazole e.g. Emtryl soluble (Rhône-Mérieux)	Oral powder for addition to drinking water 400 g/kg Licensed for use in poultry and game birds 500 g pack	p.o.	26.7 g/100 litres (poultry 1 × level teaspoonful/4.5 litres 40 mg/kg	Effective against trichomoniasis, hexamitiasis, giardiasis, histomoniasis and some anaerobes	Not as safe a drug as metronidazole. Has a low therapeutic index. Toxic for many finches. Extended therapy or overdosing easily causes toxic CNS signs and death. In lories and mynahs use $\frac{1}{2}$ normal dose.

Anti-malarial drugs licensed for human use

These may be effective against the blood protozoan parasites sometimes found in birds, i.e. *Plasmodium,* which occurs in wild birds in the UK and is transmitted to captive birds by biting arthropods; *Leucocytozoon* – probably specific. *Haemoproteus* may not be pathogenic. Trypanosomes possible in imported birds.

Generic and trade names	Formulation	Route of admin.	Dosage	Activity	Comment
Chloroquine e.g. Nivaquine (Rhône-Poulenc Rorer)	Syrup 68 mg/ml Injection 40 mg/ml 5 ml ampoule	p.o.	10 mg/kg once then 5 mg/kg at 6, 18 & 24 h	Active against *Plasmodium*	Bitter taste. Crushed tablet dissolved in fruit juice or with honey. Rapidly absorbed from GI tract. May cause mucous membranes to turn yellow. Low therpeutic index. Overdose fatal. Best used in combination with primaquine. Used in penguins, raptors and psittacines.

Generic and trade names	Formulation	Route of admin.	Dosage	Activity	Comment
Primaquine	Tablets 7.5 mg		0.03 mg/kg daily × 3 days	Active against *Plasmodium*	Used in penguins. Used in conjunction with chloroquine.
Pyrimethamine e.g. Daraprim (Wellcome) Fansidar (Roche)	Tablets 25 mg 25 mg 12.5 mg	p.o.	0.5 mg/kg q 12h. Mix tablet × 10 days in 21 ml water. Add 4 ml KY jelly to give a suspension of 1 mg/ml	Active against *Plasmodium*, *Toxoplasma, Sarcocystis*	Folic acid antagonist, therefore effects potentiated by the simultaneous administration of sulphonamides.

Prophylactic protection against viruses

Virus	Formulation	Effectiveness & comment
Pox viruses		
Fowl pox	Vaccine Freeze-dried live virus powder for reconstitution Poxine (Solvay)	Very few species specific vaccines Licensed in the UK for use in poultry: effective for turkey pox, quail pox, falcon pox. Does not protect peacocks against peacock pox virus.
Pigeon pox	Living vaccine Pigeon pox Nobilus (Intervet) Freeze-dried for reconstitution	Licensed in the UK for use in pigeons. If used in raptors may increase mortality.
Canary pox	Homologous vaccine available in USA	
Psittacine pox	Homologous vaccine available in USA	
Herpes viruses	Very few taxon specific vaccines available to the many herpes virus diseases	Note herpes viruses are intranuclear and so protected by the cytoplasm of the cell from the body's humoral defences.
Duck virus hepatitis enteritis	Duck virus hepatitis (Animal Health Trust)	Only available to members of Duck Producers Association

Infectious laryngotracheitis	Freeze-dried live vaccine ILT Vaccine (Solvay)	Licensed for use in UK in poultry, not pheasants. May be effective against Amazon tracheitis but there is a risk of undesirable reaction.
Marek's disease virus	Freeze-dried live vaccines Delvax (Mycofarm) Marexine (Intervet) MD-Vac (Solvay) Also cell associated live vaccines available	Licensed for use in UK in poultry. Before use consult manufacturers and MAFF.
Pacheco's virus of parrots	Vaccine available in USA	
Corona viruses Avian infectious bronchitis	Live virus vaccines for addition to drinking water IBMM (Sovay) IB Nobilis H-52, H-120 and Strain Ma5 (Intervet) Poulvac H52 & H120 (Solvay)	Licensed for use in UK in poultry but *may* be effective in pheasants, guineafowl, psittacines, pigeons, ostrich and Japanese quail providing an exact diagnosis has been made. Consult manufacturer & MAFF before use.
Arbo viruses Avian encephalomyelitis	Live virus vaccine for addition to drinking water. AE-Vac (Solvay) AE-Nobilis (Intervet)	Licensed for use in UK in poultry but *may* be effective in other species providing a specific diagnosis has been made. Consult manufacturer & MAFF before use.
Louping ill virus	Inactivated + oil adjuvant louping ill vaccine (Mallinckrodt Veterinary)	Licensed for use in UK in cattle, sheep & goats but may be effective in susceptible avian species, i.e. grouse, capercaillie and pheasant. Consult manufacturer & MAFF before use.
Paramyxo viruses Newcastle disease virus	Live freeze-dried vaccines: Hitchner B1 (Solvay) Hitchner B1 Nobilis (Intervet) Inactivated vaccines: Newcavac Nobilis (Intervet)	Licensed for use in the UK in poultry. Do not use live vaccines in species other than those for which licensed. The inactivated vaccine may be effective in other avian species after a specific diagnosis has been made. Consult the manufacturer & MAFF before use. A notifiable disease.

Virus	Formulation	Effectiveness & comment
Pigeon paramyxovirus	Inactivated virus Columboval (Solvay) Nobi-Vac Paramyxo (Intervet) Paramyx (Harkers)	Licensed in the UK for use in pigeons. A notifiable disease.
Circo viruses Psittacine beak and feather disease virus	Experimental vaccine available in USA	
Papova viruses Polyomavirus	Experimental vaccine available in USA	

Suggested routines for dealing with virus infections

(1) For herpes virus infections only, use *aciclovir* tablets or suspension, i.e. Zovirax (Wellcome medical) at the rate of 80 mg/kg 8h (gavage) or 240 mg/kg of feed. This drug blocks herpes virus DNA polymerase in infected cells. Occasionally causes vomiting. Most effective in aviary outbreaks before clinical signs are recognised.

May be nephrotoxic so do not use in dehydrated birds, etc. or with other potentially nephrotoxic drugs such as the aminoglycosides or sulphonamides.

Do not use the injectable formulation.

Acyclovir may help in some pox virus cases.

(2) Use *ascorbic acid* (non-proprietary) at dose rate of 20–40 mg/kg q 24 h up to 7 days. This, together with zinc, has a salutory effect on the immune response.

(3) *Ensure the diet is adequate* particularly in essential amino acids, vitamins A, E and B vitamins and also zinc, e.g. use Ace-High (Vetark).

(4) Use appropriate *treatment for secondary invaders* and treat any concomitant parasitic infection.

(5) Pay attention to *strict aviary hygiene*, noting the modes of transmission and possible latent carriers, etc.

(6) *Idoxuridine* blocks the replication of some DNA viruses.

The use of idoxuridine i.e. Idoxene (Spodefell) 0.5% eye ointment. *A little* applied to the eye of herpes virus infected birds may help to improve the condition of the eyes and encourage the bird to feed.

May also help in some pox virus cases.

Miscellaneous drugs for use in birds

Drug	Formulation	Route	Dosage	Comment
Iodine Lugol's iodine	Lugol's iodine BP	In drinking water	Dilute by adding 2 parts to 28 parts of water. Add 3 drops of this solution to 100 ml drinking water – use for 3 weeks.	Secondary thyroid hyperplasia due to iodine deficiency commonly seen in budgerigars. Often an overall general improvement in activity and plumage is seen in budgerigars after 3–4 months treatment.
Sodium iodide	20% sterile solution for injection 200 mg/ml	i.m.	0.01–0.03 ml (2–6 mg)/ 30 g bird 0.33–1.0 ml (66–133 mg)/ kg body weight	Secondary thyroid hyperplasia due to iodine deficiency. Considerable improvement to respiratory obstruction seen within 3 days in budgerigars.
Potassium iodide		In drinking water	100–200 mg/100 ml	As a palliative in the treatment of chronic respiratory disease. Should not be given for periods longer than a week.
Bromhexidine Bisolvon (Boehringer Ingelheim)	Sterile solution for injection containing 3 mg/ml bromhexine hydrochloride. Tablet containing 8 mg (Medical Product)	i.m.	3–6 mg/(1–2 ml)/kg, 0.1 ml/30 g divided into 2 or 3 doses daily	May help better penetration of the antibiotics and gamma globulins into respiratory tract. Well tolerated. The injection is water-based so can be given orally or in daily water intake (Ahlers, 1970).
Allopurinol e.g. Zyloric (Wellcome)	100 mg tablet	Oral Drinking water	40 mg/kg. Crush a 100 mg tablet, mix in 10 ml water. Use 2.6 ml of this solution to 100 ml. Give daily for life.	Treatment of gout. Reduces the level of uric acid in the plasma by reducing its production in the liver, i.e. inhibits xanthine oxidase which catalyses purines to uric acid. However can result in the deposition of crystals of xanthine and hypoxathine, the precursors of uric acid. Deposition of these metabolytes in the renal tubules may result in acute renal obstruction. Documented in red tailed hawks and may be true for other raptors. Use with caution.

Drug	Formulation	Route	Dosage	Comment
Calcuim borogluconate	10% (100 mg) ml	i.v. s.c.	0.5–2 ml (50–250 mg) per kg, by *slow* intravenous injection to effect.	Treatment of impaction of the oviduct and egg binding used *together with* oxytocin. Treatment of raptors with 'fits' due to hypocalcaemia. Advisable to give Dextrose injection at the same time.
Carprofen e.g: Zenecarp (C-Vet VP)	Injection 50 mg/ml 20 ml phial	i.m.	2 mg/kg q 24 h	An NSAID which is a weaker inhibitor of cyclo-oxygenase than either ketoprofen or flunixin and therefore safer. A potent analgesic and a useful anti-inflammatory even systemically has a marked euphorbic effect. A better choice than using corticosteroids.
Dimethyl sulphoxide (non-proprietary) DSMO	50% w/w			Solvent disolving many drugs and transporting these through the skin through which it easily penetrates. Is itself an anti-inflammatory agent helping in the dissolution of collagen. May be toxic in some species and to humans.
Ferric chloride solution BP *also powder* (non-proprietary)		Apply topically to bleeding areas		To arrest minor haemorrhage
Silver nitrate	Stick or pencil	Apply to points of minor haemorrhage		To arrest localised bleeding by chemical cautery. Flush the area with saline solution to form silver chloride when bleeding has ceased, to neutralise the cauterising action.

Drug	Presentation	Route	Dose	Comments
Hyaluronidase BP	Ampoule with 1500 IU for reconstitution	500 IU per injection site		Breaks down the polysaccharide hyaluronic acid which is part of intracellular connective tissue. Dispenses fluids.
Glibenclamide BP (non-proprietary)	2.5 mg tablets	Oral in drinking water	Dissolve $\frac{1}{4}$ tablet 0.62 mg in one litre	For non-insulin dependent diabetes melitus in psittacines, particularly budgerigars.
Propentofylline e.g. Vivitonin (Hoechst)	Small tablets containing 50 mg	Oral in food	25 mg/kg q 24 h Split tablet in half and give on alternate days	Peripheral vascular dilator used for idiopathetic dullness, lethargy in old senile parrots, also for treatment of wing tip oedema (Forbes, 1995, personal communication).
Isoxsuprine e.g. Navilox (Univet)	Oral powder 30 mg/g		5–10 mg/kg q 24 h	Arterial dilator working predominantly on skeletal muscle. Appears to work better than the above drug in the treatment of wing tip oedema (Lewis *et al.* 1993).
Vecuronium bromide e.g. Norcuron (Organon-Teknika)	Powder 10 mg ampoule for reconstitution	Topically to the eye	Reconstitute powder 10 mg in 2.5 ml water. Use one drop only every 5 min × 15 min until pupil dilates	Used as an alternative to tubocurarine as a non-depolarising muscle relaxant to cause dilation of the pupil (mydriasis), since in birds this is under the CNS and *not* the parasympathic as in mammals.
Atropine sulphate e.g. Atropine sulphate (C-Vet VP) Artrocare (Animal Care)	A sterile solution for injection containing 600 µg/ml 0.6 mg/ml	i.m. s.c.	0.05–0.1 mg/kg, 0.1–0.6 ml/kg Use higher dose for small birds only	For premedication 10 min prior to anaesthesia. As a partial antidote to organophosphorous poisoning.

Hormones for use in birds

Hormone	Formulation	Route	Dosage	Comment
Testosterone e.g. Androject (Intervet)	An oily solution for injection containing 10 mg testosterone phenylproprionate per ml	i.m. s.c.	2–8 mg/kg once	For stimulation of sexual behaviour in the male. Has been used for baldness in the canary. Should not be used in birds with liver or renal disease.
e.g. Durateston (Intervet)	An oily solution for injection containing 4 esters of testosterone 50 mg total esters/ml	i.m. s.c.	2–8 mg/kg once	Prolonged activity over 2 weeks.
Nandrolone e.g. Nandrolin (Intervet)	Sterile oily injection containing 25 mg/ml, 50 mg/ml	i.m.	0.4 mg/kg 0.02 mg/30 g once	Chronic and debilitating disease. Should not be used if there is liver disease.
Dexamethasone e.g. Dexadreson (Intervet)	A clear aqueous suspension containing 10 mg/ml	i.m. topically	0.3–3 mg/kg Mixed in 50% solution with DSMO	To reduce the inflammatory response and combat shock. Preferably given with appropriate antibiotics. Note: the action of corticosteroids is subtly different in birds compared with mammals (Westerhof, 1996). Birds are much more sensitive to their action. If possible always use NSAIDs
Dinoprost e.g. Lutalyse (Upjohn)	5 mg/ml contains naturally occurring prostaglandin	i.m. Intra-cloacal	0.02–0.1 mg/kg use once only	For egg binding, relaxes vent and increases tone in oviduct. Also useful in treating salpingitis.
Delmadinone e.g. Tardak (Pfizer)	An aqueous suspension containing 10 mg/ml	i.m.	1 mg/kg 0.02 ml/30 g once	An anti-androgen. Neurotic regurgitation in budgerigars – sometimes effective. Well tolerated. Used successfully for excessively aggressive swans.

Drug	Presentation	Route	Dose	Notes
Medroxyprogesterone e.g. Promone-E (Upjohn) Perlutex (Leo)	Aqueous suspension containing 50 mg/ml Aqueous suspension containing 25 mg/ml	i.m.	30 mg/kg once 18–50 mg/kg larger birds (over 700 g the smaller doses)	Neurotic regurgitation in budgerigars. Also some feather conditions involving excess preening. Has been used for persistent egg laying in budgerigars and in other species of psittacine birds. Side effects: obesity, polyurea, even diabetes. Cockatoos are the most sensitive to this drug.
Oxytocin e.g. Oxytocin-S (Intervet)	A clear aqueous solution containing 10 units/ml	i.m.	0.3–0.5 ml/kg	Used in conjunction with calcium borogluconate for impaction of the oviduct, see Chapter 7, p 168. See also dinoprost.
Thyroxine e.g. Eltroxin (Goldshield)	Tablets containing 0.05 mg 100 µg	In drinking water	50 g ($\frac{1}{2}$–$\frac{3}{4}$ tablet) 100 ml for 4 weeks	Hypothyroidism. Double the dose for birds that drink little. The tablets are not very soluble.
Soloxine (Vet-2-Vet)		Oral, crushed & mixed in feed Oral	Up to 100 µg/kg q 24 h every 3 days	May induce moult in some species – use only for 7 days. Toxic effects, vomiting, loss of weight, convulsions and ultimately death.
Liothyronine sodium i.e. Tertroxin (Link)	Tablets 20 µg		20 µg/kg q 24 h	
Thyroid stimulating hormone (non-proprietory)		i.m.	1–2 IU/kg	Available in USA but not in UK. The related thyroid releasing hormone can be obtained in the UK and functions for diagnostic purposes as well, providing the pituitary gland is normal.
Thyroid releasing hormone (non-proprietory)		i.m.	15 µg/kg q 24 h once	

Vitamins, minerals and nutritional supplements for use in birds

Drug	Formulation	Route	Dosage	Comment
Avipro (Vetark)	Water soluble probiotic containing *Lactobacillus* (2 species), *Streptococcus faecum* yeasts; enzymes: lipase, amylase, protease and cellulase. Electrolytes and vitamins.	Orally in drink or food	One scoop (provided with pack) i.e. 4 g/100 ml drinking water	A probiotic specifically adapted for use in birds under stress. Can be used simultaneously with antibiotics, particularly if autochronous flora is liable to be affected.
Avipro Paediatric (Vetark)	Enzymes & electrolytes as above, but less *Lactobacillus* and contains glucose	As above	Follow suggested routine on pack	Designed to mimic the effects of the parent bird's crop to aid in support of the hand reared chick.
ACE-High (Vetark)	Powdered vitamin supplement with high levels of vitamin A, C & E plus B vitamins & minerals including Zn	Orally in food	Follow directions on pack	As an aid in the treatment of stress or infectious disease particularly viral infections. Do not use with other vitamin supplements.
Nutrobal (Vetark)	Powdered vitamin/ mineral supplement with calcium phosphorous ratio of 40–50: 1	Orally in food	Follow directions on pack	Designed to balance diets low in calcium, also contains 150 IU vitamin D_3 per gram. Valuable supplement for fast growing young birds and laying hen birds. Do not use with other vitamin supplements.
Critical Care Formula (CCF) (Vetark)	Each 5 g contains 0.72 g protein, 18 kcal of energy	Orally	Make up 1:2 with water. Do not make up more concentrated and give orally by gavage	Provides easily digestible calorific support as mixture of short chain maltodextrin plus concentrated protein and amino acids to stop weight loss in severely ill birds.

Multivitamin and mineral e.g. SA-37 (Intervet) Vionate (Pfizer)	See makers' data and information sheets	Oral	500 mg/kg	May be wasteful when mixed with seed. Needs to be given in a mash.
Multivitamin injections	See makers' data and information sheets	i.m.	0.5 ml/kg supplying 7500 IU vitamin A and other vitamins	Vitamin A overdose is toxic and can produce skeletal abnormalities and damage to membranes. Use with caution in macaws and African grey parrots.
Multivitamin drops e.g. Abidec (W-L)	See maker's data and information sheets. Vitamin A approx 6500 units/ml	In drinking water	5 drops/0.3 ml/30 g bird, every third day	
Minivit drops (Univet)	Drops containing 10 essential vitamins, trace elements 7 ml dropper	In drinking water		Multivitamin supplement
'Ornimed' Vit B_{12} (L.A.B.)	Canary impregnated seed containing vitamin B_{12} 4 µg/g.	Oral	1.5 g (one capful)/30 g bird	
Duphalyte (Solvay Duphar)	An injectable solution of electrolytes, vitamins, amino acids and dextrose	s.c. i.v.	10 ml/kg q 12 h	Given in the groin or at base of neck with Hyaluronidase. Give *very slowly* i.v.
Vitamin E Vitesel (Norbrook)	Alpha-tocopheryl acetate 68 mg selenium 1.5 mg/ml injection	i.m. s.c.	0.5–0.1 mg/kg q 24 h × 14 days	Cockatiel paralysis/paresis syndrome and similar neuropathies in other psittacine species.
Vitamin C (non-proprietary)	Ascorbic acid 100 mg/ml 5 ml	i.m.	20–40 mg/kg q 24 h	Nutrition support for infectious disease.

Drug	Formulation	Route	Dosage	Comment
Vitamin K (phytomenadione) Konakion (Roche)	Injection 2 mg/ml	i.m.	0.2–2.5 mg/kg q 24 h up to 70 days	May help in cases of haemorrhage. Can be used together with sulpha drugs.
Vitamin A Ro-A-Vit (Cambridge)	50,000 IU/ml 2 ml ampoule	i.m.	5000 IU/kg q 24 h × 2–4 weeks	Supportive treatment for many infectious diseases. (See warning on p. 273.)
Lactulose Duphalac (Solvay)	Liquid containing 3.35 g/ 5 ml lactulose 300 ml	Orally	0.3 ml/kg q 24 h	Slows GI transit of ingesta. Helps to absorb enterotoxins. Mild laxative. Useful in cases of auctochronous GI flora.
Natural yogurt	Contains Lactobacillus acidophilus	Oral	2 ml/kg	May help to restore gut flora after antibiotic therapy. Controversial but will do no harm.
Invalid foods: Farlene Complan (Farley Health Foods) Build Up (Carnation Foods) Vita Food (Boots Ltd) Milupa	Human invalid foods that contain approx. 400 kcal/100 g of food / Fruit salad, tropical fruit	By crop tube	100 g/kg daily 7.5 g/30 g daily	Best results obtained in the severely debilitated bird by dividing daily dose and giving at hourly intervals. Add a probiotic, e.g. Avipro.
Collovet (C-Vet VP)	A liquid containing iron, copper, manganese, chromium, caffine, thiamine and glycerophosphates	Oral, in drinking water	1–2 drops (0.06–0.12 ml)/30 g bird in drinking water every other day.	General tonic to stimulate appetite in anorexia and debility

| Vi-Sorbin (Pfizer) | A liquid containing cyanocobalamin 8.34 µg, vit B_6 2 mg, ferricpyrophosphate 100 mg, folic acid 0.5 mg, sorbitol 4.4 ml/5 ml. | Oral | 0.6 ml/kg | As above for Collovet. |

Drugs acting on the alimentary canal

Drug	Formulation	Route	Dosage	Comment
Liquid paraffin mineral oil		Oral or per cloacum	4 ml/kg q 24 h	For impaction of the cloaca and egg binding.
Glycerine		Oral or per cloacum	5 ml/kg q 24 h	
Sucrose in water	30% solution	Oral	Up to 10 ml/kg q 12 h	Mild purgative

Antidiarrhoeals without antibiotic

Drug	Formulation	Route	Dosage	Comment
Stat (Intervet)	Light kaolin 10.8 g Aluminium hydroxide gel 1.93 g Sodium acetate 1.98 g Sodium chloride 1.81 g Potassium acetate 330 mg Magnesium chloride 100 mg Calcium chloride 100 mg in each 100 ml.	Oral	3 ml/kg q 12 h or q 8 h	Note: many birds that are anorexic have watery droppings but do not have diarrhoea
Kaogel (Upjohn)	Light kaolin 200 mg/ml Pectin 4.3 mg/ml in 15 ml			
Kaopectate (Upjohn)	Kaolin 2.6 mg/ml			
Metoclopramide Emequell (Pfizer)	Hydrochloride BP injection 5 mg/ml 2 ml phial	i.m.	0.5 mg/kg q 24 h	Increases motility of upper GI tract and reduces vomiting. Indicated in sour crop to empty crop. Do not use if obstruction suspected. Can cause restlessness and excitement in some birds.

Sedatives, stimulant drugs and drugs for behavioural modification

Drug	Formulation	Route	Dosage	Comment
Diazepam Valium (Roche)	5 mg/ml; 2 ml ampoules	i.v. or i.m.	0.5–1 mg/kg i.v. or i.m.	To control feather picking and seizures.
Ketamine Vetalar (Upjohn)	Sterile solution for injection containing 100 mg/ml	i.m.	up to 15 mg/kg	Not very reliable as sedatives. These doses are sedative doses.
Xylazine Rompun (Bayer)	Sterile aqueous solution for injection 20 mg/ml	i.m.	up to 2 mg/kg	For anaesthetic doses see pp. 135 and 136.
Primidone Mysoline (Mallinckrodt veterinary)	Tablets 250 mg Suspension 250 mg/5 ml	Oral	56 mg/kg q 24 h	Treatment of idiopathic epilepsy in parrots.
Potassium bromide	Crystals to be dissolved in water at the rate of 250 mg/ml	Oral	25 mg/kg q 24 h	Clear tasteless odourless fluid for the treatment of idiopathic epilepsy in parrots.
Doxepin Sinequan (Pfizer)	Capsules of 10, 25, 50 and 75 mg Suspension 10 mg/ml	Oral	0.5–1 mg/kg q 12 h	Human tricyclic anti-depressant, may be effective in some cases of feather pucking.
Haloperidol B.P. Haldol (Janssen)	Clear colourless and odourless liquid 2 mg/ml, 100 ml	Oral	0.4 mg (0.2 ml)/kg q 24 h Dilute 1.5 ml in a litre drinking water, double dose every 2 weeks until 6 ml is diluted in a litre, treat for at *least* 3–4 months. Tail off gradually at end of treatment.	Human antipsychotic. Sometimes quite effective in self feather pucking. Anti-dopamine side effects, reversible on withdrawal of the drug.

Drug	Formulation	Route	Dosage	Comment
Doxapram hydrochloride Dopram-V (Willows Francis)	Oral drops and injection, multidose phials containing 20 mg/ml doxapram hydrochloride	Oral i.m. s.c.	One drop in a small bird's mouth. 7 mg/kg (0.3 ml/kg) 0.01 mg/30 g	Respiratory stimulant when apnoea occurs. To stimulate breathing in newly hatched chicks. Use once. Neurotoxic with excessive dosage.
Respirot (Ciba)	A syrup containing crotethamide 75 mg/ml cropropamide 75 mg/ml	Oral	One drop in the mouth of a pigeon-sized bird, 2 drops/kg	Do not use in small birds below 100 g. Side effects as for doxapram but potentially more toxic.
Sodium calciumedetate	A sterile solution containing 25% w/v 250 mg/ml	i.v. i.m. s.c.	62.5 mg (0.25 ml)/kg for swans q 24 h (Cooke, 1984) Also 20–40 mg/kg q 8 h May be able to increase dose to 80–100 mg/kg for smaller birds.	For lead and other heavy metals poisoning. If given i.v. give slowly, s.c. may cause some slight reaction. Can be nephrotoxic if bird is dehydrated or signs of polydipsia/polyurea. May need to give for prolonged periods up to 6 weeks.
Dimercaprol BP (non-proprietary) BAL (British Anti Lewisite)	2 ml ampoules 50 mg/ml in arachis oil	Oral i.m.	25–35 mg/kg q 12 h × 5 days per week, rest 2 days and recommence for 3–5 weeks.	May be more effective as a chelating agent than EDTA also less toxic. Can be used together with EDTA.

APPENDIX 2: INFECTIOUS DISEASES OF BIRDS: BACTERIAL DISEASES

This table does not include all the diseases affecting poultry.

The Enterobacteriacae

These bacteria are mostly Gram-negative rods. Pathological strains all produce endotoxins and most can produce a septicaemia.

Disease	Cause	Species susceptible	Relative occurrence	Principal clinical signs*	Confirmation of diagnosis	Differential diagnosis
Salmonellosis An important *zoonosis* from infected carrier companion birds	Over 2000 species of *Salmonella* commonly *S. typhimurium*. Carried by rodents, insects, water, wild birds. Most strains motile under right conditions. Propagate outside host. Egg transmission from day-old infected chicks	All species. Wild birds often infected and carriers, particularly winter flocks. Species without caeca apparently more susceptible. Owls	Common except in raptors. Human carriers can infect companion birds. Parrots in quarantine stations may have unusual strains	Non-specific signs of illness and diarrhoea. Sudden death or subacute septicaemic disease with enteritis. Chronic disease. PM signs depend on which stage died. White focal hepatic necrosis, caseous impaction of caeca localised necrosis of intestine. In pigeons and some parrots often localises in joints producing arthrosynovitis. Also localised dermatitis on some parrots.	Isolation and culture of the organism. Serology – simple O&H agglutination tests	A notifiable disease in the UK. Public health hazard. *E. coli* Other enteric pathogens *Chlamydia* *Pasteurella sp.* *Pseudomonas sp.*

Disease	Cause	Species susceptible	Relative occurrence	Principal clinical signs*	Confirmation of diagnosis	Differential diagnosis
Avian typhoid 'Pullorum disease'	*Salmonella gallinarum.* *Salmonella pullorum.* Carrier birds	Mainly diseases of poultry but can affect game birds and occasionally other birds including wild birds	Common in insanitary conditions	General malaise anorexia enteritis. In chronic form drop in egg production. At PM in *pullorum* infection disease localised in the ovary with misshapen ova. PM of *gallinarum* cases shows septicaemic signs with enlarged liver and spleen	Rapid slide agglutination. Test for *S. pullorum*. Otherwise as for other *Salmonella*	
Coli bacillosis	*Escherichia coli.* Genus contains many species. Motile, some non-motile. Primary or secondary invader	All species	Very common. Hjaerr's disease or coli-granulomatosis is most common in Galliformes	Often an acute septicaemic disease with no premonitory signs. In subacute or chronic form, dullness, anorexia, diarrhoea. PM shows air-sacculitis, fibrinous pericarditis with ecchymosis, a perihepatitis with enlarged liver. There may be hepatic granulomas. Enlarged necrotic spleen, caseous peritonitis. Organism often found in salpingitis and bumblefoot infections	Isolation of the organism by culture from infected tissue. Serotyping is academic. Histology indicates serofibrinous inflammation with plasma cells in liver and kidney	*Mycobacterium avium* infection

| *Pseudomonas aeruginosa* and *Aeromonas hydrophilia* | Both common avian pathogens, also both types of organism can propagate in cool water particularly if contaminated by organic waste, also contaminated food | All species of birds but particularly aquatic birds. Free ranging waterfowl | Widespread. These organisms are usually secondary pathogens producing potent extracellular toxins | Although *Pseudomonas* and *Aeromonas* are unrelated infection, either can produce similar signs: (1) Localised upper respiratory tract infection, dypsnoea, dirrhoea (2) Septicaemia → death. PM: widespread haemorrhages, necrosis of the liver, spleen and kidney together with enteritis, either catarrhal or haemorrhagic | Both Gram-negative rods. Cultural isolation from diseased tissue and possibly contaminated food or water supply | Other pathogens causing enteritis together with respiratory signs. |
| *Alcaligenes faecalis* and *Bordetella avium* and *B. bronchiseptica* | Both organisms shed in faeces Ingestion of the *Alicaligenes* organism and ingestion of *Bordetella* | Many species of birds susceptible but particularly Psittaciformes, turkeys and many species of finches | Both widespread in the environment, *Alcaligenes* particularly in water | Both organisms cause upper respiratory tract infection, often as secondary invaders after other primary bacterial or viral infections. *Alcaligenes* may also produce necrotic lesions in the liver | Isolation and culture of the causative specific organism | Other pathogens causing similar ante- and post-mortem signs plus necrotic liver lesions. |

Disease	Cause	Species susceptible	Relative occurrence	Principal clinical signs*	Confirmation of diagnosis	Differential diagnosis
Camylobacter sp. Several species and many serovars of varying pathogenicity (Note: *C. jejuni* often confused with *Vibrio* spp.)	Pathogenic strains of *C. jejuni* in faeces. Dogs may act as carriers and possibly also other mammals. Ingestion of animal and human sewage. Contaminated food or water	Probably all species, but particularly Galliformes, gulls, crows, waders, waterfowl, some Passeriformes	Fairly widespread. Not very stable in the environment	May act as a secondary invader to other enteric pathogens. Lethargy, marked weight loss, anorexia, diarrhoea (often yellow faeces), subacute → chronic hepatitis → death. PM often enlarged focal necrotic liver with prominent liver lobules, mucoid haemorrhagic enteritis. Many birds die of chronic liver damage	Culture from affected tissues and faeces. Must use transport medium for swabs	Other organisms causing a hepatitis together with enteritis.
		Ostriches *A zoonosis*	Can be a serious problem in young ostriches which pass typical green urine			
Klebsiella pneumoniae K. oxytoca	Non-motile Enterobacteriacae often encapsulated so survives well in the environment and resistant to many disinfectants	Pigeon, finches, waterfowl, raptors, parrots. May be transmitted to humans	Often primary pathogens particularly in some finches. Often isolated as a local infection of upper respiratory and alimentary tracts	Non-specific sick bird → septicaemia. Polydipsia/polyuria due to renal failure. Chronic respiratory signs	Isolation and culture of the causal organism	Other pathogens causing respiratory signs with polydipsia/polyuria. See DD for *Salmonella*.

Enterococcosis	*Enterococcus faecalis* Opportunistic pathogens triggered by immunosuppression and other debilitating factors. *Citrobacter* sp. Can cause secondary infection in some birds	Probably most species	Thought to be part of the autochthonous flora of avian skin, and all mucous membranes	(1) Acute post-hatching septicaemia as a result of infection through the yolk sac. (2) Respiratory infection of all species especially Passeriformes, and particularly canaries. Dyspnoea, râles (due to tracheitis), loss of normal voice	Culture and isolation. Although not strictly belonging to the Enterobacteriacae since they are Gram-positive, they grow on selective culture media for Enterobacteriacae	Air sac mites and tracheal mites which are usually the cause in Gouldian finches
Spirochaetacea Borreliosis	Biting arthropods, principally ticks act as vectors for: *Borrelia anserina (Spirochaeta gallinarum* i.e. in *Gallinarum* species)	Water-fowl, Galliformes, pigeons, Corvidae, sparrows and starlings, African grey parrots, raptors.	May be fairly common where the incidence of ticks is high. Tick bites can cause subcutaneous haemorrhage and oedema for 2–3 cm which may easily be missed at PM. Tick saliva may be toxic. Not common	Young chicks particularly susceptible, signs 4–8 days post-infection. Acute bacteraemia → fever, anorexia, depression, cyan blue congested heads. Yellow diarrhoea, ataxia → paralysis. High mobidity. Mortality up to 100%. Chronic anaemia, dyspnoea, paralysis PM. Heptomegally with haemorrhage and necrotic foci	Culture of the organism difficult. Stain blood smears with Giemsa. Gram-negative helical organism	
Non-classified spirochaetes		Sporadically occurs in the upper respiratory tract of cockatiels			Agglutination, immunofluorescence can be used	

Disease	Cause	Species susceptible	Relative occurrence	Principal clinical signs*	Confirmation of diagnosis	Differential diagnosis
Pseudo-tuberculosis	*Yersinia pseudo-tuberculosis* (Formerly called *Pasteurella pseudo-tuberculosis*). Can replicate outside host at very low temperatures if organic nitrogen available. Motile at high temps. Organism carried by rodents and wild birds which contaminate food supplies. Many soil invertebrates including molluscs act as mechanical vectors *Y. enterocolitica. Zoonotic*	All species. Wild birds, particularly those flocking in winter. Falciformes. Toucans, barbets, turacos very susceptible Birds that inhabit sewage farms	Not uncommon, particularly at the end of a severe winter Rare Mainly a human pathogen	Non-specific clinical signs in the live bird. At PM in the acute case the liver and spleen are enlarged. In the chronic condition there are yellowish white milliary necrotic foci on the liver, spleen and pectoral muscles. There may be a severe enteritis.	Bacterial isolation by culture. May take up to 2 weeks to grow. May need to store culture in fridge first. No acid fast organism on Ziel-Neelsen stained smear.	Tuberculosis. Subacute fowl cholera. *E. coli* (can produce similar milliary abscesses in liver)

Disease	Organism / Epidemiology	Species affected	Incidence	Signs / Pathology	Diagnosis	Differential
Avian cholera	Pasteurella multocida organism. P. gallinarum organism can survive and propagate in environment if conditions are favourable e.g. large volumes of water. Large numbers excreted in droppings and nasal discharge. Aerosol infection & from blood-sucking mites acting as mechanical vectors. Birds bitten by cats often develop Pasteurella infection and die in 12–24 hours	Most species / Wild Passeriformes. Owls / Diurnal raptors / Anseriformes, wild ducks concentrated by agricultural development on to small ponds or lakes may suffer high losses. / Galliformes Columbiformes	Can cause epidemics in aviaries / Sporadic epidemics, Occasional. / Uncommon / Common / Common	A highly infectious and virulent disease often producing sudden death. Dyspnoea, mucoid oral and nasal discharge, diarrhoea. PM septicaemic changes with multiple petechia. In chronic cases white serositis + necrotic foci in viscera. In raptors and pigeons – granulomatous dermatitis	Stained smear of liver imprints. Giemsa, Leishman's or methylene blue show bipolar stained rounded end rods. Culture and animal inoculation. Serological tests	E. coli. Septicaemia. Pseudo-tuberculosis (Yersiniosis). Erysipelas. Other pathogens causing respiratory or septicaemic signs
New duck disease (Anatipestifer infection)	Pasteurella (organism now reclassified as Cytophaga) anatipestifer probably from the egg and respiratory route	A specific infection of ducklings. Very occasionally other species of poultry, waterfowl and parrots	Not uncommon	Ocular discharge, diarrhoea. Signs of central nervous disease. Often just found dead. 75% mortality, survivors stunted. PM congestion of lungs, enlarged liver and spleen. Fibrinous membranes on the viscera. Pericarditis and perihepatitis. Inspissated caseation in the air sacs.	Stained smear from lesions shows Gram-negative pleomorphic rods often in long filaments. Bacterial culture and isolation of the organism. ELISA	Duck plague. Viral enteritis. Duck viral hepatitis, Coccidiosis and as above for P. multocida.

Disease	Cause	Species susceptible	Relative occurrence	Principal clinical signs*	Confirmation of diagnosis	Differential diagnosis
Actinobacillosis	*Actinobacillus* transmission by the egg	Many species	Not uncommon	Acute death → chronic cases with joint lesions. PM necrotic liver, salpingitis, peritonitis and fibrinous arthritis.	Isolation by culture stained smear polymorphic pods with bipolar staining as for *Pasteurella*	*E. coli* New duck disease (*Cytophaga*) Other bacterial infections.
Erysipelas	*Erysipelothrix rhusiopathiae* can propagate outside host in environment even in sea water and reservoirs. Carried by rodents, pigs	All species, but most common in waterfowl and fish-eating birds. Pigeons. Occasionally parrots	Only occasionally seen but can cause epidemics in aviaries, particularly in winter	Usually acute death. Dullness inappetence. Loose droppings. Septicaemic in a subacute form. Conjunctivitis may be seen in budgerigars. May see bruising of non-pigmented skin. PM widespread petechiae	Stained smear shows a Gram-positive pleomorphic slender rod-like bacterium, which is sometimes beaded. Culture liver and spleen or bone marrow if carcass is autolytic	As for avian cholera
Listeriosis	*Listeria monocytogenes*. Can survive in environment and propagate outside host. Non-pathogenic species of *Listeria* do occur	Many species. Canaries may be most susceptible	Rare, tends to be localised.	Often a peracute septicaemia, occasionally there is opisthontonus and other CNS signs. Sometimes produces a wasting disease. Often sporadic deaths in a group of birds. PM may be no gross lesions even in brain.	Stained smear from liver and brain. Shows a Gram-positive coccobacillus. Culture. Swabs require special transport medium.	CNS signs may be caused by a variety of bacterial infections, e.g. *E. coli*, *Salmonella*, *Staphylococcus*, *Klebsiella*. Also trauma and cardiopathy in old parrots.

Tuberculosis	*Mycobacterium avium*. A number of subspecies and serovars. Shed in faeces and urine → soil and water. Very resistant. Can remain up to 7 years in environment. Usually route of infection is oral.	All species. Wild birds, particularly starlings, sparrows woodpigeons	Not uncommon	Adults often maintain appetite. Debility, emaciation and diarrhoea. Anaemic. At PM tubercles can be found on and in any of the viscera, particularly the liver, which may be studded with foci.	Stained smear from tubercles. Faeces. Stained smear for acid fast organisms in bone marrow aspirate. Acid fast organisms shown by Ziel-Neelsen method, but note non-pathogenic acid fast organisms do occur. The tuberculin test is used in poultry for elimination of infected birds. Culture/biopsy. ELISA Haematology. Agglutination test. Wildfowl Trust at Slimbridge, Glos, UK will carry out test on wildfowl	Pseudo-tuberculosis (*Yersiniosis*). Possibly confused with salmonellosis or *E. coli* at PM
		Ostriches	Chronic problem in farms			
		Raptors	Not uncommon	Raptors may show persistent ulcerated and thick skin on thigh or shank and arthritis. Suspect any persistent ulceration or granuloma of the head. Not all species of birds form tuberulous granulomas		
		Anseriformes. White winged wood duck (*Cairina scutulata*) much more susceptible, little natural immunity.	Common in all birds living in aquatic environments			
		Potential zoonotic disease, particularly for immunosuppressed humans. Treatment of avian patients not recommended.				
		Parrots have contracted disease from human contacts.	Not common nowadays.			
	Mycobacterium genavense (Hoop *et al.*, 1995)	Pet birds	*Also a zoonosis*			

Disease	Cause	Species susceptible	Relative occurrence	Principal clinical signs*	Confirmation of diagnosis	Differential diagnosis
Anthrax	*Bacillus anthracis.* Vultures and scavenging raptors may act as mechanical vectors.	All species probably susceptible except vulture. Occurs if birds feed on infected meat or carrion.	In most species very rare. Usually in zoos. Occurs in ostriches	No clinical signs. Sudden death. Enlarged liver, spleen and kidneys. Areas of haemorrhage throughout carcass	Stained smear with methylene blue shows typical rod-shaped bacilli	
Botulism (Limberneck) 'Western duck sickness'	*Clostridium botulinum* 'C' toxin found in rotting carcasses and rotting vegetable and invertebrate matter. Maggots act as mechanical vectors	Particularly Anseriformes also gulls and raptors feeding on carrion. Vultures are resistant to the toxin	Not uncommon in hot, humid weather of late summer in UK, particularly in gulls. In periods of drought, particularly in shallow water	A progressive flaccid paralysis of the neck, the tongue, the legs and wings. Greenish diarrhoea due to anorexia. No PM signs. Death due to respiratory failure or drowning	Mouse protection inoculation test using specific antitoxin. Sample liver and kidney, also food or water or mud/ sewage. Deep freeze all samples	Lead poisoning. Poisoning with chlorinated hydrocarbons. Newcastle disease. In raptors hypocalcaemia. Listerosis Also during hot dry late summer, blue-green or red algal toxin. Also *Aeromonas hydrophila*

Disease	Cause	Species	Occurrence	Clinical signs	Diagnosis	Differential diagnosis
Clostridial enterotoxaemia other than caused by *Clostridium botulinum*	*Cl. perfringens* an opportunistic pathogen. Ingestion of organism from contaminated food together with: (1) Reduced gut motility (impaction) (2) Change of diet or (3) Food items inhibiting trypsin production e.g. peas, cereals, lentils, some beans (4) Diets with high sugar levels	Game birds (grouse, quail) Galliformes pigeon, captive and free ranging lorikeets	Widespread	Acute form in young birds. Diarrhoea possibly sanguinous polydipsia → death in a few hours. Chronic in older birds weight loss → death. Ulcerative necrotic enteritis of upper intestine	Gram smear from necrotic mucosa Short Gram-positive rod Spores if present central or subterminal, large and oval producing a 'safety-pin' like image Anaerobic culture ELISA for alpha beta & epsilon toxins Culture and demonstration of toxin	Newcastle virus *E. coli* *Salmonella* & other Enterobactericae Enteritis due to coccidiosis
		Ostriches	A not uncommon disease in ostriches of all ages	May be swelling and necrosis of liver and spleen Often ulcerative gastritis in ostriches		
Clostridial gangrenous dermatitis	*Cl. perfringens* *Cl. septicum* *Cl. novyi* Triggering factors: damaged skin secondary to pox virus, trauma, staphylococci, immunosuppression	Probably all species but particularly birds which are attacked by cage mates or rivals	Uncommon Birds tend to be relatively resistant to wound infection	Localised loss of feathers together with dark pigmentation of skin. May be oedematous. Death within 24 hours. PM emphysema, oedema, haemorrhage beneath skin and in muscle – also in heart muscle		

Disease	Cause	Species susceptible	Relative occurrence	Principal clinical signs*	Confirmation of diagnosis	Differential diagnosis
Haemophilus	'Contagious coryza' *H. paragallinarum*	Chickens	Not uncommon	Mainly an upper respiratory disease causing coryza, rhinitis (serous) mucoid → fibrinous exudate. Conjunctivitis and sinusitis.	Culture of organism but often not the definitive cause	Other pathogens causing respiratory signs *Chlamydia* *Pasteurella* Entero-bacteriacae (see ILT, p. 296)
	H. avium *H. paravium*	Pigeons Some parrot species Some Anseriformes Some Galliformes		Occasional pneumonic signs often as a secondary invader after other pathogens (?virus infections)		
Tularaemia	*Francisella tularensis* Rodents act as a resevoir	Pheasants, daylight and night raptors, raven. A zoonotic infection	Birds inhabiting northern and subarctic regions	PM signs as for *Pasteurella* or *Yersinia*	Short Gram-negative rod	
Megabacteriosis	*Megabacterium*	Budgerigars canaries, finches, cockatiels, lovebirds, chickens, ostriches	World-wide very common.	'Going light' syndrome Occasional blood in faeces, sporadic deaths.	Large Gram-positive rod	*Leucocytozoon*
	Possible carrier birds. Organism may be an opportunistic pathogen		In British exhibition budgerigars and incidence increasing.	X-ray shows dilation and filling defects of proventriculus, sometimes extensive.	Stain faeces, 85% of cases can be diagnosed from faecal smears.	
			Young birds lose weight and die	PM ulceration and haemorrhages in the proventriculus and gizzard.	Stain impression smears from liver and spleen.	
				Latter bile stained with degerated koilin pads	Culture difficult	

| Avian mycoplasmosis | Mycoplasma (PPL organisms) Pleuropneumonia like organisms, many strains may be commensals. Acholeplasma sp. A number of species. Infection of all Mycoplasmatodes occurs through close contact so that densely concentrated birds confined to restricted air space are most at risk | All species Turkeys Poultry and pheasants Pigeons, parrots, Passeriformes Diurnal raptors | Very common Common Not uncommon Occasional | An upper respiratory infection, coryza, sneezing, sinusitis, blepharitis. In poultry affects the joints causing lameness. Clinical signs and PM are not pathognomic. Often associated with other organisms such as staphylococci, streptococci and E. coli | Culture of the causative organism. Serology only really applicable to poultry. Intracytoplasmic inclusions in impressions stained with Giemsa | Often associated with other upper respiratory infections: ornithosis, trichomoniasis |

*In many infectious diseases of birds, both bacterial and viral, the clinical signs are not pathognomic and the disease can only be diagnosed on post-mortem and subsequent laboratory examination. In the case of viruses, infection may have occurred some considerable time previously (months) although damaged cells and immune responses may remain impaired so that the bird is open to secondary infection, but the initiating virus has disappeared from the body systems. When making a diagnosis please refer to the relevant organ system in Chapter 4 on post-mortem examination.

Other bacterial organisms such as Staphylococcus, Streptococcus, Proteus, Pseudomonas and Corynebacterium species act as secondary invaders but are not usually the prime cause of disease.

APPENDIX 3
INFECTIOUS DISEASES OF BIRDS: VIRAL/RICKETTSIAL INFECTIONS

Only the more important viruses found in avian tissues are listed, not those found only in poultry. For a more comprehensive description of avian viruses see Gerlach (1994), Ritchie (1995). See also p. 382.

Disease	Cause	Species susceptible	Relative occurrence	Principal clinical signs	Confirmation of diagnosis	Differential diagnosis
Ornithosis, psittacosis, chlamydiosis	Various strains of *Chlamydia*, rickettsia-like organisms	All species, particularly psittacines. Anseriformes. Columbiformes But also in wild owls and raptors An important *zoonotic*	Not uncommon Common	Unthriftiness. Ocular and nasal discharge dyspnoea, enteritis. These signs are not pathognomic. PM hepatomegaly – patchy faint necrosis. Mottled enlarged spleen, airsacculitis, pericarditis, sometimes serosal haemorrhage. One cause of 'one-eyed cold' in pigeons	Impression smears from liver. Stain modified Ziehl-Neelsen or Macchiavello stain. Isolation by culture of the organism from faeces and tissues. Organism can be isolated from faeces of apparently healthy birds. Polymerised chain reaction for *Chlamydia* DNA carried out by Central Veterinary Laboratories	Pacheco parrot virus. Herpes virus of other species. Pox infection. Mycoplasmosis. Trichomoniasis often together with ornithosis. Salmonellosis. Avian influenza

Herpesviridae

Thought to be a well established old group of viruses. Often produce latent and persistent infections. Replicate in the nucleus of epithelia, B and T lymphocytes and nerve tissue.

Disease	Cause	Species susceptible	Relative occurrence	Principal clinical signs	Confirmation of diagnosis	Differential diagnosis
Pacheco's parrot disease	Herpes virus. Asymptomatic carriers. Possibly at least 3 different serotypes	All Psittacines. But Old World parrots are more resistant. Conures may be asymptomatic carriers.	Not often diagnosed. May be more common than realised. World-wide.	Often peracute, may be just found dead with no premonitory signs. Acute infection, lethargy, anorexia, diarrhoea, bright green biliverdin stained faeces and urates. Occasionally conjunctivitis and tremors → convulsions. PM faintly mottled, swollen liver with saucer-shaped necrotic areas. Sometimes necrotic foci in kidney and spleen which are swollen	Isolation of causal organism by culture in embryonated eggs. Antibody titres may produce false negatives. Virus identification with VN, ELISA and immunofluorescence	*Chlamydia* infection. Bacterial hepatitis. *Salmonella*. Paramyxo virus

Disease	Cause	Species susceptible	Relative occurrence	Principal clinical signs	Confirmation of diagnosis	Differential diagnosis
Falcon inclusion body hepatitis	Herpes virus. Contaminated food or water or infected pigeons	The virus is specific for diurnal raptors, but experimentally can infect some owls, some pigeons and immature budgerigars	Widespread in northern hemisphere	Usually acute with severe depression and anorexia. A non-specific generalised disease. But the incubation period of 7–10 days is longer than for other herpes viruses. PM focal diffuse necrosis of the enlarged liver and spleen. May show signs on the lungs and kidneys and lymph follicles of intestine.	Haematology shows leucopaenia in all cases	It is possible there may be some cross infection between falcon, owl and pigeon herpes viruses
Owl herpes virus (infectious hepatosplenitis)	Herpes virus. Contaminated food or water or infected pigeons	Believed to occur only in the owls except the barn owl which is in a separate genus *Tyto*	May be more common than generally realised	May be peracute with sudden death. Necrotic foci in the oropharanx may look like trichomoniasis which can also be a secondary invader. Necrotic foci in liver, spleen, intestine and lungs.	All these viruses are closely related serologically. The viruses can be isolated in embryonated eggs.	Avian tuberculosis. Newcastle disease. Trichomoniasis. Candidiasis. *Salmonella*. Listeria. Avipox

					Histopathology	
Pigeon herpes virus (infectious oesophagitis)	Herpes virus. Contaminated feed of water	Specific for pigeons, but falcons might be susceptible by contact with infected pigeons. Also budgerigars are susceptible	Periodic epizootics in some lofts. Squabs most at risk.	Up to 15% mortality. Mainly respiratory, dyspnoea, rhinitis, conjunctivitis. Sometimes CNS signs with tremors and ataxia → paralysis. PM may show faint necrotic foci in liver and other viscera. Focal diphtheroid membrane in pharynx and larynx.	Histopathology shows intranuclear inclusion bodies from the areas of necrotic foci of liver and spleen	Paramyxo virus in pigeons
Pigeon herpes encephalomyelitis (contagious paralysis of pigeons)	A pigeon herpes virus			Progressive CNS signs. Circling, torticollis. Ataxia → paralysis. PM signs similar to those for paramyxo virus		
Crane herpes / Cicioniae herpes (stork herpes)	Two distinct unrelated viruses. Latent virus in captive birds	Cranes / Storks, both black and white	World-wide	Usually acute. Apathy and diarrhoea. Both viruses cause swelling and lesions in the liver, spleen, kidney and intestine, i.e. milliary necrotic foci. Diphtheroid membranes in upper GI tract and throughout gut in crane.		As above. Visceral coccidiosis in cranes

Disease	Cause	Species susceptible	Relative occurrence	Principal clinical signs	Confirmation of diagnosis	Differential diagnosis
Amazon tracheitis	Herpes virus. Probably a mutant strain of ILT. Probably aerial transmission. May be latent carrier birds with active infection triggered by stress	Amazon parrots. ? Bourke's parrot	More common in new imports	Peracute death. Acute and chronic (up to 9 months). Pseudomembranous tracheitis with ocular, nasal or oral exudate. Chronic dyspnoea with rales and coughing. Death due to blocked trachea.	Isolation of the causal organism in chicken embryo-chorioallantois. Swabs from oropharynx in special transport medium.	Influenza virus. Avitaminosis A. Avipox. Newcastle disease. *Candida*. Trichomoniasis.
Infectious laryngotracheitis	Herpes virus	Chickens Pheasants Peafowl Canaries May also be another separated herpes strain affecting canaries	World-wide Not common because of vaccination	*Acute form*: respiratory signs with death in 2 to 3 days. PM haemorrhagic tracheitis. *Sub-acute form*: respiratory signs less severe. Conjunctivitis, sinusitis. *Chronic form*: cough only if stressed. PM mucoid diphtheritic membranes on the upper respiratory tract with a cheesy like necrosis.	Eosinophilic intranuclear inclusion bodies found in diseased tissue in the early stages. Growth of virus in chick embryo. Virus neutralization, immunofluorensce and ELIZA tests.	Chronic fowl pox. Avitaminosis A. Newcastle disease. Infra-orbital sinusitis. *Syngamus*. Mycoplasmosis. Infectious coryza

	Cause	Species	Distribution	Clinical signs / PM	Diagnosis	Differential
Duck plague. Duck viral enteritis.	Herpes virus. Reservoir in wild waterfowl. Virus survives in pond water. Vertical transmission through the egg. Adverse climate acts as a trigger.	Ducks Geese Swans Mallard fairly resistant. Carriers shed virus for up to 5 years	World-wide Sporadic outbreaks. Epizootics result in high concentrations of virus in the local environment	Peracute – often just found dead. Blood from natural orifices. Acute form polydipsia, photophobia, ocular and nasal exudate, paralysis of the phallus, can't fly, extended neck, may drown. PM haemorrhagic eruptive lesions of the GI mucosa. Diphtheritic oesophagitis which is diagnostic.	Growth of the virus in chick embryo. VN test	Bacterial septicaemia. Avian cholera. Erysipelas. Duck picorna. Virus hepatitis. Influenza virus
Marek's disease	Herpes virus living in cells of feather follicle. Remains in feather debris for a long time. Direct and indirect transmission	Common in gallinaceous birds also in swans and ducks. Occurs in domestic fowl in birds as young as 6 weeks. Pigeons, possibly canaries, toucans. Has been reported in some wild birds. Not confirmed in raptors	World-wide. Prior to vaccination, very common in domestic poultry. Rare and sporadic in other birds	Progressive paresis and paralysis leading to emaciation. PM lymphoid infiltration of viscera, thickening of the peripheral nerves. Tumours in skin eyes and muscle	Clinical signs combined with PM picture	Avian leukosis Riboflavin deficiency causes thickening of the nerves in young chicks. If suspected in a raptor consider 'Goshawk cramps' (Forbes and Simpson, in press)

Other less important and well known herpes viruses

Disease	Cause	Species susceptible	Relative occurrence	Principal clinical signs	Confirmation of diagnosis	Differential diagnosis
Budgerigar herpes virus	Herpes virus transmitted in feathers shed in dropping	Budgerigars, double yellow headed Amazons, pigeon		Acute in some flocks, 3–5 days after initial case. Reduced hatchability. Often associated with feather duster syndrome which is a genetic problem (see Plate 10)	Isolation of virus in cell culture from feathers, blood, faeces, viscera VN or ID tests	
Lovebird herpes virus		Lovebirds		May be the cause of malformed feathers		
American bald eagle herpes virus		Bald eagle possibly other eagles	Only two cases recorded			
Lake Victoria cormorant virus		Little pied cormorant (*Phalacrocorax melanolencos*)	One isolate			
Bob white quail herpes virus	Colinus herpes virus	Bob white quail	Probably only occurs in North America	Necrotic hepatitis		
Turkey herpes virus		Turkeys, chickens		Asymptomatic in turkeys		

		Some other finches and some small Passeriformes		Apathy → dyspnoea Eyelids swollen and sealed with exudate → death. PM fibrinoid thickening of air sacs, apparently has a predilection for epithelial tissue		
Gouldian finch herpes virus						
Localised dermal disease virus	Herpes virus plus possible immunosuppression	Cockatoos, macaws		Causes wart-like lesions on the feet, but birds otherwise normal	Electron microscopy	
Conure papilloma virus	Herpes virus	Conures	One case demonstrated with cloacal papilloma			

Retroviridae

Disease	Cause	Species susceptible	Relative occurrence	Principal clinical signs	Confirmation of diagnosis	Differential diagnosis
Avian sarcoma/leucosis complex	A number of RNA viruses of the leucosis/sarcoma group. Vertical and horizontal transmission	All species, but mostly domestic poultry. Birds over 14 wks old	Rare. Incubation period may be months	Viruses can induce a whole range of neoplasms including leucosis. Tumours particularly of the liver (big liver disease) but also of the kidney, spleen and skin and other organs including long bones	PM macroscopic lesions. Usually multiple. Isolation of virus. Samples frozen	Marek's disease With other types of neoplasm the tumours are usually single. Marek's usually in birds 6–24 wks old

Disease	Cause	Species susceptible	Relative occurrence	Principal clinical signs	Confirmation of diagnosis	Differential diagnosis
Haemorrhagic conure syndrome	Ill-defined viral cause, possibly a retrovirus which may be related to sarcoma/leukosis virus	Many species of conures (*Aratinga*)		Periodic bleeding from nasal passages, dyspnoea, weakness, diarrhoea, PCV ↓ 50%. Marked heterophilia. Polychromasia and anisocytosis. Rubricytes in blood. Erythremic myelosis of bone marrow. Hypocalcaemia may trigger disease. PM multiple haemorrhages particularly in lungs		
Reticulo-endotheliosis virus	These viruses are oncogenic. Virus shed in faeces. Transmitted by biting insects. Immunosuppressive (i.e. B & T-lymphocytes affected)	Turkeys	Mostly young birds	Relatively long incubation. Diarrhoea, dilated liver, lameness. Mortality up to 60%. PM grossly enlarged liver and multiple small tumours in parenchymatous organs + cloacal bursal, thymus and bone marrow	Heparinised blood for viral isolation. Homogenate of tumourous tissue. Consult laboratory on transport media and storage and package of sample ELISA, IF or ID tests	

Disease	Cause	Species	Occurrence	Clinical signs
		Japanese quail	Young birds which have just reached sexual maturity	Depression, anorexia, dyspnoea. Mortality up to 100%. Multiple small tumours particularly along GI tract
		Pheasants and guinea fowl		Compact nodules in skin of head and oral mucosa. Caseous infra-orbital sinusitis. PM small tumours in many viscera and skeletal muscles
		Ducks, both domestic and free ranging	Disease in ducks in Australia	Non-specific signs. PM similar to that in pheasants except no skin or head lesions. Mortality 40%
		Domestic geese		
Infectious anaemia of ducks	Reticulo-endotheliosis virus. Transmitted by *Plasmodium* (avian malaria)	Ducks	Very rare	

Paramyxoviridae

Disease	Cause	Species susceptible	Relative occurrence	Principal clinical signs	Confirmation of diagnosis	Differential diagnosis
Newcastle disease (*A notifiable disease in the UK*)	Paramyxo virus serotype Group 1. Other serotypes 1–9. Infection orally, via respiratory tract. Shed in faeces. Mechanical vectors. Reservoirs in many wild bird which may carry a latent infection	All species – variable susceptibility. Galliformes – very susceptible Anseriformes – not very susceptible Raptors – not very susceptible Passeriformes, psittacines – both have a variable susceptibility. Columbiformes – fairly resistant to serotype Group 1. Ostrich – moderately susceptible, 30% mortality	World-wide Not uncommon Often latent infection Rare. Often only show mild signs but can be severe Not very common True Newcastle disease is rare	Respiratory signs with rhinitis and conjunctivitis; gastrointestinal signs with greenish, watery diarrhoea. Central nervous signs – torticollis, opisthotonos, dropping of a wing, paralysis. PM sometimes petechiae on viscera and green staining around the vent. Sometimes haemorrhagic necrotic enteritis. *Clinical signs vary with species of bird and virulence of different strains of virus. Severe conjunctivitis in humans*	Virus isolation and haemaglutination – inhibition test. Swabs from faeces, respiratory tract, in *special transport medium and ice.* PM specimens for lab, trachea, lung, spleen, liver, brain	(1) Avian pox (2) Laryno-tracheitis. (3) Falcon, crane, pigeon, owl, ciconiae herpes virus infections. A notifiable disease in the UK. B vitamin deficiencies. Listerosis Paramyxo virus disease of pigeons. *Chlamydia. Salmonella.* Lead toxicity Other infectious diseases of GI and respiratory tract

Disease	Cause/vector	Host	Distribution	Clinical signs	Diagnosis	Notes
Paramyxo disease	A mutant strain of PMV-1 (pigeon). Carried by house sparrows, blackbirds, feral pigeons	Mainly in pigeons, also in chickens, some wild raptors, parrots, pheasants, peafowl and turacos	World-wide. Common if not vaccinated. Has infected kestrels (Harcourt-Brown, 1995)	Rather vague clinical signs which, when seen, are similar to those of Newcastle disease with the central nervous signs (flaccid wings, torticollis, lameness and paralysis) being often seen first before diarrhoea. However some cases have been seen with just loose droppings and loss of weight. Adults may recover in 3–4 weeks	Haemaglutination inhibition test and virus isolation. Histopathology of brain but this may be negative	Pigeon herpes virus. Ornithosis/ Chlamydia. A notifiable disease in the UK
Paramyxo virus-(2)	Possibly carried by free ranging wild birds	Some Passeriformes (endemic) Some Galliformes	World-wide	Mostly a latent infection, sometimes a mild upper respiratory infection	As for PMV-1	
	Passeriformes, many of which are migratory	Ducks Railes Homing pigeons Some birds of prey Psittaciformes	Especially African grey parrots	These birds may just exhibit loose droppings with no CNS signs. PM young birds may have persistently enlarged bursa. Quite a severe infection with signs of weakness, loss of weight and respiratory disease, death		

Disease	Cause	Species susceptible	Relative occurrence	Principal clinical signs	Confirmation of diagnosis	Differential diagnosis
Paramyxo virus– (3)	Probably occurs in free ranging wild birds	Galliformes Some imported Passeriformes Australian finches Psittaciformes particularly *Neophema* sp. *Platycercus* sp. Domestic pigeon	Northern hemisphere Not uncommon	Conjunctivitis in finches → yellow diarrhoea, dyspnoea → some deaths, some recover. CNS signs not usually seen in finches. Parrots develop CNS signs like Newcastle disease, eye lesions and bloody nasal exudate, particularly. Torticollis. Yellow/white chalky stool containing a lot of starch and with increased appetite. Some birds emaciated → die. Mortality 30%	Histopathology of liver, kidneys and haemorrhagic enteritis Pancreatitis in parrots Check for starch with iodine (p. 27)	*Salmonella* *Chlamydia* Mycotoxin *E. coli* Avitaminosis E (van der Hage *et al.*, 1987) Psittacine adenovirus
Paramyxo virus– (5)	Kumitachi virus	Carried by free ranging budgerigars & rainbow lories	Localised area of Australia	Acute diarrhoea, dyspnoea, CNS signs → death. Mortality 50%. PM congestion of parenchymatous organs necrotic ulceration of mucosa of GI tract		

Paramyxo virus-(7)		Pigeons and doves	USA & Japan ⎫		
Paramyxo viruses-(4) (6) (8) & (9)		Waterfowl	USA & Asia ⎬	No clinical signs	
Twirling syndrome	Suspected PMV virus	Some imported old world finches		Some torticollis and circling. Emaciation. Mortality 20%. Some birds remain disabled, others recover completely	
Borna disease (Ashash *et al.*, 1995)	A single stranded negative RNA neurotrophic virus	Ostriches only. Infects many mammal species particularly horses & sheep. *A zoonotic disease.* Horizontal transmission from faeces	Young up to 90 days of age. Diagnosed in Jordan valley of Israel	Acute paresis (chicks 14–42 days old). Incordination → recumbancy. Death due to secondary infection. Morbidity & mortality up to 20%	Histopathology of lumbo sacral spinal cord. ELISA and IF tests

Avipox viridae

Disease	Cause	Species susceptible	Relative occurrence	Principal clinical signs	Confirmation of diagnosis	Differential diagnosis
Avian pox *Avipox* spp.	Avian pox viruses. At least 17 distinct viruses identified. Mostly adapted to different families of birds so that some are species specific. Crosta *et al.* (1995) recorded an outbreak confined to Neophema parakeets in a mixed collection. These viruses often transmitted by biting arthropod vectors. Mites, ticks, mosquitoes retain viruses for up to 8 weeks	Most species susceptible to a species specific virus. Including ostrich, mortality 10–15% in young birds	Common in Passeriformes more common in S. American parrots than Australian parrots. Uncommon in raptors and generally mild. Localised when mosquitoes about in late summer. Geographically important in the Middle East (see Plate 6).	*Acute form*: septicaemic sudden death. Usually in canaries. Due to pneumonia. *Sub-acute to chronic form*: yellowish papules changing to brown appear on the skin of head and legs. *Dry form*: usually in Passeriformes and raptors. Conjunctivitis, erythrema, oedema, lachrymation, dysphagia because diphtheric lesions appear in oropharynx, if diphtheric membranes removed – bleeding. This often seen in parrots, pheasants, pigeons and starlings, some pigeons and Passeriformes which survive subsequently develop wart-like neoplasms	Histopathology. Bollinger bodies – intracytoplasmic inclusions seen in the epithelium of the skin, respiratory tract, oral cavity. Viral culture from faecal samples ID or VN tests but serology often not a lot of help	Avitaminosis A. Pigeon herpes (infectious oesophagitis). Newcastle disease. Laryngo-tracheitis. Amazon tracheitis. Trauma. Trichophyton. Chemidocoptes. Trichomoniasis. Candidiasis. Aspergillosis.

Orthomyxoviridae

Disease	Cause	Species susceptible	Relative occurrence	Principal clinical signs	Confirmation of diagnosis	Differential diagnosis
Avian influenza Fowl plague	Influenza 'A' virus. A number of serotypes. Free living water-fowl reservoir of infection. 25–30% latent infection. May release very large amounts of virus in summer and be related to human pandemics	Mynahs Passeriformes Turacos Galliformes Ducks and other Anseriformes Sea birds Psittacines Not seen in pigeons *A zoonosis*	World-wide Not uncommon. Spread by migratory birds (Bourne, 1989) Rare	An inapparent sinusitis to a severe respiratory disease. In parrots may cause CNS signs	Virus isolation and serology. Swabs from cloaca and upper respiratory tract. PM samples from viscera in ice. ELISA or ID test	Ornithosis Newcastle disease Fowl cholera Mycoplasma

Picornaviridae

Disease	Cause	Species susceptible	Relative occurrence	Principal clinical signs	Confirmation of diagnosis	Differential diagnosis
Duck virus hepatitis Type I	Picorna virus spread in faeces. Rats may act as a mechanical vector	Ducklings from 2 weeks of age. Mallard ducklings infected but not susceptible to the disease. May attack duck species in zoos	Not uncommon. World-wide	Peracute. Sudden death within hours. Maybe sluggishness then CNS signs, e.g. opisthotonos PM. Liver enlarged and shows petechial haemorrhages. Mortality may be 100%	Inoculation of the embryonated chicken egg	Often secondarily infected with *Salmonella* or *Chlamydia*. Duck enteritis. Bacterial septicaemias. Coccidiosis. Mycotoxicosis

Type II	An astro-virus probably spread by free ranging wild gulls		Localised in East Anglia	Mortality 10–50%	
Type III		Mallards and domestic ducks only susceptible	Only in USA	Mortality up to 30%	
Specific avian encephalomyelitis. Epidemic tremor	Picornavirus. Vertical transmission. Latent carriers	Mainly a poultry disease, can affect pigeons and Anseriformes. Pheasants, partridge, quail, black grouse, capercaillie	World-wide. Affects young chicks 1–6 weeks	CNS signs – epidemic tremors paralysis, incordination. Fall in egg production in older birds (5–10%). Survivors develop eye lesions	Inoculation of embryonic eggs and serology. ID and ELISA test. Histopathology of brain, proventriculus, pancreas and heart	Newcastle disease. Marek's disease. Vitamin E and selenium deficiency. Lead poisoning
Viral enteritis of cockatoos	Not vertically transmitted	Free ranging rose breasted cockatoos, sulphur-crested cockatoos and galahs 6–9 weeks	Australia	Birds affected just after they have left the nest. Profuse yellow-green faeces. Anorexia, weight loss, death. Mortality 10–20%	Histopathology of intestine

Parvoviridae

Disease	Cause	Species susceptible	Relative occurrence	Principal clinical signs	Confirmation of diagnosis	Differential diagnosis
Goose virus hepatitis Goose influenza Goose plague	Parvo virus Lateral transmission Oral and nasal exudate	Goslings of domestic goose, Canada goose, Muscovy ducks	Europe/Asia Not uncommon	Anorexia, polydipsia, coryza, diarrhoea, ataxia. PM fibrinous exudate of viscera. *Enlarged liver* petechiae haemorrhages. Up to 100% mortality	Virus identification. VN and ELISA tests	Gosling reovirus which is predominantly a respiratory infection. Goose adenovirus infection

Togaviridae and Flaviviridae (i.e. Arboviruses)

Disease	Cause	Species susceptible	Relative occurrence	Principal clinical signs	Confirmation of diagnosis	Differential diagnosis
Eastern and western equine encephalitis and other encephalitis. Encephalomyelitis	Arboviruses transmitted by biting insects. Mainly in the Americas but also in other parts of the world	Birds may act as important hosts. All species including ratites. Galliformes, Passeriformes, house sparrows in N. America, Anseriformes most susceptible. *A zoonosis*	Possibly common carriers in birds. Clinical disease in birds rare. *Mainly* in Western hemisphere	May cause CNS signs in birds, i.e. paralysis, incoordination. Torticollis. Mortality up to 80%. Sometimes haemorrhagic enteritis.	Virus isolation from brain homogenate. HI, ELISA tests	

Disease	Cause	Species susceptible	Relative occurrence	Principal clinical signs	Confirmation of diagnosis	Differential diagnosis
Avain viral serositis	An arbovirus May be related to neuropathic gastric dilatation	Parrots, i.e. macaws & rose ringed parakeets	Only identified in USA	Acute death or weight loss + distended abdomen with ascites. PM hepatomegally oedema of lungs intestinal and hepatic serosa congested	Histopathology of proventriculus & gizzard, spleen, brain, heart & skeletal muscle	
Louping ill virus	Arbovirus spread by ticks	Grouse species (Duncan et al., 1978) & pheasants. A zoonosis	Northern hemisphere Shown to cause considerable reduction of black grouse on Welsh uplands Birds most at risk inhabit moorlands	CNS signs		
St Louis encephalitis Japanese B-encephalitis Murray valley encephalitis	All caused by Arboviruses spread by mosquitoes Resevoirs in wild birds	Carried by more than 30 species of birds including house sparrow, heron, ibises & cormorants. A zoonosis	USA Japan Australia	Asymptomatic in birds		

There are at least 7 other aboviruses in various parts of the world which are transmitted by mosquoties and ticks and which are spread by migratory birds (Jericová, 1993) and guillemots. They have a zoonotic potential causing CNS signs in humans although they are asymptomatic in the infected birds. Although they have not yet been documented as occurring in ostriches they may yet be found to do so.

Rhabdoviridae

Disease	Cause	Species susceptible	Relative occurrence	Principal clinical signs	Confirmation of diagnosis	Differential diagnosis
Rabies virus	Many species of birds, particularly raptors & scavengers are documented as carrying the virus and also as reservoirs of the infection	Birds do not usually develop active infection because of their rapid production of antibodies. *Zoonotic* but not from birds	World-wide (except UK) Birds are not documented as spreading the disease to humans	Occasionally after an incubation period of 2–42 days affected birds may show a change in behaviour towards human contacts & develop epileptiform fits as well as other CNS signs → die	VN antibodies can be detected in nerve tissue	

Circoviridae

Disease	Cause	Species susceptible	Relative occurrence	Principal clinical signs	Confirmation of diagnosis	Differential diagnosis
Black spot canary disease (Goldsmith, 1995)	Circo virus unrelated to the circovirus of cockatoo beak and feather disease	Canary chicks up to 7–20 days	Not uncommon in Europe, also in USA	Abdominal enlargement due to swollen gallbladder. Mortality 90%	Necrosis of bursa. Yellow fluid in air sacs. Electron microscopy	*Plasmodium.* Atoxoplasmosis also called 'black spot' (p. 333)

Disease	Cause	Species susceptible	Relative occurrence	Principal clinical signs	Confirmation of diagnosis	Differential diagnosis
Psittacine beak and feather syndrome. An immuno-suppressive disease (see p. 34)	A recently discovered new type of virus. Circo virus. Endemic in free ranging cockatoos of Australia and SE Asia. Transmission through faeces, crop epithelium (feeding chicks), feathers and dust, probably also vertical transmission	Probably all old world psittacines. Also documented in Janday conure and green-winged macaw, pionus parrot, Amazons	Originally from Australia. Not uncommon in captive parrots. Usually fatal in 6–12 months but can live up to 10 years	Loss of normal contour feathers, replaced by abnormal plumage, i.e. short club-like feathers, fret lines in the vane, constrictions on the shaft, curled feather. Feather retained in blood-filled sheath. Beak becomes more shiny, elongated, shows fault lines, surface flakes off. Tip necrotic. In vasa parrots black plumage replaced by white feathers. African greys may develop red instead of grey feathers (see Plate 12)	Histopathology. Feather biopsy in 10% formal saline. Intracytoplasmic basophilic inclusion bodies in feather pulp and follicular epithelium. DNA probe 0.5 ml blood. Lesions usually bilaterally symmetrical and involve head feathers (see p. 70)	Polyoma virus. May also cause 'French moult' in budgerigars. Also adenovirus, bacterial and fungal feather follicle infections. Suspect all feather abnormalities particularly in neonates and fledglings

Papovaviridae

Disease	Cause	Species susceptible	Relative occurrence	Principal clinical signs	Confirmation of diagnosis	Differential diagnosis
Papova viruses I Polyomavirus (budgerigar fledgling disease)	A papova-like agent reported by Bernier et al. (1981) Horizontal and vertical transmission from feeding chicks. Feather dust. Sub-clinical carriers. Intermittently shed in droppings. Environmentally stable virus	Nestling budgerigars 1–15 days of age. Similar syndromes seen in other psittacines and in some finches	May be more common than realised. World-wide	Abdominal distension lack of down feathers on back and abdomen. Hydropericardium. Enlarged heart. Enlarged liver. Ascites. Liver shows multiple white or yellow spots. Mortality 30–100%. Some die suddenly without signs. Survivors become 'runners' (one cause of 'French moult'. Symmetrical feather lesions in other Psittaformes. Feather dystrophy less evident. Much more a GI disease with subcutaneous and other haemorrhages. CNS signs. Occasionally surviving finches may show lower beak abnormalities	DNA probe 0.5 ml blood or cloacal swab or swab from cut surface of liver, spleen. Intranuclear inclusion in epidermis and feather follicles	Birds which have feather dystrophy Cockatoo beak and feather disease Other bacterial infections Strains of virus may be different in (1) budgerigars, (2) finches, (3) other psittacines. Sudden death even in adult birds

Disease	Cause	Species susceptible	Relative occurrence	Principal clinical signs	Confirmation of diagnosis	Differential diagnosis
II Benign papillomas	Papilloma virus. May be carried by wild chaffinch, although this may be a distinct strain	Parrots (see Plate 7) Some finches (Fringillidae) Canaries (Dom *et al.*, 1993)	Not uncommon	Wart-like growths on legs and feet of finches. Also on many other unfeathered skin areas of parrots. Also papillomas of GI tract. Particularly, cloaca, oesophagus and bile duct	Application of 5% acetic acid will turn papilloma lesions white. Histopathology. Many Amazons also have malignant bile and pancreatic duct carcinomas	Avian pox. Herpes virus in cockatoos. Dysphagia from other causes. Haemorrhagic cloacal prolapse particularly in Amazon parrots (see p. 169)

Adenoviridae

Infection of birds other than poultry. The situation is complex, often these viruses cause CNS signs as well as hepatitis, nephritis and respiratory signs.

Disease	Cause	Species susceptible	Relative occurrence	Principal clinical signs	Confirmation of diagnosis	Differential diagnosis
Adenovirus infection. All adenoviruses are environmentally persistent	Usually an opportunistic pathogens. Latent carrier birds shed virus in faeces & susceptible birds ingest virus. Also vertical transmission	Many species are known to be susceptible and in the future many more are likely to be found to be so	World-wide. May act as a trigger for other diseases, e.g. bacterial, fungal, protozoa. Also required by parvoviruses to complete their replication	There is often reduced hatchability without other clinical signs. Gross PM often non-specific	*All adenoviruses* Histopathology of liver, kidney, pancreas. Usually basophilic but sometimes eosinophilic intranuclear inclusion bodies. Upper respiratory tract, VN, viral culture, DNA probes, ELISA, electron microscopy	

GROUP I FOWL ADENOVIRUS
12 serotypes and a number of subgroups of varying pathognicity

Disease	Cause	Species susceptible	Relative occurrence	Principal clinical signs	Confirmation of diagnosis	Differential diagnosis
Guinea fowl		Guinea fowl	Young chicks very susceptible	Main clinical signs necrotic pancreatitis		
Japanese quail		Japanese quail	Isolated from chicks	Showed CNS signs		
Adenovirus chick diseases	Vertical and horizontal transmission	Chickens	Chicks 5–7 wks	Anorexia, white pasty faeces → death		
Quail bronchitis		Quail bronchitis (Bob white quail)	Young birds up to 6 weeks. Game farms in USA	Acute death or severe respiratory distress. Occasional CNS signs. PM respiratory system & hepatic necrosis, excess mucus in airways, cloudy air sac membranes		
Pigeon inclusion body hepatitis & inclusion body enteritis	May be more than one virus type involved in adenovirus infection of pigeons	Pigeons	All ages affected but usually young birds under a year. Fairly common in spring & summer when they are breeding & racing (i.e. enclosed in transporter trucks)	Dull, anorexia, mucoid green droppings, polyipsia, vomiting, dyspnoea. PM hepatospleno- mengally & haemorrhagic enteritis	Paramyxo I hexamitiasis	

Disease	Cause	Species susceptible	Relative occurrence	Principal clinical signs	Confirmation of diagnosis	Differential diagnosis
Raptor adenovirus disease	Possible source dead hatchery chicks (both chicken & turkey)	Goshawk	One isolated case	CNS signs, clonic fits		
		American kestrel	One isolated case	Haemorrhagic enteritis, anaemia, high mortality		
		Merlin	One isolated case	Hepatitis		
		Mauritius kestrel (Forbes *et al.*, in press). Bengalese eagle owl, white bellied sea eagle (Forbes *et al.*, in press)	Two isolated epizootics	Peracute Collapse anaemic → death. PM mucohaemorrhagic enteritis, hepatosplenomegally 100% morbidity & mortality		
Psittacine adenovirus infection		Psittaciformes Lovebirds		Blepharitis & nephritis 30% mortality. Pancreatitis & nephritis. PM distended proventriculus & duodenum		
		Eclectus parrots		Mild diarrhoea sometimes acute death		

Disease	Cause	Species susceptible	Relative occurrence	Principal clinical signs	Confirmation of diagnosis	Differential diagnosis
		Pionus parrots Neophema parakeets		Enteritis + CNS signs also pancreatitis Similar to paramyxovirus infection		Paramyxovirus infection
		Budgerigars	One documented chronic epizootic (Gassman et al., 1981)	CNS signs Hepatitis, enteritis, pancreatitis		
Adenovirus disease of waterfowl		Muscovy ducks		Lameness & emaciation, mortality about 10–15%, some have bronchitis & pneumonia		
		Goslings Free ranging herring gulls		Hepatitis, with a high mortality	Adenovirus-like particles in hepatocytes	Goose parvo virus infection
Ostrich fading chick syndrome (Raines et al., 1995)	Untyped adenovirus	Ostriches		Weight loss, anorexia, chalky faeces, ascites, death in 2–3 weeks		

Group II adenovirus

Disease	Cause	Species susceptible	Relative occurrence	Principal clinical signs	Confirmation of diagnosis	Differential diagnosis
Marble spleen disease	Latently infected birds' faeces	Pheasants, guinea fowl & chickens, possibly in blue grouse	Global	Acute death grossly enlarged spleen, mottled grey. Subacute anorexia dyspnoea and diarrhoea	DNA probe virus isolation	

Disease	Cause	Species susceptible	Relative occurrence	Principal clinical signs	Confirmation of diagnosis	Differential diagnosis
Turkey haemorrhagic enteritis	Shed in faeces	Turkeys, chickens, pheasants	Global	Rapid spread through flock chicks 4–12 wks. 60% mortality	Elisa	

Group III adenovirus

Disease	Cause	Species susceptible	Relative occurrence	Principal clinical signs	Confirmation of diagnosis	Differential diagnosis
Turkeys, domestic geese, Muscovy ducks, chickens, cattle egrets all asymptomatic carriers			Europe & Asia	Causes soft shelled eggs		
Guinea fowl						

Coronaviridae

Disease	Cause	Species susceptible	Relative occurrence	Principal clinical signs	Confirmation of diagnosis	Differential diagnosis
Infectious bronchitis	Coronavirus carried by chickens possibly wild birds (owls & Passeriformes)	Pheasants	World-wide, common in UK. Chicks most susceptible	Moderate respiratory signs Reduced egg production 40% mortality in chicks PM swollen kidney and visceral gout, egg peritonitis	Specimens to the laboratory for virus isolation must be in 50% glycerol and deep frozen	
		Guinea fowl	Chicks most suceptible	Respiratory signs only mild otherwise clinical signs similar to those in pheasants plus enteritis and pancreatitis		
		Psittaciformes including budgerigars	Only two instances of recorded natural infection	Necrotic hepatosplenitis		
		Pigeons	One documented instance	Respiratory signs with mucopharyngitis plus ulcerated crop and oesophagus		

Disease	Cause	Species susceptible	Relative occurrence	Principal clinical signs	Confirmation of diagnosis	Differential diagnosis
		Ostrich chicks, Rhea (Kennedy and Brenneman, 1995)		Anorexia, loss of weight, enteritis Low mortality Proventriculus thin walled and enlarged filled with food		
		Japanese quail	One documented instance	Respiratory signs.		

Reoviridae

Disease	Cause	Species susceptible	Relative occurrence	Principal clinical signs	Confirmation of diagnosis	Differential diagnosis
Reovirus diseases	Sub-group orthovirus. Probably immunosuppressive virus. Latent carriers. Shed in faeces. Virus ingested. Some reovirus strains not pathogenic. Virus occurs in Galliformes, raptors, pheasants as well as those species which are susceptible	Psittaformes, probably old world parrots are more susceptible than those from the Americas	World-wide	Reovirus is immunosuppressive therefore signs often complicated by secondary infections. Often non-pathognomonic. Eyes swollen, enteritis, emaciation, incoordination. PM swollen liver, kidney & spleen, necrotic areas and fluid in lungs. Mortality 70–100%	Cloacal swabs or at PM swabs from viscera, liver, spleen, kidney for virus isolation. Electron microscopy. May get false negatives	

Cause	Host	Distribution	Clinical signs and post-mortem	Virus/Disease
	Pigeons	Approximately 10% of pigeons in Europe	Diarrhoea and dyspnoea PM mucoid enteritis	
	Muscovy ducks and their hybrids	Affects ducklings in France	Stunted growth and feather dystrophy. Mortality up to 90% PM inflammation of pericardium and air sacs	Adenovirus disease of waterfowl
	Geese	Goslings	Peracute death or dullness, anorexia, mild respiratory signs and grey/white diarrhoea, weakness and tremor. PM grey dilated heart and respiratory and liver lesions	Goose parvovirus. Adenovirus disease of waterfowl
	Finches		Enteritis and obviously swollen liver PM multiple areas of necrosis throughout viscera	
Orbivirus (i.e. a sub-group of the reoviruses). Transmitted by biting insects	Budgerigars and cockatiels		Acute death. Myocarditis Hepatosplenomegaly, enteritis	

Disease	Cause	Species susceptible	Relative occurrence	Principal clinical signs	Confirmation of diagnosis	Differential diagnosis
Reovirus diseases	Reovirus (sub-group rotavirus). Ingestion of virus shed in faeces. Asymptomatic in ducks and one lovebird	Occurs in Galliformes	World-wide	Stunting	Electron microscopy	
		Pheasants	Chicks	Diarrhoea and stunting Mortality 30%		
		Pigeons	Fairly common	Watery diarrhoea		
		May occur in other species		PM signs non-specific.		

Other diseases which may have viral causes

Disease	Cause	Species susceptible	Relative occurrence	Principal clinical signs	Confirmation of diagnosis	Differential diagnosis
Neuropathic gastric proventicular dilation of Psittacines (Macaw wasting disease, Psittacine myoenteric-ganglioneuritis, encephalomyelitis of parrots)	Suspect virus-like particles seen in spinal cord and coeliac ganglion electron microscopy. Destruction of intramural ganglia (Auerbach's plexus), of proventriculus, ventriculus & first part of duodenum. Also affects autonomic gangia of heart, brain and spinal cord. Possibly carried by some free ranging wild birds	Documented in many Psittacine species	Probably world-wide. An increasingly common problem in North and South America. Has been epidemic in some aviaries. Not uncommon in Europe	A chronic disease with possibly a long incubation period of up to 2 years. Usually in young birds. Depression, progressive loss of weight, vomiting, undigested seed in droppings, anorexia, weakness, possible lameness (CNS involved), marked leucocytosis (heterophilia and monocytosis). Death after prolonged disease. PM emaciation, distended and impacted proventriculus and crop. Muscle layers of gizzard white and atrophied → may ulcerate and rupture.	Barium contrast radiograph. Very reduced emptying time of proventriculus. Biopsy of crop or better still proventriculus but difficult surgically and risky on debilitated patient. Also may produce false negatives	Vitramin E and selenium deficiency. Neoplasia of upper GI tract. Foreign body in proventriculus. Pyloric obstruction → gastric impaction. Megabacterial infection. Nematode infection. Visceral larval migrans

Disease	Cause	Species susceptible	Relative occurrence	Principal clinical signs	Confirmation of diagnosis	Differential diagnosis
Similar disease		Free ranging Canada geese				
Runting and stunting syndrome	May have a similar cause	Broiler chickens Goshawk (Forbes and Simpson, in press)	Suspected case in 4-week-old bird			See pp. 321 and 322

APPENDIX 4:
INFECTIOUS DISEASES OF BIRDS: MYCOTIC DISEASES

Disease	Cause	Species susceptible	Relative occurrence	Principal clinical signs	Confirmation of diagnosis	Differential diagnosis
Aspergillosis. Can be a primary or a secondary infection	*Aspergillus* sp. e.g. *fumigatus, flavus, niger, tenens* At least 200 species, all of which are normally saprophytic and found in damp, mouldy straw, hay, wood chips, etc. The spores are ubiquitous	All species captive and wild including ostrich chicks. More common in diving birds, possibly because of air recirculation when diving. Also not uncommon in parrots and raptors	Common predisposing causes: (1) hypovitaminosis A, (2) stress, (3) challenge by massive dose of spores, (4) age i.e. young birds or aged birds, (5) injudicious use of antibiotics, steroids, etc., (6) ammonical fumes in poorly ventilated aviaries and poor hygiene	Can be sudden death, particularly in young, if organism is spread haematogenously. More usually debility and emaciation, resp. signs (10% of acute resp. obstruction cases caused by aspergillosis), post-paralysis, due to lesion in spine. PM appearance of lesions variable. Yellow miliary nodules in lung, disc-like plaques of grey or white + necrosis in resp. and GI tracts. Granulomata	Often heterophilia and monocytosis + non-regenerative anaemia. Examine lesions for signs of hyphae and fruiting bodies, look for typical 'foot' cell and septate banches. Use 20% KOH and stain with lactophenol cotton blue or new methylene blue. Radiography, laparoscopy, tracheal swab, abdominal swabs for culture and cytology. ELISA not very reliable or agar gel diffusion test	Tuberculosis *Yersinia* Avipox Trichomoniasis *Candida* *Syngamus* *E. coli* Hypovitaminosis A in parrots. Also *Salmonella* can produce granulomatous plaques

Disease	Cause	Species susceptible	Relative occurrence	Principal clinical signs	Confirmation of diagnosis	Differential diagnosis
Candidiasis (Moniliasis) A primary or secondary infection	*Candida albicans* (*Monilia*). May occur in normal gut flora and overgrow after indiscriminate use of antibiotic and bad hygiene or stress.	Pigeons, turkeys, partridges, grouse, budgerigars, psittacines, Passeriformes	Not uncommon, particularly in young birds. Said to be common in nectar-feeding birds.	Vomiting, delayed crop emptying, loss of condition, anorexia, sporadic deaths. PM mucosa of crop and oesophagus thickened and covered in a soft, whitish cheesy material under which the mucosa is velvet-like. Occasionally in proventriculus. Also of cloaca, resp. tract and skin.	If possible examine the crop in a live bird with a laparoscope. Wet mount smears stained with lactophenol blue, Gram strain, methylene blue or Giemsa show budding, yeast-like organisms. Occasionally hyphae. Histopathology.	Trichomoniasis (Macroscopically *Candida* lesions are indistinguishable from trichomoniasis). Sour crop causing a bacterial necrosis. *Salmonella typhimurium* in passerines can infect the crop. In psittacines neuropathic gastric dilation formerly known as macaw wasting disease. Other mycotic disease. Hypovitaminosis A. Foreign bodies (see p. 38).

	Organism/Source	Host	Clinical signs	Diagnosis	Differential
Cryptococcosis (Torulosis) (Blastomycosis)	*Cryptococcus neoformans* A common saprophytic yeast found on plant and organic material often excreted and found on faeces. *Potentially a serious and fatal zoonosis,* particularly from sick birds kept in insanitary conditions in old wooden aviaries. Inhalation of dust containing spores	Probably all captive species	Ubiquitous but particularly in faeces of Passeriformes, *Galliformes* and pigeons	In birds can cause dyspnoea, debility, emaciation, non-regenerative anaemia and generalised necrotising gelatinous granulomata in viscera.	Impression smears. Stain or use Indian Ink. Look for thickly encapsulated yeast-like organisms.	Other mycotic infections.
Histoplasmosis	*Histoplasma* sp. Another soil saprohyte found in bird faeces. Can build up in aviaries with earthen floors. *Potentially zoonotic.* By inhalation	Probably all species. May be carried as a latent infection by many wild birds particularly pigeons.	Ubiquitous, but much more common in geographically local areas particularly some river valleys. May only be pathogenic in immuno-suppressed birds	May be some respiratory signs accompanied by loss of condition, diarrhoea and hepatopathy	Histopathology particularly of liver and spleen	Other mycoses

Disease	Cause	Species susceptible	Relative occurrence	Principal clinical signs	Confirmation of diagnosis	Differential diagnosis
Dermatomycosis (ringworm) (favus)	*Trichophyton* sp. *Cladosporium* sp.	Probably occurs in all species but particularly Passeriformes. A zoonosis	Uncommon	Loss of feathers. Skin thickened; greyish-white, lifeless. Skin has tendency to be corrugated and encrusted. White crust on comb or wattles causing 'fowl favus'.	Microscopical examination of skin scrapings. Stain with Gram strain. Histopathology, culture.	Mange mite infection.
Actinomycosis	*Actinomyces* spp. Reported by Coffin in parrots. One case seen by the author in a Moluccan cockatoo which formed a granuloma caudal to the vent.	Possibly all species can become infected via an open wound	Uncommon in birds	Except when sub-cutaneous signs rather vague. Loss of bodily condition causes granulomata of subcutaneous tissue and viscera	Histopathology	Aspergillosis and other mycoses

Other rare mycotic infections of birds are caused by *Penicillium, Nocardia, Rhinosporidium* (from sprouted seed), *Mucor* sp. (hyphae in vascula endothelium of finches).

APPENDIX 5:
PARASITIC DISEASES OF BIRDS: PROTOZOAL PARASITES

Coccidiosis and related parasitic diseases

The coccidia comprise an extremely variable and large group of protozoan parasites, all of which are in the family Eimeriidae. Many species are host specific and all propagate both asexually (which in some genera of coccidians takes place in an intermediate host) and sexually (in the definitive host). The latter results in the production of an environmentally resistant oocyst formed in the enteric/mucosal cells of the definitive host. After maturation (i.e. sporulation) the oocyst produces infectious sporozoites. Often severe disease does not result in the definitive host in contrast to often fatal disease caused in the intermediate host.

All parasites within this group thrive in batches of stressed and crowded birds kept under insanitary conditions. The young are particularly vulnerable with adult birds acting as latent carriers.

Disease	Cause	Species susceptible	Relative occurrence	Principal clinical signs	Confirmation of diagnosis	Differential diagnosis
Cyst forming protozoan parasites causing classical coccidiosis	*Eimeria* sp. (at least 160 species infect birds) A host genera specific parasite	Poultry, pigeons, game birds, toucans	Common	Can vary from being apathogenic to disease with vague signs to severe mucoid sanguinous diarrhoea. Sometimes just acute death	In most species infected with coccidians, faecal exam. shows oocysts characteristic for each genera. Sporolation outside the host may require several days. Identification of individual species of coccidian is important to indicate the range of susceptible species, including possible intermediate hosts: *Eimeria* sp. oocyst has 4 sporocysts each with 2 sporozoites	
		Budgerigars	Common in Australia, elsewhere more rare	*Eimeria truncata* infects the kidneys of geese and some other Anseriformes. Kidneys are swollen and covered in white patches. Oocysts seen on impression smears.		
		Parrots (except lories)	Uncommon			
		Anseriformes	Not uncommon			
		Raptors	Occasional			

world-wide

Disease	Cause	Species susceptible	Relative occurrence	Principal clinical signs	Confirmation of diagnosis	Differential diagnosis
In these coccidians the life cycle is completed in one host and infection is by ingestion of the sporulated oocyst.	*Isospora* sp. Not so host specific as *Eimeria* and often not so pathogenic	Infects many avian species including ratites, canaries, finches and other Passerines	Common	Signs as for *Eimeria*	*Isospora* sp. oocyst has 2 sporocysts each with 4 sporozoites.	
	Dorisiella sp.	Passeriformes	Common	Signs as for *Eimeria* but may not be very pathogenic	*Dorisiella* sp. oocyst has 2 sporocysts each containing 8 sporozoites	
	Tyzzeria sp.	Ducks		Quite pathogenic. Haemorrhagic white lesions in caudal intestine.	*Tyzzeria* oocyst contains no sporocyst only 8 freely separated sporozoites	
	Wenyonella sp.	Ducks and Passerines			*Wenyonella* oocyst contains 4 sporocysts each with 4 sporozoites	

world-wide

Related coccidian parasites with an indirect lifecycle

Predators act as the definitive host while prey species are often the intermediate host in which asexual reproduction occurs

	Host	Distribution	Signs / pathology	Diagnosis	Notes
Cryptosporidium sp. Not so host specific as *Eimeria* and may be opportunistic invader infecting immuno-suppressed birds	Infects a wide range of avian species including Galliformes, Anseriformes, Psittaciformes, raptors and the ostrich	World-wide	As well as lesions in the alimentary canal the parasite invades the whole body but particularly the bursa of fabricus, the kidneys and upper resp. tract causing excess mucus with marked resp. signs both premonitary and PM as well as signs in GI tract. Parasite replicates *on the surface* of epithelia	Very small oocyst often difficult to find by faecal exam. Also intermittently shed. Stain faeces with Giemsa. Oocyst similar to *Isospora* but is already sporulated when shed, often releasing sporocysts directly into faeces.	Not often epizootic. Note reovirus infected birds
Caryospora sp. (over 100 species) some species may not be strictly host specific	Raptors including owls. Rodents are the intermediate host	May be more common in wild raptors than so far documented	Dependent on the host species infected. The parasite may or may not be pathogenic. Pathogenisis shows listlessness, anorexia, mucoid haemorrhagic diarrhoea, muscle cramps or acute death without premonitary signs.	Faecal exam. shows large oocyst containing 8 non-encysted stubby sporozoites.	
Frenkelia sp. (only 2 species recorded)	Both species occur in buzzards including the red tailed hawk	N. America	Non-pathogenic in the definitive host but causes severe and fatal illness in the intermediate host (rodents)	Sporulated oocyst contains 2 sporocysts each with 4 sporozoites	

Disease	Cause	Species susceptible	Relative occurrence	Principal clinical signs	Confirmation of diagnosis	Differential diagnosis
	Sarcocystis sp. very many species Invertebrates may act as mechanical vectors	Documented in a broad range of vertebrate species including many birds. Raptors (including owls) may act as both definitive and intermediate host. Captive old world parrots in USA particularly at risk. Native opossum is definitive host	World-wide although some species of *Sarcocystis* have restricted geographical range. Carried by many raptors and their prey species, e.g. Passerines, rodents, deer, etc.	Dependent on the species of sarcocyst, the host and the circumstances, the parasite may or may not be pathogenic even fatal. Sarcocysts (i.e. encysted schizonts) sometimes found incidently in muscle when host has died of unrelated disease. When pathogenic in parrots causes dullness, dypsnoea, hepatopathy, sudden death. PM hepatosplenomegally and pneumonic histopathology.	Sporulated oocyst contains 2 sporocysts containing 4 sporozoites. Although schizongony occurs throughout the body sarcocyst formation takes place primarily in the muscle and may cause severe tissue reaction	
	Hammondia sp. *Besnoitia* sp. Similar parasites to *Sarcocystis*			Schizonts of *Besnoitia* sp. documented in muscle of parakeets.		

| Other cyst forming protozoan parasites | *Toxoplasma gondii* Not a host specific parasite. Can invade most if not all vertebrate species which act as the intermediate host, only the Felidae act as the definitive host. Birds become infected from food contaminated by cat faeces or in carnivorous birds by ingestion of carcase tissue containing cysts. A zoonotic disease | Toxoplasma cysts (i.e. resting stage of parasite) documented as found throughout the tissues of many vertebrate species including birds Pathogenic: in parrots in Anseriformes in Passeriformes | World-wide and ubiquitous   Not common Quite common Occasional | In birds the parasite may or may not be pathogenic. Pathogenesis is caused by asexual multiplication within the intermediate host's tissues causing focal necrosis resulting in anorexia, weight loss, diarrhoea, resp. signs, conjunctivitis and CNS signs. Can be fatal in many parrots and cause severe disease in Anseriformes | The oocyst is only found in the faeces of cats (the definitive host). Diagnosis in birds is by histopathology and use of various serological tests | Any other disease causing CNS signs, e.g. Newcastle, paramyxo, listerella. |
| | *Atoxoplasma* sp. (formerly *Lankesterella*). Infection by ingeston of oocyst in faeces of infected bird. Direct life cycle originally thought to be transmitted by red mite – possible mechanical vector. Oocyst quite resistant to disinfection | Probably all species of Passeriformes. In canaries causes disease in hatchlings 'black spot' due to enlarged liver seen through the skin. May be cause of 'going light' in greenfinch. | Global distribution | Usually non-pathogenic but very heavy infection may be fatal in nestlings. Depression, anorexia, diarrhoea. PM hepatomegally with white spots | Examine Giemsa stained smear from blood, liver, spleen, bone marrow. Intracytoplasmic parasite may cause indentation of nucleus of mononuclear blood cells which it invades. Difficult to locate in peripheral blood, use the buffy coat of haematorcrit sample. Oocyst may be found in faeces | Plasmodium. See 'black spot' canary disease, p. 311 |

Disease	Cause	Species susceptible	Relative occurrence	Principal clinical signs	Confirmation of diagnosis	Differential diagnosis
	Microsporidium sp. An opportunistic pathogen which may act as a *zoonotic hazard to immunocompromised humans* in contact with pet birds housed in insanitary conditions	Documented in lovebirds and budgerigars (7–10 days of age)	Probably global	Can cause unthriftiness and stunting in nestlings. Yellow pasty droppings. Mortality 75% PM distended alimentary canal and necrotic liver.	Histopathology	Polyoma virus. See reovirus, pp. 320 and 322
Trichomoniasis 'Frounce' in raptors 'Canker' in pigeons	*Trichomonas gallinae* Variable pathogenicity, direct transmission (1) Adults feeding young (2) Contaminated food (3) Raptors from infected prey. Possibly many healthy carriers occur.	Probably all species. Raptors Pigeons Parrots Nestlings Budgerigars Cockatiels Ostrich chicks	May be more common than realised. Not uncommon Common Often undiagnosed Common	Sometimes acute death. Inappetence, dyspnoea unthriftiness, loss of weight, diarrhoea. PM cheesy material often thick anywhere from the oropharanx to GI tract also resp. system. Initially lesions quite small but become gross.	Microscopical examination of the lesions for highly mobile parasites. Use: (1) wet cotton bud on oesophageal mucosa, squeeze out onto warm slide, (2) crop wash, (3) impression smear of lung of dead chick, stain with Giemsa to see 4 anterior flagellae. If in doubt culture in a special liquid medium overnight, before examining on a warm slide.	Candidiasis (gross lesions of Trichomonas are indistinguishable). Hypovitaminosis A Avipox Pigeon herpes 'Sour crop' Air sac mite (Passerines) Scalds in gavaged chicks. See capillariasis, p. 38

Disease	Organism / life history	Host / epidemiology	Clinical signs / PM	Diagnosis	Differential / associated
Giardiasis Parasite related to *Hexamita*	*Giardia* spp. Opportunistic pathogen of small intestine. Latent carriers irregularly shed encysted parasites in faeces, remain viable several weeks in moisture	Reported in many species of birds and mammals including man but probably not zoonotic. Different species of parasite occur in man	May be more common than previously recognised.	Chronic diarrhoea, unthriftiness due to malabsorbtion. Possible high mortality in young birds. Overcrowding and insanitary conditions predispose. Organism lives on surface of mucosa therefore few PM signs.	Identification of the mobile parasites can be difficult. Tick walled cysts can be seen by using flotation methods. Also serology IF and ELISA. Does not survive more than few minutes outside host. Stain faeces with Lugol's iodine or carbolfuchsin to identify 8 flagellae, large sucking disc and 2 nuclei	May be associated with concurrent: *E. coli* coccidiosis *Hexamita*
Hexamitiasis	*Hexamita* sp. Life history similar to *Giardia*. May encyst outside host. Wild pigeons may be latent carriers. Ingestion of infective cysts	Young birds Pigeons { Important: often undiagnosed 50% of young pigeons can be carriers & causes 10% of clinical cases of diarrhoea More common in summer } Galliformes Not very common Documented in a few Psittaciformes	Diarrhoea, bright green with unpleasant odour, and unthriftiness. PM catarrhal inflammation of the intestine with dilation of the small intestine.	Histopathology Demonstration of relatively small, quick moving parasites in faeces or deep scrapings of mucosa in fresh PM specimens, or cloacal swab fresh wet, mount at body temperature or stain with Giemsa. Trophozoite similar to *Giardia* without sucking disc	Trichomoniasis and girdiasis Coccidiosis *Salmonella* *E. coli* Paramyxo Herpes virus Helminths Check husbandry.

Disease	Cause	Species susceptible	Relative occurrence	Principal clinical signs	Confirmation of diagnosis	Differential diagnosis
Histomoniasis 'Blackhead'.	*Histomonas meleagridis* organism carried by ova of the worm *Heterakis gallinae* which acts as a vector (see p. 340).	Turkeys and other gallinaceous birds, chickens, pheasants, quail, peafowl, grouse.	Common, particularly if the birds associate with the domestic fowl which carry the vector.	Dullness – diarrhoea with yellowish droppings. PM Caeca enlarged, filled with caseous necrotic material. Characteristic cream-coloured circular lesions on the liver the centre of which is darker and haemorrhagic.	PM lesions and histopathology.	All diarrhoeas, particularly salmonellosis, campylobacteriosis, chlamydia

Avian haematozoa

Mostly benign or latent infections of their natural hosts but stress, migration, breeding, trapping, captivity together with concurrent infection by other non-related pathogens may all precipitate a clinical parasitaemia. Simultaneous infection with more than one haematozoon is not uncommon. Wild birds may act as reservoirs of infection for domestic or captive birds.

Disease	Cause	Species susceptible	Relative occurrence	Principal clinical signs	Confirmation of diagnosis	Differential diagnosis
Avian malaria At least 25 spp.	*Plasmodium* sp. invade red blood cells of the bird. Transmitted by various spp. of mosquitoes. Wild passerines may act as latent carriers for pathogenesis in some captive species	Probably most species of birds. The parasite is not always host specific and can infect related species. Canaries, penguins, waterfowl, raptors, pigeons, parrots	May be more common than realised, although not always pathogenic. Not confined to the tropics	Swelling of the eyelids reported in some species. Depression, fluffed up, haemolytic anaemia. Death within hours. Dyspnoea, vomiting, bright green faeces due to increased biliverdin. PM subcutaneous haemorrhage hepatosplenomegaly	Examination of stained smear for the *pigmented* parasites within both erythrocytes and leucocytes, nucleus often displaced	*Haemoproteus* Leucocytozoonosis Avipox Ornithosis Atoxoplasma

Disease	Parasite	Hosts	Prevalence	Pathogenicity / Clinical signs	Diagnosis	Related
Leucocytozoonosis	Leucocytozoon species. Transmitted by biting flies (Simulium) and midges (Culicoides).	Very pathogenic to young of: Galliformes. Anseriformes Passeriformes Psittacines Owls Raptors	Common in right weather and environmental conditions Rare but can be fatal Common but not pathogenic Common	Anorexia, anaemia. Disease only occurs if conditions are right for build-up of flies. Important disease of ducks and geese in N. America where the black fly (Simulium) is prevalent	Examination of stained blood. *Large* parasites may be seen to have invaded usually the leucocytes but sometimes RBCs. PM hepatosplenomegaly. Schizonts in impression smears of viscera	Avian malaria. *Haemoproteus.* Parasite also large but pigmented and does not distort host cell. *Leucocytozoon* parasite non-pigmented and so large distorts host cell
Haemoproteus	Haemoproteus sp. Each species probably has a definitive host range of species. Species transmitted by hippoboscid flat flies, midges (Culicoides). (Transmits sub-genus Parahaemoproteus)	Galliformes Passeriformes Columbiformes Many wild sp. are latent carriers. Psittacines Owls Falconides	Global Common Common Common Quite common	Not usually pathogenic except in a heavy infection or in stressed birds. Haemolytic anaemia, weakness. Schizonts cause white streaks in cardiac and skeletal muscle. Occasionally hepatosplenomegaly	Examination of stained blood smear shows large pigmented parasites *within* the RBCs. May be confused with plasmodium infections. Schizonts found in imprints of many viscera	Avian malaria. *Haemoproteus* may occupy $\frac{2}{3}$ of host cell but does not distort it. *Plasmodium* also large but displaces nucelus. Leucocytozoonisis
Trypanosomiasis	Trypanosoma species. Transmitted by biting arthropods including hippoboscids and red mite	Passeriformes Galliformes Anseriformes Columbiformes Strigiformes Falconides	Probably not uncommon	Probably not pathogenic	Examination of a stained smear of blood or bone marrow. Parasite occurs in the plasma.	

Other protozal parasites that occur in birds: *Babesia*; *Heptatozoon*; *Aegyptianella* species causing piroplasmosis. A tick-transmitted rickettsia occurring in passerines, lovebirds, raptors, pigeons, Anseriformes, Galliformes. *Cocklosoma* (similar to *Giardia*) occurring in young ornamental finches, the adults being more resistant. An unnamed relatively large slow moving flagellate in the crop of canaries (documented by van der Hage and Dorrestein, 1991).

APPENDIX 6:
PARASITIC DISEASES OF BIRDS: HELMINTH PARASITES

Note: (1) Pseudoparasitism. During the faecal examination of birds of prey for helminth parasites the eggs of parasites infecting the prey species may occasionally be found. (2) Parasitism in imported birds. Many imported species may have been infected in their country of origin and the parasite may remain undetected for years.

Disease	Cause	Species susceptible	Relative occurrence	Principal clinical signs	Confirmation of diagnosis	Differential diagnosis
Ascaridiasis	*Ascaridia* (a) *galli* (b) *hermaphrodita* (c) *columbae* (d) *platycerci* Eggs resistant to disinfection. Budgerigars are coprophagic	Psittacines. Domestic fowl and game birds. Passeriformes. Falconides. Columbiformes.	Not uncommon. Quite common. Rare. Not uncommon. Common	Loss of condition. Sudden death due to impaction of the bowel said to cause paralysis of the legs because of impaction of the intestine in parakeets. Visceral larval migrans of CNS documented in USA. In many avian species in contact with racoon faeces. Racoon is definitive host of *Baylisascaris procyonis*	Examination of the droppings by normal flotation methods shows typical worm eggs	
Gizzard and intestinal worms	*Porrocaecum* species.	Passeriformes ducks. Raptors	Global	Unthriftiness. PM larvae found under horny lining of gizzard and worms may cause tumours in serosal surface of intestine.	PM signs. Eggs in faeces look like ascarid eggs. Thick-walled, oval egg $1\frac{1}{2}$ size ascarid egg	

Condition	Parasite	Hosts	Occurrence	Pathology	Diagnosis
Proventricular and gizzard worms	*Microtetrameres* sp. *Hatertia* sp. *Dispharynx* sp. *Spiroptera* species (*Habronema*). Intermediate host ground-living arthropods, cockroach and some 'bugs'	Galliformes. Passeriformes. Psittacines. Raptors. Owls	May be more common than realised. Not always pathogenic	Parasite burrows beneath the horny lining of the gizzard and into the mucosa of oesophagus and intestine. General unthriftiness and sudden death. Cause nodules and ulceration in proventriculus	Examination of droppings for embryonated eggs. Oval egg, thick-walled and $\frac{1}{2}$ size of ascarid egg
	Streptocar sp. Intermediate host crustaceans	Anseriformes	Not uncommon	Mucosa of upper GI tract may be ulcerated – possible haemorrhage	
Eyeworms	*Thelazia* sp. has invertebrate intermediate host.	All found in psittacines. Also in raptors		Occur under nictatating membrane and adjacent structures. Irritation, chemosis, ulceration	
	Ceratospira sp. *Annulospira* sp. *Oxyspirura* sp. Cockroach is intermediate host	Also in Galliformes S. USA			
Gizzard worms of ducks and geese	*Amidostomum anseris* Adult birds act as carriers. Direct lifecycle. Eggs hatch in water, larvae ingested	Ducks and geese domestic and wild.		Anorexia, emaciation in goslings and ducklings – death. Erosion (and necrosis) of lining of gizzard, larvae found beneath koilin. May attack proventriculus and oesophagus.	PM signs. Oval eggs in faeces, thin-walled, usually embryonated, slightly larger than ascarid egg

Disease	Cause	Species susceptible	Relative occurrence	Principal clinical signs	Confirmation of diagnosis	Differential diagnosis
Capillariasis (Threadworms) (Hairworms)	Capillaria sp. Sometimes pass through the transport host the earthworm. Embryonation of the egg takes 3 weeks	Galliformes. Passeriformes. Strigiacines. Falconides. Pigeons	Not uncommon. Common Common	Dysphagia. Loss of condition, lack of appetite, mucoid diarrhoea, sometimes with blood, eventually death. PM in heavy infection anaemia. Worms found in lumen of intestine, oesophagus and buccal cavity, worms burrow into mucosa. Throughout GI tract particularly upper GI tract.	Examination of droppings shows eggs of the parasite with typical bi-polar plugs. Eggs shed sporadically, therefore, examine serial specimens.	Trichomoniasis in raptors. Both Capillaria and Trichomonas can produce similar white necrotic lesions. Examine scrapings of mucosa of oropharanx for eggs (see p. 38 and Plate 9)
Caecal worms carriers of the parasite Histomonas	Heterakis gallinarum Earthworms act as a vector.	Domestic fowl and all gallinaceous birds Anseriformes.	Common.	The worm by itself is probably not pathogenic unless there is heavy infestation when there is unthriftiness and diarrhoea. Pin-point haemorrhages and nodules in mucosa of caeca.	Examination of the faeces for the ova which are not unlike those of Ascaridia galli, but the egg wall is slightly thinner and also smaller	
Proventricular worms	Acuaria (Echinuria) sp. Intermediate host water flea (Daphnia sp.)	Ducks, swans, occasionally geese	Very high mortality in signets during hot summer on shallow warm water	Parasites cause nodules in proventriculus and gizzard. Results in partial obstruction, weight loss and diarrhoea. PM excessive mucus in proventriculus	Small elliptical embryonated egg containing single larva	Thorny headed worms, gizzard worms, pp. 338 and 339 (Amidostomum and Porrocaecum)

Trichostronglyosis	*Trichostrongylus tenuis*	Galliformes and water-fowl but particularly grouse on the moor	On grouse moors cyclical yearly variation in epizootics	Large numbers of worms in the caecae cause typhlitis, haemorrhage and death	Elliptical embryonated eggs in faeces	
Syngamiasis (Gapes)	*Syngamus* species Direct transmission or may pass through a transport host such as earthworms, slugs, snails and beetles	Probably can infect all species and naturally occurs in many species.	Not uncommon. Very easy to find in many wild Paseriformes.	Dyspnoea – gaping, cough, shaking head. Anorexia, loss of condition, death. PM parasites found in the trachea which may be completely blocked. Tracheitis, bronchitis, pneumonia.	Examination of the droppings for the typical egg with operculum at each end like a *Capillaria* egg but larger. Endoscopy in large birds of the trachea. Sometimes worms can be seen by naked eye.	*Capillaria* in raptors. Trichomoniasis. Candidiasis. *Aspergillus.* Avian pox
Cyanthostomiasis helminth infection by a genus closely related to *Syngamus*	*Cyanthostoma lari* Possible direct prey–predator transmission or from intermediate host – earthworm in GI tract of host	Raptors (Simpson and Harris, 1992). Also gulls, waders, herons, crows.	May be more common than documented.	Parasitic in orbit and nasal cavity, localised inflammation. Occasional anaemia, weakness, death. PM remove eye and examine orbit	Faecal examination. Use saturated sugar flotation or sedimentation techniques	
	C. america *C. brodskii* *C. bronchalis* *C. sp.*	Raptors Owls Geese Cockatoos	N. America, Russia, E. Europe, Central Asia	Parasite in bronchi, trachea, air sacs causing pneumonia		

Disease	Cause	Species susceptible	Relative occurrence	Principal clinical signs	Confirmation of diagnosis	Differential diagnosis
Filiariasis	Larvae of *Serratospiculum* sp. Found as microfilariae in blood stream. Biting arthropods act as vectors. Weather conditions may favour increase in vector, i.e. gnats.	Falcons. Other species found in Passeriformes, psittacines and ostrich chicks	Common in the tropics. Occasionally may be found in imported birds. Not uncommon.	The larvae in the blood stream. Pathogenicity varies. During body migration the larvae can cause quite a severe reaction in the lung and air sacs. The adult worm is found in the body cavities and the intestine, beneath the serosa, it is long thin and coiled. Also adult and larvae subcut, in fluid swellings around metatarsal area of parrots. Occasional microfilaria in antechamber of eye removed by author. In ostrich chicks causes CNS signs	Examination of a stained blood smear or a wet mount unstained blood smear to see the living microfiliarae. Most easily recovered from buffycoat. Examine the droppings for the embryonated thin-walled egg which is oval-shaped like that of *Syngamus*.	In the blood. Do not confuse with trypanosomiasis
Thorny headed worms	Various species of acanthocephalids. All have intermediate invertebrate hosts. *Polymorphus* sp. *Prosthorhynchus* sp. *Centrorhynchus* sp. *Fillicollis* sp.	Waterfowl. Passeriformes. Raptors, including owls. Also pigeons and lorikeets	Not very common. Can be geographically localised and common in such areas	Found in the mucosa of the intestine causing enteritis and unthriftiness if they are present in large numbers.	It may be possible to find the spindle shaped embryonated egg in the droppings. The embryo contains a circlet of hooks on the head. Difficult to identify for the non-specialist.	

		Host species	Occurrence	Clinical signs / pathogenicity	Diagnosis	Notes
Tapeworms	A very large number of species of *Cestoda*. All require a secondary host – usually an invertebrate but may be fish – which is usually only found in the country of origin	Probably all species. Less common in the seed- and fruit-eating birds except in nestlings. Raptors and owls. Occasionally imported birds	Occurrence variable Not common	Not often pathogenic. General debility and diarrhoea, anorexia. PM varying degrees of enteritis together with the worms. If much mucus is present scrape the mucosa and examine the scrapings microscopically.	Finding the proglottids in the faeces. Examine more than one sample of droppings. Focus down with microscope and look for hook on larva within the egg	*Railietina* species can produce nodules in gut wall which can be seen from the serosal surface and look like TB
Flukes	Numerous trematode species. Complex lifecycle. Always require a secondary host such as a mollusc which is usually but not always aquatic. Sometimes involves water snail eaten by fish etc. Possible insect vector	Passeriformes. Waterfowl and aquatic birds, including penguins. Columbiformes. Falconiformes. Psittacines. Occurs in imported birds	Not very common. Not uncommon. Not common. Most common in tropical areas and tend to be regionally located.	Clinical signs indefinite. General unthriftiness. Anaemia. Signs depend where the flukes are located in the body. At PM they can be found in almost any part of the body, sometimes located in liver and bile ducts causing an obvious hepatopathy and severe enteritis	Finding fluke eggs in the droppings. PM signs.	

APPENDIX 7
PARASITIC DISEASES OF BIRDS: ARTHROPOD ECTOPARASITES.

Wild birds migrating from tropical to temperate climates may pick up parasites (e.g. *Amblyoma* sp. of ticks in the tropics which do not normally occur in temperate zones. Ectoparasites are also the transport hosts of many avian parasites such as the haematozoa. The parasitic load of birds tends to increase during the breeding season, affecting egg production and chick mortality.

Disease	Cause	Species susceptible	Relative occurrence	Principal clinical signs	Confirmation of diagnosis	Differential diagnosis
Lice	All bird lice are biting or chewing lice (Mallophaga).	Probably most species of lice are host specific. More than one louse species may be found on the same bird but in different locations	Very common particularly in birds debilitated from other causes.	Most lice feed on feather debris and not blood. But some species of louse feed on feathers 'in blood' and therefore ingest blood. Cause irritation and restlessness. Healthy birds keep lice in check when preening, but heavy louse infection may lead to feather plucking.	Finding the lice or the eggs in the feathers. Often seen in anaesthetised birds and in recently dead birds.	Pruritis may be caused by hippoboscids or mites
Hippoboscids (flat or louse flies).	Arthropods related to the 'Sheep Ked' e.g. *Pseudolynchia* sp. *Icosa* sp. *Ornithomyia* sp. Some species complete lifecycle on host others lay eggs in environment	Probably all species. Seen particularly in raptors, pigeons, swifts, martins, swallows. Not particularly host specific	Common on many wild birds.	Cause pruritis and suck blood and transmit *Haemoproteus* and trypanosomes Often jump onto human handler and can get into clothing and hair and remain some time. Has been recognised as a problem for sometime in nestling pigeons.	Recognition of the dorsoventrally flattened stout flies which may or may not have wings depending on the species.	Because of shape and size unlikely to be confused with other ectoparasites. Can transport parasitic mites

Fleas.	Many species of the order Siphonaptera. Probably all species. Not as host specific as lice		Not often seen. Can build up in nesting areas and nest boxes.	Irritation, restlessness. Although they suck blood they are of doubtful pathogenicity. They are not host specific so that birds can become infected with mammalian species from domestic pets. Can live on humans. Bird fleas from nesting starlings can build up in roof space of houses	Identification of adult eggs and larvae in nesting sites. Adult fleas may only remain on host for short periods when feeding	
Sticktight fleas	*Echidnophaga gallinacea*	Mainly on poultry but also on game birds, pigeons, passerines and raptors	Common in tropics and subtropics. May be seen on imported birds	Adult fleas attached in large numbers around the head particularly the eyes → hyperkeratinisation, anaemia, irritation, death in young birds		
Red mites	*Dermanyssus* sp. Breeds off host in e.g. woodwork. Lifecycle completed in a week. Can survive off host for months	Domestic poultry.	Global distribution Common.	Cause intense irritation and restlessness. Suck blood and cause anaemia and debility. Fatal to young birds. *D. gallinae* only found on the bird at night. Hide in crevices during the day. Ornithonyssus causes more irritation because feeds throughout 24 hours	Examine perches and woodwork by torch light at night. Keymer (1969) suggests covering cage with a white cloth at night when mites can be seen on or under surface in the morning. Mites and their eggs are occasionally found during faecal examinations after they have been ingested by the bird during preening	Other ectoparasites. Other causes of anaemia. In passerines trichomoniasis air sac mite
Northern fowl mite.	*Ornithonyssus* sp. Completes lifecycle on host which the mite doesn't leave	Passeriformes. Columbiformes. Psittacines. Raptors.	Not uncommon.			

Disease	Cause	Species susceptible	Relative occurrence	Principal clinical signs	Confirmation of diagnosis	Differential diagnosis
Harvest mites.	Larvae of *Trombicula* species, during spring and autumn.	Most ground living species.	Widespread but clinical infection uncommon, localised.	Irritation may show vesicles where a bird has been biting together with loss of feathers. The adult mites may be quite large and are free living in woods, scrubland and old pasture. They feed on invertebrates and plants.	Identification of larvae on the skin.	Red mite and northern fowl mite infection.
Feather mites	Various species inhabit different parts of the feather and different body feathers. Most are surface scavengers			Usually not pathogenic unless very heavy infestation → pruritis and feather loss, occasional thickening of the skin	Microscopy of feathers	
Feather follicle mites	Probably occur in all species of birds and not particularly host specific			May cause feather loss. Mites in powdery material of feather stumps	Express contents of blood feathers and examine with magnification	
Epidermoptic mites	*Myialges* sp. and others cause 'depluming mange'. Burrow into stratum corneum of skin. Transported by hippoboscids and lice	Documented in passerines, psittacines and owls	May be more common than recognised	Pruritis, scaly dermatitis, brown scabs, desquamation of skin. Mostly affects covert feathers, mostly head, cere, neck and body coverts. May also look like sarcoptic mange	Skin scrapings	Psittacine beak and feather disease

Forage mite	Many species. Free living in foodstuffs. Distributed by transport on insects and by wind. Scavengers in nests	Anywhere where food is badly stored in humid conditions.	Very common. May occur in huge numbers.	Not pathogenic but may be confused with the pathogenic mites. Causes considerable spoiling of grain and seed foods. May cause allergic reaction and very occasionally death after eating infected food. The author has seen a massive infestation of grain fed to over 100 quail with no deaths in the birds. Very small. Off-white in colour.	*Dermanyssus.* *Ornithonyssus.* *Trombicula*
Air sac mites.	*Sternostoma* species. Complete lifecycle on host. Adults infect young when feeding them	Mostly reported in Passeriformes, particularly gouldian finches. Can be rapidly fatal. Occasionally psittacines.	Global. Possibly more common than realised.	Loss of condition, dyspnoea, loss of voice, sneezing, gasping, death. Nasal exudate. PM mites black in colour seen in trachea and upper air passages and in the air sacs + mucus + pneumonia. They have been seen in the air sacs by laparoscopy and by transillumination of the trachea. Eggs can be found in faeces	*Syngamus.* Aspergillosis. Avian pox
Scaly face and scaly leg mites. 'Depluming itch' or 'Feather rot' in pigeons.	*Knemidokoptes* species.	Budgerigars.	Common.	Grey-white encrustations around the cere, the beak, the commissures of the upper and lower beak often gross distortion of the beak. Tassle foot lesions on canaries and other passeriformes. May infest cloaca. Mites easily identified in powdery scrapings. Clear slide with 10% KOH.	Carcinoma of beak. Avian pox. Papillomas of the legs
		Crossbills.	Common on legs.		
		Passeriformes.	Causing depigmentation		
		Other species of psittacines. Canaries. Domestic poultry. Wild birds	Occasional		

Disease	Cause	Species susceptible	Relative occurrence	Principal clinical signs	Confirmation of diagnosis	Differential diagnosis
Bugs	Order Hemiptera, e.g. *Cimex* sp., *Oeciacus* sp. Can survive off host for some time. Eggs laid in environment	Pigeons, poultry, swallows – host specific		Heavy infestation causes anaemia. Can be fatal in young birds	Tend to feed on host at night	Body size larger than mites
Ticks	Hard ticks. *Ixodes ricinus* and a number of other species. *Argas* sp. Soft ticks. *Rhipicephalus*, *Amblyomma*	Probably all species, including ostrich. Migrating raptors in Israel	Attack grouse. Localised. Most likely to be seen in aviaries or tethered falcons near sheep or poultry	Irritation, loss of condition, anaemia and death if the infestation is severe. Small birds do not need many ticks to lose quite a lot of blood. Transmit haematoprotozoa including *Aegyptianella* sp, arboviruses, e.g. louping ill virus (grouse on British uplands) also may carry *Borrelia* spp. Tick bites can cause oedema and haemorrhage and result in acute death		
Dipterous flies	*Calliphora, Lucilia Phormia* species. All cause blow fly strike	All species	Not common but can invade gangrenous wound or chicks in a dirty nest.	Typical signs myiasis		

Mosquitoes, gnats, midges and black flies all bite and suck avian blood and often transmit blood parasites and can cause anaemia particularly in hatchlings.

APPENDIX 8:
POISONS LIKELY TO AFFECT BIRDS

General comment. This list is not comprehensive and is only a guide. A specific diagnosis of poisoning is not often possible – much depends on circumstantial evidence. The analysis of samples can be expensive and the analyst must be given a good idea of what to look for. One should collect samples of liver, kidney and the contents of proventriculus and gizzard. Collect pancreas if zinc is suspected or brain for organophosphates. Wrap all samples in aluminium foil and freeze. Contact the laboratory to ascertain if analysis is possible. Many poisons do not cause acute death but in sub-lethal doses may be responsible for lower fertility, reduced resistance to infection and non-specific symptoms such as sporadic nervous tremors. Few cases of poisoning are malicious; most are due to carelessness of thoughtlessness.

Type of poison	Comments
Agricultural and gardening chemicals. Seed dressings and storage preservatives. Organomercury compounds. Lead arsenate. Sodium chlorate used as a weed killer. Paraquat and diquat – herbicides	Many substances are used to control infection of the seed and growing plants by micro-organisms. They may also be used to control weevils in stored grain. The chemicals may be used at the wrong dose or the treated seed inadvertently fed to birds. Supplies of many seeds come from countries where the control of these chemicals is not strict enough.
Insecticidal and herbicidal sprays. Agricultural fertilisers. Ammonium sulphate, phenoxyacid herbicides, carbamates. Phosphorothionates and malathion.	Most notorious of the insecticides in the past has been DDT, and the other organochlorines, lindane (BHC) and dieldrin, and the polychlorinated biphenyls. Nowadays many organophosphates are used to spray growing crops including fruit crops. The cloud of spray may be blown by wind. The insects killed and contaminated with the insecticide may be eaten by birds. Nitrogenous fertilisers may leach into water supplies. Roadside and garden herbage may be contaminated by many chemicals. Water supplies of birds may become contaminated. Diesel fuel leaking from a farm into a waterway killed many ducks.
Insecticides used to control pests in domestic animals	Sheep dips and preparations to control fly strike in sheep may be misused. Many organophosphates used on domestic pets as sprays and baths are toxic if misused on birds. Dichlorvos organophosphate strips if misused. Birds must not have direct contact. Must be in well ventilated room. Minimum air space $30\,\mathrm{m}^3$ per strip. Use for 3 days only. Avoid use in high temperatures.

Type of poison	Comments
Rodenticides	In the past strychnine, aresenic, thallium, zinc phosphide and phosphorus were widely used and are still used in some countries. Warfarin and related compounds together with the organophosphates are now commonly used and birds may gain access to treated bait. Sodium fluoroacetate and fluoroacetamide are also widely used in many parts of the world and are very poisonous. Strychnine can still be used under licence in the UK for killing moles and rodents.
Tea, coffee, cocoa (drinking chocolate), chocolate to eat	All contain theobromine which can cause hyperexcitability, cardiopathy and death.
Crude oil	Ingested by birds after oil spillage at sea. Also some wild birds nest in and around oil refineries.
Molluscicides	These are used to control garden and agricultural pest and the vectors of many helminth infections. Metaldehyde and copper sulphate are both toxic to birds.
Alphachloralose	These are used to control pigeons in urban areas. Affected pigeons are narcotised and may be eaten by raptors. Also used as a rodenticide.
Wood preservatives	Bitumen paint, pentachlorophenol, creosote and naphtha compounds may be used to preserve the woodwork or aviaries. This may be chewed by psittacines which may acquire sublethal doses.
Disinfectants	Phenols and cresols and hyperchlorites are often used far more concentrated than the manufacturers' recommendations. Can lie in pools in the bottom of aviaries and dry on perches, etc. The quaternary ammonium antiseptics are relatively non-toxic.

Lead

In waterfowl the differential diagnosis is botulism.

Cage or aviary birds may be exposed to old lead paint, window leaded lights, linoleum, lead toys, curtain weights, discarded lead pipes, solder, golf balls. Water-fowl and gamebirds may pick up lead from ground which has been heavily shot over. Water-fowl, particularly swans, may gradually accumulate lead from discarded fisherman's lead weights lying in the bottom mud of watercourses. Lead poisoning has also been seen in water-fowl near a rubbish tip containing lead car batteries. Old lead mining areas, lead smelting and industrial areas may be heavily contaminated. Plants and insects become contaminated and may be eaten by birds.

Raptors may pick up subclinical lead levels from the tissues of prey species and also intact lead shot from their gizzards (Reiser and Temple, 1980). The latter may or may not be voided in the casting of the raptor. Also possible chronic exposure to automobile exhaust fumes. Radiographs of affected birds may be negative but plasma levels raised.

Carbon monoxide

These fumes can come from a car left running in a garage or from a gas central heating boiler or gas water heater which is not functioning properly. Birds may be transported in the rear 'boot' or 'trunk' or a vehicle with faulty exhaust system.

Fumes from a Teflon non-stick cooking utensil

If this dries and overheats toxic fumes can be produced. Other plastics if burnt can produce toxic fumes. In the industrial process of plastic coating metal sheets, faulty controls resulted in toxic effluent downwind of the plant and many bird deaths. In humans only moderate upper respiratory distress. PM of affected birds shows intense red coloration of all tissues particularly the lungs. A similar picture is seen in carbon monoxide poisoning.

Type of poison	Comments
Naturally occurring toxins	*Botulism:* mentioned under infectious diseases. Blow flies often attack meat infected with *Clostridium botulinum*, the maggots pick up the toxin and they may then be eaten by birds. Another cause is dead aquatic invertebrates in rotting vegetation. Sometimes associated with poisoning by blue green algae (Cyanophyceae) and other algal blooms occurring in static shallow water in hot weather.
	Many *plants* or parts of plants are poisonous to birds, but many plants poisonous to one species are not necessarily poisonous to another species of bird, e.g. parsley (*Petroselinum* sp.) is toxic to ostriches but not parrots. Insects which eat poisonous plants may contain the toxin which, if they are themselves eaten by birds, poison the bird. E.g. the milkweeds (*Asclepias* sp.) of the Western hemisphere are eaten by monarch butterflies (*Danaus plexippus*) and these contain cardiac glycosides produced by the plant. If the insect is eaten by a bird it is poisoned.
	Listed are a few plants that may be toxic to birds: lily of the valley (*Convallaria majalis*), oleander (*Nerium oleander*), Virginia creeper (*Parthenocissus quinquefolia*), dumb cane (*Dieffenbachia* sp.), Swiss cheese plant (*Monstera* sp.), *Philodendron* sp., poinsettia (*Euphorbia* sp.), clematis (*Clematis* sp.), foxglove (*Digitalis* sp.), lupin (*Lupinus* sp.), croton (*Codiaeum* sp.), castor oil plant (*Ricinus communis*), cherry laurel (evergreen, *Prunus laurocerasus* sp.) (clippings of laurel trees if stored in a plastic bag overnight in a warm atmosphere can accumulate toxic cyanide fumes), bay tree (*Laurus nobilis*), avocado (*Persea* sp.) (toxicity of different species is variable), tobacco plant (*Nicotiana affinis*). Ingestion of tobacco products (e.g. cigarette ends), direct contact or indirect contact through tobacco stains on a smoker's hands can be toxic to household pets.
	Hemlock (*Conium* sp.): seeds eaten by pigeons have caused fatalities.
	Yew (*Taxus* sp.): eaten by game or aviary birds. All parts of the plants are very poisonous.
	Aflatoxins and other mycotoxins: first discovered in groundnuts affecting turkeys. The toxin is a metabolite of an *Aspergillus* fungus which can grow in badly stored grain or seed. Toxicity of aflatoxins variable. Aflatoxin B1 is a hepatotoxin.
	Ergot (*Claviceps purpurea*) infected grain. If eaten in large amounts they cause necrosis of the extremities.

Salt poisoning

Brackish water consumed in drought.
Peanuts (salted) and potato crisps fed to parrots. Some birds are able to excrete salt through nasal salt gland.

Tannins and alkaloids contained in plants

The leaves and twigs of rhododendron, azalea, laburnum and many other plants are toxic to herbivorous mammals and the bark may be toxic for birds. The leaves and bark of many trees contain low grade toxins such as tannins. These are bitter tasting and are part of the plants' natural defence systems against insects and vertebrates feeding on them. Perrins (1979) has shown that blue tit nestlings fed on mealworms containing tannins grow more slowly than nestlings fed on mealworms which do not contain tannins. This phenomenon could occur with many other plant substances taken directly or indirectly by birds

For a full discussion of the subject of poisoning in birds the reader is referred to three publications: *Bird Disease* by Arnall and Keymer; *Veterinary Aspects of Captive Birds of Prey* by Cooper; *First Aid and Care of Wild Birds* edited by Cooper and Eley. See further reading list. Also see Coles, B.H. 'Cage and Aviary Birds', in *The Manual of Exotic Pets*, published by the British Small Animal Veterinary Association.

Poisons information services in the UK:
London Tel. 0171 635 9195 Fax 0171 635 1053
Leeds Tel. 0113 243 0715 Fax 0113 244 5849

In case of wildlife poisoning contact the Wildlife Officer of the local Agricultural Development and Advisory Service.

APPENDIX 9:
SOME SUGGESTED DIAGNOSTIC SCHEDULES

All the procedures listed may not be necessary to reach a diagnosis.

Schedule 1: Basic investigation of the sick bird

This will be carried out as a sequel to the initial clinical examination and anamnesis after which there is still no clear indication of the cause of the problem. If some more definite clinical signs are present to indicate which body system or systems are involved then it might be more appropriate to commence with one of the other schedules listed. If a number of birds are affected, euthanasia of the worst and subsequent post-mortem examination may enable a more rapid diagnosis to be made.

Clinical procedure	Comment
(a) Full haematological examination	This may indicate an inflammatory reaction. However, serial (24–48 hours apart) total white cell count (TWCC) and red cell count (RCC) are more useful than one sample alone. Differential white cell count (WCC) may not be very helpful in making a diagnosis in birds. Take into account any previously administered steroids. Haematology may indicate haemoparasite infection. Also, it may indicate anaemia and its type.
(b) Basic biochemical profile to include: Total protein ⎫ Albumen: globulin ratio ⎬ Fibrinogen ⎭	In most cases, this data will only provide a rough guide to the problem. For in-depth interpretation of the results see the relevant sections in Chapter 3, Aids to Diagnosis. These parameters provide some information on the overall state of health and the presence or absence of an inflammatory response.
AST, CPK ⎫ Bile acids ⎭	Those parameters may indicate a hepatopathy or solely tissue trauma.
If the blood sample is lipaemic estimate the plasma cholesterol	A cholesterol estimation will indicate possible hypothyroidism which will also be indicated by hypoglycaemia. Alternatively, a hypercholesterolaemia may be associated with fatty liver and kidney syndrome.
Plasma calcium	Latent hypocalcaemia can be an important debilitating condition in some parrots (particularly African grey parrots – *Psittacus erithacus*) and also in raptors.

Uric acid	Increased levels of uric acid do not necessarily indicate nephropathy. Uric acid should be considered in conjunction with the plasma levels of albumen, glucose and CPK together with the haematology. Changes in these parameters may indicate starvation (also indicated by loss of pectoral muscle), or extensive trauma accompanied with haemorrhage. These conditions may also result in an increase of plasma uric acid.
(c) *Whole body radiography* *Both* ventro-dorsal and lateral projections IF the equipment is available supplement by ultrasonography	This may indicate neoplasia, latent respiratory disease (e.g. airsacculitis), skeletal disease, tuberculosis, aspergillosis, splenomegally (which with haematology and biochemistry) may indicate an increased immune response (e.g. *Chlamydia*), changes or displacement of the GI tract (e.g. neuropathic proventricular dilatation of psittacines) or possible cardiopathy.
(d) *Faecal screen* To include enteroparasites (also stain with carbolfuchsin for giardia) and differential Gram stain for assessment of total Gram-negative or Gram-positive bacteria. Also always check for *Chlamydia* with polymerised chain reaction (PCR), DNA (see pp. 69 and 70).	Apart from disease due to specific Enterobacteriacae many sick birds exhibit a shift in faecal bacterial flora to predominantly Gram-negatives. A primary search for *Chlamydia* is important in any sick bird particularly parrots because of possible zoonosis and the veterinarian's legal liability.

Schedule 2: For the investigation of respiratory signs

To carry out some of the following procedures light isoflurane anaesthesia may be required. If respiratory disease is severe an air sac cannula will be needed. The clinician should try to decide if upper or lower systemic disease is present.

Clinical procedure	Comment
(a) *Whole body radiography* Both ventro-dorsal and lateral	Apart from indications of disease in the respiratory tract (airsacculitis granulomata of the lungs, air trapping etc.) space-occupying lesions (neoplasmas, egg peritonitis etc.) may be responsible for respiratory signs.
(b) *Full haematological and biochemical profiles* always including cholesterol	For the same reasons as in Schedule 1. A hypercholesterolaemia may indicate hypothyroidism with associated hypertrophy of the gland and pressure on the syrinx.

Clinical procedure	Comment
(c) *Endoscopy* of the oropharynx, trachea, syrinx, choanal aperture and posterior nares	Together with both these procedures collect cytological and bacteriological samples. Apart from overt airsacculitis and aspergillomata etc., parasites such as *Serratospiculum* (this should also show microfilaria), *Syngamus* and sternostoma may be seen. Air sac mites in small finches are more easily seen by transillumination of the trachea via the skin of the neck.
(d) *Laparoscopy* of the coelomic air sacs, the caudal surface of the lung and in larger birds entry into the mesobronchus.	
(e) *Microbiology* of all exudate and solid lesions	A variety of organisms may be isolated, some of which will be secondary viral infection or hypovitaminosis 'A'. Lesions of trichomoniasis may be confused with owl herpes virus infection. Mycobacteria isolated may include *Aspergillus* spp. *Candida* spp, and *Cryptococcus* spp. They may take time to culture so cytology is important.
(f) *Serological examination*	This may confirm the presence of *Chlamydia*, *Aspergillus*, mycobacteria, *Salmonella* (sometimes a systemic infection), *Borrellia*, *Mycoplasma* and a variety of viruses. Among the latter are paramyxo (including Newcastle), avian influenza, laryngotracheitis and goose parvo virus. Which test is used will depend on the particular circumstances.
(g) *Virus isolation*	Some viruses can be isolated and identified by cell culture. However, special transport media must be used. Check with the laboratory first. Such viruses are Amazon tracheitis, infectious bronchitis and pigeon herpes.
(h) *Cytology*	This can be carried out by either the clinician or the laboratory. Sample exudate or solid material from the paraorbital sinuses, the choanal space, tracheal washings etc. as well as specimens obtained by endoscopy or laparoscopy. Don't forget the use of Indian ink if searching for *Cryptococcus* (see pp. 72, 75 and 327).

(j) *Faecal examination*	When investigating respiratory signs perhaps faecal examination may not be such an obvious part of the search. However, some parasites (e.g. *Syngamus, Capillara, Sarcocystis* and cryptosporidia produce ova or encrusted larvae shed in the faeces. These may not be released regularly so that more than one sample should be examined. Don't forget use of Giemsa stain for cryptosporidia.
(k) *Consideration of toxins*	Industrial effluent, crop and forestry sprays, tobacco smoke. Teflon, carbon monoxide, creosote and other timber treatments, ammonia from insanitary aviaries or cages and aerosols may all be responsible for respiratory signs

Don't forget hypovitaminosis A or iodine deficiency (particularly in budgerigars) can cause respiratory signs. Also respiratory disease may be the most obvious sign of an overall systemic infection particularly viral in origin.

Schedule 3: Investigation of gastro-intestinal problems including hepatopathy

Clinical procedure	Comment
(a) Complete *faecal examination* for evidence of parasites and bacterial culture	Not all birds with loose droppings have diarrhoea or a GI problem. They may be just anorexic. Take note of any abnormal colour for that particular species. Bright green caused by excessive biliverdin usually indicates a hepatitis, often viral but may be caused by *Chlamydia* or even *Plasmodium.* Clay coloured faeces may be due to maldigestion or paramyxo III in *Neophema* parakeets. Chalky faeces in ostrich chicks may be caused by adenovirus. Overt blood may be due to neoplasms, TB, bacterial enteritis (often with mucus) or lead or faecaliths. Take into account what the bird may have eaten (e.g. elder or blackberries). Some drugs (e.g. B vitamins) may colour droppings. Absence of or reduced faeces may be due to mechanical obstruction, parasites, cloacal impaction, intussusception or just water deprivation.
Stain faeces sample with Giemsa.	To detect *Cryptosporidia* or *Giardia.*
Stain sample with iodine	Detection of excessive starch.
Stain sample with Sudan III	Detection of fat.
Stain with Gram stain	Differential assessment of Gram negatives and Gram positives
Stain with acid-fast stain	Detection of mycobacteria
Examine fresh (within 10 min of being voided) faecal sample on warm slide.	Detection of *Giardia* or *Hexamita*; often difficult to confirm.

Clinical procedure	Comment
(b) *Microbiological and cytological examination of crop washings*	Particularly important for the detection of trichomonads, yeasts and fungi. Use Gram stain and lactophenol cotton blue and examine unstained fresh sample on warm slide to detect moving trichomonads.
(c) *Microbiological examination of fresh castings from raptors*	Note some other species may produce regurgitated castings or pellets.
(d) *Radiography using both ventro-dorsal and lateral projections. Plain and contrast media techniques. Possibly via enema. May be supplemented by using ultrasonography*	May indicate foreign bodies, neoplasia, ulceration, proventricular dilatation, undigested seed in the intestine and occasionally parasitic nematodes.
(d) *Endoscopy of the upper alimentary tract as far as the proventriculus. Also of the cloaca and rectum. If necessary inflate with air or water.*	
(f) *Complete haematology*	For the same reasons as in the basic Schedule 1.
(g) *A biochemical profile* As in Schedule 1 but in addition to include lactate dehydrogenase (LDH), glucose and alkaline phosphate (AP).	This should give an indication of hepatopathy but this may need to be associated with radiographic (and/or ultrasonographic) interpretation, liver biopsy, haematology and microbiological examination (via laparoscopy) to confirm the aetiology. There may be a need to investigate toxins. Hyperglycaemia may indicate a pancreatitis, diabetes mellitus or lead toxicosis. Increased AP may be a sign of aflatoxicosis.
(h) *Laparoscopy/laparotomy* For biopsy of liver or proventriculus	If a hepatopathy is suspected and a liver biopsy is contemplated, give a prior injection of vitamin K. Biopsy of proventriculus may confirm neopathic proventricular dilatation.
(i) *Plasma T4 estimation*	Reduced thyroid hormone may indicate thyroid dysplasia in an enlarged thyroid. Possible retching, change in vocalisation. Also note any increased cholesterol.

Schedule 4: The investigation of renal disorders

It is important to appreciate that renal disease in birds is usually not suspected during the initial examination. Nephropathy is much more likely to be revealed during the subsequent laboratory examination or during the investigation of other body systems. It may be indicated by other apparently unrelated signs such as unilateral or bilateral lameness or paresis of the legs or by gross abdominal changes resulting in dyspnoea. The classical early signs of nephropathy in mammals (polydipsia, polyurea, oliguria) are not usually notable signs of avian renal disease. The avian kidney is proportionately larger than in mammals so that most of it will have to have become diseased before plasma uric acid levels rise significantly or gout is seen. Also uric acid is much less toxic than urea. The physiology of avian kidneys varies considerably between species and also quite differently from that in mammals and is not well documented.

Clinical procedure	Comment
(a) *Complete haematology*	As for the same reasons in Schedule 1. The kidneys are involved in approximately 50% of all cases of multisystemic diseases and also many renal disease cases are anaemic.
(b) *A biochemical profile* as in Schedule 1 with the addition of plasma urea	Although not hitherto considered an important parameter in the diagnosis of nephronpathy, Lumeij (1987) has demonstrated that *a rise in plasma urea* is the single most important factor for diagnosis of prerenal failure, see the relevant section in Chapter 3, Aids to Diagnosis, p. 61. Note the normally high levels of postprandial uric acid in peregrine falcons and red tailed hawks which may also occur in other raptors. Also note a hypoalbinuria may be the result of protein loss due to glomerulonephritis.
(c) *Urine analysis* of a sample aspirated by syringe and needle from waxed paper or the clean plastic tray at the bottom of the cage. Birds, especially parrots, when stressed in a clinic often pass fluid excreta, the urinary fraction of which can be harvested. In ostriches the urine is voided first and separately from faecal matter. Use multistix dip sticks tests. However, the test for protein is unreliable. Examine the urine sample for castes and/or cell types which may give an indication of renal disease.	It is most important to carefully collect only urine uncontaminated by faeces – this may not be easy. Persistent proteinuria together with hypoalbineamia and glucosuria with hyperglycaemia may indicate a glomerulonephritis, also often with ascites or oedema of feet. Red pigmentation of the urine may be due to haemoglobinuria or haematuria or porphyrinuria urea (an indication of lead toxicity). Urine positive for porphyrins fluoresces red under UV light but blue if negative. Haematuria may be from the reproductive tract or caused by Amazon or conure bleeding syndromes. Haemoglobinuria may be the result of a coagulopathy, *Plasmodium*, bacterial or chemical toxins.
Check the specific gravity. Check the pH. This should be between 4.7 and 8.0	This should be between 1.005 and 1.020. In birds laying eggs the pH becomes acid (4.7). Calcium deposited in the shell results in a plasma excess of hydrogen ions. Bicarbonate is reabsorbed from the urine to buffer this, so that the urine becomes acid.

Clinical procedure	Comment
(d) *Radiography* Note ultrasonography is not a lot of help in the investigation of renal disease. Barium contrast radiography of the GI tract. This may indicate displacement caused by an enlarged kidney. Contrast radiography can be used but needs very careful timing and correct exposure. It is probably of more use in an academic institution.	This may indicate an increase in the renal shadow, often quite subtle so correct exposure is essential. Enlargement of the kidneys may indicate neoplasia or amyloidosis (particularly in water birds, gulls and shore birds) indicating a chronic inflammatory reaction. Nephrocalcinosis together with generalised increased density of skeletal tissue is usually the result of prolonged and excessive vitamin D_3 supplementation. However, differentiate this from polyostotic hyperostosis due to gonadal dysplasia (common in budgerigars). Radiography may also reveal a marked urolithiasis (possible salt poisoning, any *sudden* rise in plasma uric acid, use of toxic drugs, urinary tract infection: bacterial, virus or mycotic, acid urine due to metabolic acidosis or heavy metal poisoning). However, all these causes mentioned may only result in anuria or oliguria without urolithiasis.
(e) *Endoscopy* of the cloaca and *laparoscopy*	This may reveal a cloacal impaction not always seen at the initial examination. Alternatively, a cloacal neoplasm may be seen. Laparoscopy and examination of the surface of the kidney may show any of the following: the pale waxy appearance of amyloidosis, the irregular surface texture of glomerulonephritis, neoplastic change, uric acid deposits in the parenchyma or on the surface together with signs of gout on the surface of heart or liver.
(f) *Faecal examination*	Some parasites notably *Eimeria truncata* of geese, cryptosporidia and occasionally trematodes infect the kidneys.

In addition, in any bird exhibiting signs of hypovitaminosis A, i.e. pustules in the oropharynx (particularly African grey parrots), hyperkeratosis of the feet, paraorbital sinusitis or bilateral epiphora should be suspected of having an underling nephropathy caused by metaplasia of the epithelium of the kidney tubules. This may reduce active excretion of uric acid or affect urea excretion. Other renal toxins not already mentioned under (d) radiography, are aflatoxin, other mycotoxins, ethylene glycol and carbon tetrachloride.

Schedule 5: Signs of polydipsia/polyuria

These are generally not indications of nephropathy in birds. These signs are most likely to indicate a hormonal problem, hepatopathy, the use of corticosteroids or they may be psychogenic. Also excessive fruit or high protein or toxic drugs or the use of progesterones may all precipitate this condition. Some infections, particularly paramyxo virus in pigeons, chronic chlamydiosis, or *klebsiella* may all be responsible for a marked and prolonged polydipsia and polyuria. Always take into account any concurrent and primary alimentary tract disease which may account for substantial fluid loss.

Clinical procedure	Comment
(a) *Urinary glucose*. See schedule 4 (c) for method of sampling. Use dipstix for testing.	This should be negative but if the sample is *slightly* contaminated with faeces there may be a false positive. Only if there is a hyperglycaemia should a diagnosis of *diabetes mellitus* be *diagnosed*, otherwise the cause may be glomerulonephritis if other signs are present.
(b) *Glucose tolerance test* for the confirmation of diabetes mellitus	First blood sample for plasma glucose, then starve the bird for 2–3 hours. Administer glucose orally (2 g/kg) blood sample again in 7 min and again in 90 min. In the diabetic bird plasma glucose remains elevated. Note glucogan not insulin is the principle hormone controlling plasma glucose in most birds (see p. 59).
(c) *Water deprivation test* Collect urine samples as described in Schedule 4 (c).	This test must *only* be carried out on normally hydrated birds (first check the PCV) and those in good bodily condition. Starve the bird 12 hours if a small bird or up to 20 hours for pigeon sized birds, to reduce the risk of faecal contamination. Measure the urinary specific gravity at the start and after 24 hours without water. Specific gravity should increase to above 1.025 in the normal bird which if polydipsic/polyuric may be psychogenic in origin. If no increase occurs and the sp. gr. of the sample remains between 1.008 and 1.012, this could indicate nephropathy, rectal disease (an important region of water conservation) or central diabetes insipidus. Psychogenic polydipsia may be related to stressors and increased secretion of corticosteroids. It is not uncommon in recently weaned parrots, cockatoos and African grey parrots.
(d) *The use of antidiuretic hormone*	Arginine vasotocin is the principle hormone regulating water balance in birds. However, mammalian vasopressin does have some effect but is not so potent.

Clinical procedure	Comment
	Using a dose of 0.5 units/kg body weight of vasopressin. The urinary specific gravity should increase with the water deprivation test. If this occurs, a diagnosis of central diabetes insipidus involving the pituitary gland can be made. There may be other signs such as exophthalmus or episodic seizures if a neoplasm is involved (see pp. 111 and 367).
(e) Radiography	Barium enema with air contrast of the coprodaeum and rectum may indicate pathology of these areas which are important in water conservation.

Schedule 6: The investigation of dermatological problems including skin, feathers, beak, claws, feet, wattles and comb

As in mammals, the diagnosis of some of these problems can sometimes be very difficult and they are often complex and multifactorial.

Before considering the use of any ancillary aids or laboratory tests, it is essential to obtain a thorough clinical history which should include enquiry about the duration of the condition and the relation of this to the breeding history and breeding cycle of the bird. Also information should be sought on any previous illness and any relevant vaccine status. Also husbandry practices should be considered, the type and size of caging since this affects physical fitness and behaviour, the humidity of the ambient atmosphere, if too dry leads to brittle feathering. How much natural and artificial light the bird is subjected to, since prolonged periods beyond what is normal for the species or decreasing or increasing periods of light affect the pineal/hypothalamus/pituitary complex which has an important influence on moulting. Diet received by the bird is most important and many pet and captive birds are deficient in one or more fractions of their diet. Hypovitaminosis A is easy to recognise by its other signs. In sexually dimorphic species any abnormal changes in secondary sexual characteristics or behaviour may indicate an underlying sex hormone problem. Other abnormalities of behaviour particularly in household parrots may be stress related to changes in the routine or life style of the owner. Next a thorough visual examination of the affected part or parts, if necessary using magnification and good lighting, should be carried out and much of what to look for has been described in Chapter 2. However, when examining feathers, note further if they look worn and frayed (i.e. not just chewed as with some parrots). Are new feathers emerging and do they look normal? Some parrots which have been self-plucking for months or years may have so damaged the epidermis of the follicles that they will never regenerate. A simple but good routine is to carefully pluck a damaged feather, use it for testing, note the exact position then watch the new feather gradually emerge over the next 2–4 weeks. If the epidermis and dermis have not been damaged, regrowth of a new normal feather should occur.

The observer should look to see if the uropygial gland is functional in those species which have one. It is absent in ratites, rudimentary or absent in most pigeons and many parrots. However, it is present in the African grey parrot and the budgerigar. When examining the beak, note if there is any lesion of the germinative layer and note if the claws look normal.

Clinical procedure	Comment
A full health check including those procedures described in Schedule 1	Feather plucking particularly in African grey parrots can be due to chronic chlamydosis. They look just like psychogenic feather pluckers. Also, chronic hypocalcaemia can cause self-trauma in these birds. Giardia may cause self-plucking in cockatiels. Underlying neoplasms and traumatic arthritis may also initiate self-trauma. Hepatopathy may result in changes to the colour of plumage from green to yellow or black or dark brown to black. Particularly dark coloured or black feral pigeons often have an underlying health problem.
Cytology of the pulp of affected feathers together with scrapings of cere and skin lesions. *Microscopy of feathers.*	This may reveal some ectoparasitic infections, other ectoparasites may need special techniques. See Appendix 7. Excessive dirt and debris may be seen trapped between the barbules indicating the bird is not preening or able to bath.
Biopsy of the skin. Preserve in buffered normal saline as for other biopsies.	Always include at least one feather follicle. A biopsy punch or scapel can be used. Biopsy may be necessary to confirm a suspicion of avipox virus infection.
Microbiology together with antibiotic sensitivity. If the sample is dry, small pieces harvested aseptically can be placed in the transport medium of the swab tube. Squeeze feather pulp in the swab tube with sterile forceps.	Microbiological pathogens may be either primary or secondary causes of skin problems always search for an underlying cause. A great variety of pathogens both bacterial, yeast and fungi have been documented as having been isolated from avian skin and feathers. Clostridial dermatitis is documented as causing a localised loss of feathers together with a dark pigmentation of the skin. See Appendix 2.
PCR DNA laboratory check for psittacine beak and feather disease and polyoma viruses. See p. 70 and Appendix 3, pp. 312 and 313.	
Faecal culture of avipox virus	May be difficult to find a laboratory to carry this out. Use histopathology.

Other viruses causing skin lesions for which histopathology may be appropriate are papilloma virus of the feet of some Passeriformes, localised dermal virus of the feet of cockatoos, macaws and mallard ducks and a herpes virus of lovebirds. The feather duster syndrome of budgerigars is probably not caused by a virus but is genetic in origin (Plate 10).

If the facility is available, the use of *electronmicroscopy* of newly emerging and growing pin feathers.	This has been used (courtesy of J.E. Cooper) to identify PBFD virus in vasa parrots (*Coracopsis vasa*) (see Plate 12).

Clinical procedure	Comment
Thyroxin plasma T4 estimation. In cases of hypothyroidism there is usually symmetrical feather loss and some pruritis.	Two estimations are made on a blood sample. One before an injection of thyroid stimulating hormone and one 32 hours later. There should be a 2–5-fold increase if the thyroid gland is functional. If thyroid stimulating hormone is not available, thyroid releasing hormone (TRH), which is more readily obtainable, can be used. A dose of 15 µg/kg body weight can be used. No adverse side effects of overdosage has been recorded in humans. For TRH to be effective, both pituitary and thyroid must be functionally intact. In uncomplicated cases of hypothyroidism due to iodine deficiency diluted. Lugol's iodine can be used (see Formulary, Appendix 1). In other cases of hypothyroidism, use *L*-thyroxine, 20 µg/kg p.o. 12 hours.
Trial use of haloperidol for self-plucking parrots – see Formulary (Appendix 1) for dosage (p. 277)	If all the above tests are negative, a presumptive diagnosis of psychogenic self-feather-plucking may be made. Some species of parrot are particularly prone to this condition, e.g. African greys, occasionally cockatoos and macaws, rarely budgarigars or cockatiels. The latter is more prone to self-trauma of the prepatagium. All psychogenic cases need nutritional support, spraying or bathing facilities, attention to light levels and other husbandry improvements. Overall complete resolution can only be expected in 20% of cases and 30% show no improvement at all.

Schedule 7: For the investigation of neurological signs

Many infectious diseases, toxins and traumas are responsible for neurological signs. In many cases, because of the species affected and the circumstances, the experienced clinician will have a fair idea of the cause. Tests will then be needed to confirm the tentative diagnosis. Of course, in all cases, it is necessary to obtain a thorough clinical history including the duration of the problem, whether the bird has been recently purchased or received by the owner, whether the signs are constantly present or occur sporadically. It is important to obtain in-depth information on the husbandry and whether any medicaments have been recently administered.

Listed are those conditions commonly responsible for neurological signs.

Disease/disorder	Comment
(a) *Viruses* (see Appendix 3) Newcastle disease (paramyxo serotype I) Also PMV-1 mutant stain, PMV-3	All species can be affected and can exhibit a variety of neurological signs. Common in feral pigeons. Not uncommonly seen in *Neophema* sp. grass parakeets.
A suspected PMV virus	Twirling syndrome in some finches.
Polyomavirus (one cause of budgerigar bleeding disease)	Occasional CNS signs can sometimes affect finches
Duck virus hepatitis (picorma virus)	May have extended necks and drown.
Duck virus enteritis (duck plaque) a herpes virus	Paralysis of the phallus.
Marek's disease	Mainly Galliformes but also waterfowl and occasionally in some other species
Pigeon herpes virus (infectious eosophagitis)	
Pigeon herpes virus (contagious paralysis)	
Eastern and western equine encephalomyelitis	Occurs mainly in the western hemisphere
Avian encephalomyelitis (epidemic tremor)	Mainly Galliformes but can affect water-fowl and pigeons.
Louping ill (an arbo virus)	Grouse sp. and pheasants.
Rabies virus	Rare but can occur in many species
Borma disease	Ostrich chicks
Adenoviruses	Quail, raptors, Psittaciformes and water-fowl
Reovirus (orthovirus)	Psittaciformes and geese
Reticuloendotheliosis virus	Young turkeys – may cause lameness.
(b) *Other infectious diseases* (see Appendices 2 and 5) Mycobacteriosis Aspergillosis	All species. Both pathogens can cause granulomata which may start in the vertebral column and cause paralysis.
Listeriosis	Rare, geographically localised, all species but mostly canaries.
Chlamydia	Occasional CNS signs
Filiariasis	Raptors, Passeriformes, Psittaciformes and ostrich chicks.
Toxoplasmosis	All species but particularly water-fowl.
Sarcocystis and the related *Hammondia* and *Besnotitia* spp.	In the case of a very heavy infection, the encysted parasites may cause muscle damage and atrophy, weakness and paresis.
Giardia	May be associated with hypovitaminosis in cockatiels resulting in weakness, paresis and paralysis. Occasionally in other psittacines.
Caryospira sp.	May be the cause of muscle cramps in raptors.

Disease/disorder	Comment
(c) Metabolic and nutritional causes Hypocalcaemia Seizures in African grey parrots Ataxia in conures	Particularly common in the African grey parrots due to nutritional secondary hypereparathyroidism. Precipitated by oxytetracycline. Can also occur in conures with conure haemorrhagic syndrome.
Hypoglycaemia	Raptors kept by falconers on a reduced diet. Weakness, dullness and fits. Also possible in parrots secondary to hepathopathy and starvation.
Hepatopathies	May result in hepatic encephalopathy due to raised plasma ammonia.
Hypovitaminosis B	Reduced dietary vitamins B_1, B_2, B_6 and B_{12} may all cause neuropathy. So called 'star gazing' or opisthotonos due to hypovitaminosis B_1.
Hypovitaminosis E	Particularly in cockatiels but also documented in other psittacines and possible in other species.
Hypovitaminosis D_3, calcium deficiency	As for hypocalcaemia (above).
(d) Toxins – see Appendix 8 Lead and other heavy metals such as zinc.	Common in swans due to bottom feeding fishermen's waters. Also other water birds. Differentiate botulism. Also household and aviary parrots.
Agricultural sprays drifting into aviaries	All species.
Industrial 'smoke' from temporarily uncontrolled manufacturing process.	All species.
Leakage into waterways of badly stored agricultural chemical Household pet aerosol sprays	All species.
Botulism	Particularly water birds but also raptors. Most common in hot weather but can occur at any time.
Household plants and aviary pot plants	Usually pet parrots.
Medical drug overdosage	Some drugs which might be implicated include aminoglycosides, flouroquinolones, some 'azole' antifungals, levamisole, ivermectin, metronidazole, dimetridazole, xylazine and medetomidine.
Aflatoxins	All species feeding on grains, seeds or peanuts.
Algal toxins	Warm, shallow, static water. Most water birds but any others drinking the water.

(e) *Miscellaneous causes*

Hypothalamic/pituitary tumours in budgerigars	Usually occurs in birds under 4 years. A well recognised and not uncommon syndrome results in a variety of CNS signs including episodic seizure. Often with polydip/polyuria, sometimes obesity or small size, cere may change colour (see pp. 111 and 362).
Idiopathic epilepsy	A tentative diagnosis can be assumed after ruling out other causes. Documented in parrots (particularly Amazon parrots) and mynah birds. Can be petit mal or grand mal in type. Response to phenobarbitone 0.5–6.0 mg/kg. p.o. 12 hours.
Cerebrovascular episode, strokes	May result from fat embolism during egg laying.
Nephropathy, coelomic tumours and egg impaction	Can all cause pressure on the sacral plexus causing lameness, paresis or paralysis.
Trauma	Gunshot wounds, not always obvious. Aggression from cage mates, wild conspecifics during breeding, predators, road traffic or railway injuries. Healed fractures but still paralysis due to avulsion of peripheral nerves.

If none of those causes listed above could be the reason for any of the neurological signs or these have not been confirmed with subsequent tests, then a systemic examination commencing with a thorough health check including those tests detailed in Schedule 1 will need to be carried out. A systemic assessment of the nervous system may also have to be implemented.

The bird's alertness, signs of hyperactivity, signs of sleepiness or any abnormal behaviour will given an indication of the general stage of the brain and central nervous system.

The cerebrospinal fluid. Although this is present, its collection from the subarachnoid space is not very practical because of the considerable haemorrhage from the venous sinuses in this area.

(f) *Examination of the cranial nerves.* This can be carried out in the same way as in mammals although there are some important differences in physiology between the two classes of vertebrates.

Overall examination of the cranial nerves may help to localise a neoplastic or traumatic lesion. It may also indicate unilateral or bilateral lesions. Note, apart from cranial nerves I, II and IV, all other cranial nerves emerge from the ventral or ventrolateral surface of the brain so that lesions located here are most likely to affect more than one cranial nerve. Thus the more nerves exhibiting a defect the graver the prognosis.

Cranial nerve I – the olfactory	Olfaction varies considerably between species and checking this nerve's function is difficult and often not very practical. Note noxious odours used for testing could be toxic.

Disease/disorder	Comment
Cranial nerve II – the optic	Checking this nerve is not difficult but make sure the bird does not have a cataract or intra-ocular haemorrhage from the pecten. If a bird persists in keeping one particular eye on the observer be suspicious of defective vision in the other eye. In birds, there is almost complete decussation of the optic fibres so a defect on one side indicates a brain lesion on the opposite side. Total blindness may indicate a lesion in the region of the optic chiasma, e.g. budgerigar pituitary neoplasm. Decussation of the optic fibres also results in there being no consensual pupillary light reflex. In any case, this reflex is difficult to assess in birds because the iris muscles are striated and partially under voluntary control. So a bright light directed at the eye may not evoke a response because of voluntary inhibition. Because there is no tapetum lucidum of the fundus, ophthalmic examination does not help in the diagnosis of brain lesions.
Cranial nerves III and IV – the oculomotor and trochlear	In most birds, except for the toucans and hornbills, the extra-ocular eye muscles are considerably reduced and eye movement is minimal (compensated by the highly mobile neck) consequently assessment of the function of cranial nerves III and IV is often not very practical. However, ptosis or paralysis of the upper eyelid indicates a lesion of the dorsal branch of III.
Cranial nerve V – the trigeminal	Function of this nerve is easy to assess since it is both sensory to all the structures of the head and is motor to both the lower and upper jaws.
Cranial nerve VI – the abducent	Along with the lateral rectus muscle of the eyeball, it inervates the nictating membrane. Although this is controlled by two striated muscles and is to some extent under voluntary control, touching the cornea with a moist cotton bud usually produces a marked response providing of course the afferent nerve in cranial nerve V is intact.
Cranial nerve VII – the facial	Separate assessment of this cranial nerve is difficult and not always practical.

Cranial nerve VIII – the vestibulocochlear nerve	Hearing may be difficult to check but head tilt, ataxia and spontaneous nystagmus may all indicate dysfunction of this nerve. Check for signs of exterior auditory disease. These signs may be more common in the night hunting owls due to increased size of external ear and auditory nuclei in the medulla.
Cranial nerve IX – the glossopharyngeal	Paralysis of the tongue and lack of sensation indicate dysfunction.
Cranial nerves X, XI and XII	Independent assessment of these nerves is not easy.
(g) *The remainder of the peripheral nervous system*	The withdrawal reflexes in both wings and legs are segmental reflexes but should elicit a conscious response if the spinal cord is intact. Similarly, the cloacal reflex is segmental. Lesions of the thoracolumbar vertebrae are not uncommon and are indicated by conscious appreciation of intact wing withdrawal reflex but no response by the bird to an intact leg withdrawal reflex together with a cloacal reflex. Check by radiography. Knuckling of the legs or an inability to grip the perch may be either an upper or lower motor lesion.

APPENDIX 10:
WEIGHTS OF BIRDS MOST LIKELY TO BE SEEN IN GENERAL PRACTICE

Common name	Scientific name	Weight range in grams
Order: **Psittaciformes**		
Lesser sulphur-crested cockatoo	*Cacatua sulphurea*	228–315
Greater sulphur-crested cockatoo	*Cacatua galerita galerita*	500–1250
Moluccan cockatoo	*Cacatua moluccensis*	670–800
Roseate cockatoo	*Eolophus roseicapillis*	340–480
Umbrella cockatoo or great white cockatoo	*Cacatua alba*	530–610
Blue and gold macaw	*Ara ararauna*	850–2000
Scarlet macaw	*Ara macao*	810–1100
Hahns macaw (noble macaw)	*Ara nobilis*	150–180
Orange winged Amazon	*Amazona amazonica*	440–470
Blue fronted Amazon	*Amazona aestiva*	275–510
Yellow fronted Amazon	*Amazona ochrocephala*	260–460
Double yellow headed Amazon (Levaillant's)	*Amazona ochracephala oratrix*	545
Mealy Amazon	*Amazona farinosa*	600–685
Yellow billed Amazon	*Amazona collaria*	215–270
Festive Amazon	*Amazona festiva*	358–500
Hispaniolan Amazon	*Amazona ventralis*	268
African grey parrot Three main varities with different average weights	*Psittacus erithacus*	310–460
Orange bellied Senegal parrot	*Poicephalus senegalus*	125–150
Dusky headed conure	*Aratinga acuticaudata*	155–185
Red masked conure	*Aratinga erythrogenys*	158–168
Jendaya conure	*Aratinga jandaya*	118–128
Yellow rosella parakeet	*Platycercus flaveolus*	100–120
Pale headed rosella parakeet	*Platycercus adscitus palliceps*	100–120
Blue bonnet	*Psephotus haematogaster*	100–120
Port lincoln	*Barnardius zonarius*	170–180
Blue headed parrot Pionus parrot	*Pionus menstruus*	238–278
Cockatiel	*Nymphicus hollandicus*	70–108

Budgerigar	*Melopsittacus undulatus*	35–85
Bourke's parakeet	*Neophema bourkii*	50
Turquoisine parakeet	*Neophema pulchella*	50
Blue winged grass parakeet	*Neophema chrysostoma*	38–50
Fisher's lovebird	*Agapornis fischeri*	40–50

Order: **Columbiformes**

Racing pigeon ⎫ Feral pigeon ⎬	*Columba livia*	230–540
Wood pigeon	*Columba palumbus*	454–680
Collared dove	*Streptopelia decaocto*	150–220
Diamond dove	*Geopelia cuneata*	40

Order: **Gruiformes**

Moorhen	*Gallinula chloropus*	278
Coot	*Fulica atra*	520

Infraorder: **Charadriides**

Lapwing plover	*Vanellus vanellus*	200–235
Common sandpiper	*Tringa hypoleucos*	50
Herring gull	*Larus argentatus*	750
Lesser black backed gull	*Larus fuscus*	675
Common gull	*Larus canus*	300–500
Black headed gull	*Larus ridibundus*	175–295
Common/Arctic tern	*Sterna hirundo/paradisaea*	90–100
Heron	*Ardea cinerea*	1362

Infraorder: **Ciconiides**

Gannet	*Sula bassana*	2750
Shag	*Phalacrocorax aristotelis*	1700–2200
Fulmar petrel	*Fulmaris glacialis*	800

Order: **Anseriformes**

Mute swan	*Cygnus olor*	8000–13,000
Canada goose	*Branta canadensis*	4540
Domestic goose ⎫ Grey lag goose ⎬	*Anser anser*	3100–4090
Bean goose	*Anser fabalis*	2700–3600
Muscovy duck	*Cairina moschata*	3500–5000
Domestic duck ⎫ Mallard duck ⎬	*Anas platyrhynchos* *platyrhynchos*	975–3500
Shelduck	*Tadorna tadorna*	682

Common name	Scientific name	Weight range in grams
Infraorder: Falconides		
Sparrow hawk	*Accipiter nisus*	♂ 150–210 ♀ 190–300
Goshawk	*Accipiter gentilis gentilis*	♂ 634–880 ♀ 980–1200
Buzzard	*Buteo buteo*	680–1100
Red-tailed hawk	*Buteo jamaicensis*	♂ 698–1147 ♀ 1000–1350
Harris' hawk	*Parabuteo unicinctus*	574–1000
Peregrine falcon	*Falco peregrinus*	♂ 560–850 ♀ 1100–1500
Kestrel*	*Falco tinnunculus*	♂ 145–167 ♀ 193–282
Saker falcon	*Falco cherrug*	♂ 680–990 ♀ 970–1300
Lanner falcon	*Falco biarmicus*	♂ 500–600 ♀ 700–900
Laggar falcon	*Falco jugger*	515
Merlin	*Falco columbarius*	♂ 160–170 ♀ 220–250
Order: Galliformes		
Pheasant	*Phasianus colchicus*	♂ 1300–1600 ♀ 500–1135
Domestic chicken	*Gallus gallus*	1000–4000
Order: Strigiformes		
Tawny owl	*Strix aluco*	330–465
Short eared owl	*Asio flammeus*	325–440
Long eared owl	*Asio otus*	210–325
Little owl	*Athene noctua*	150–175
Eagle owl	*Bubo bubo*	1600–2500
Barn owl	*Tyto alba*	262–600
Order: Passeriformes		
Carrion crow	*Corvus corone corone*	358–650
Rook	*Corvus frugilegus*	335–460
Jackdraw	*Corvus monedula spermologus*	145–210
Song thrush	*Turdus philomelos*	80
Blackbird	*Turdus merula*	57
Robin	*Erithacus rubecula*	20–30

Pekin robin	*Leothrix lutea*	26
Starling	*Sturnus vulgaris*	64
Purple glossy starling	*Lamprotornis purpureus*	74–82
Great Indian hill mynah	*Gracula religiosa intermedia*	180–260
House sparrow	*Passer domesticus*	25–30
Zebra finch	*Poephila guttata*	10–16
Java sparrow	*Padda oryzivora*	24–30
Goldfinch	*Carduelis carduelis*	15–20
Cross bill	*Loxia curvirostra*	41
Great tit	*Parus major*	17.5–20.72
Blue tit	*Parus caeruleus*	10–13.75
Green singing finch	*Serinus mozambicus*	10
Canary	*Serinus canaria*	12–29

Order: **Musophagiformes**

| Hartlaub's touraco | *Tauraco hartlaubi* | 248–380 (mean 308.8) |

Order: **Coraciiformes**

| Lilac breasted roller | *Coracias caudata* | 95–120 (mean 105) |

APPENDIX 11:
INCUBATION AND FLEDGING PERIODS OF SELECTED BIRDS

Common name	Scientific name	Incubation period in days	Fledging period in days
Order: **Psittaciformes**			
Budgerigar	*Melopsittacus undulatus*	16–18	22–26
Australian parakeets in general	*Genera Neophema, Platycercus, Psephotus*	18–19	30–45
Cockatiel	*Nymphicus hollandicus*	About 18	28
Ringneck parakeet	*Psittacula krameri*	23–24	55–65
Lorikeets	Genus *Trichoglossus*	25–26	62–70
Lovebirds	Genus *Agapornis*	About 18	30–35
Amazon parrots	Genus *Amazona*	23–24	45–60
Order: **Columbiformes**			
Domestic pigeon	*Columba livia*	17–19	35–37
Wood pigeon	*Columba palumbus*	17–19	16–38
Collared dove	*Streptopelia decaocto*	14	18–21

Common name	Scientific name	Incubation period in days	Fledging period in days
Infraorder: **Charadriides**			
Herring gull	*Larus argentatus*	20–34	42
Common gull	*Larus canus*	24–27	35
Black headed gull	*Larus ridibundus*	22–24	35–42
Order: **Anseriformes**			
Mute swan	*Cygnus olor*	34–40	Leave nest in 24–48 h. Dependent on parents for 100–120 days
Greylag goose ⎱ Domestic goose ⎰	*Anser anser*	24–30	Post fledging period: 53–57 days
Shelduck	*Tadorna tadorna*	28	45
Mallard	*Anas platyrhynchos*	28	52
Pochard	*Aythya ferina*	23–29	49–56
Infraorder: **Falconides**			
Sparrow hawk	*Accipiter nisus*	32–35	24–30
Goshawk	*Accipiter gentilis gentilis*	36–38	41–43
Buzzard	*Buteo buteo*	34–38	42–49
Red tailed hawk	*Buteo jamaicensis*	32–35	43–48
Harris' hawk	*Parabuteo unicinctus*	33–36	40
Peregrine falcon	*Falco peregrinus*	35–42	35–42
Kestrel	*Falco tinnunculus*	28–31	27–30
Lanner falcon	*Falco biarmicus*	32–34	44–46
Golden eagle	*Aquila chrysaetos*	41–49	about 77
Order: **Galliformes**			
Pheasant	*Phasianus colchicus*	21–28	Fly at 12–14 days
Domestic chicken	*Gallus gallus*	21	
Order: **Strigiformes**			
Tawny owl	*Strix aluco*	28–30	30–37
Short eared owl	*Asio flammeus*	24–28	24–27
Long eared owl	*Asio otus*	27–28	about 23
Little owl	*Athene noctua*	28–29	35–40
Barn owl	*Tyto alba*	32–34	64–86
Snowy owl	*Nyctea scandiaca*	32–34	51–57

Order: **Passeriformes**

Carrion crow	*Corvus corone corone*	16–20	26–38
Rook	*Corvus frugilegus*	16–18	28–30
Jackdaw	*Corvus monedula*	17–18	30–35
Magpie	*Pica pica*	17–18	22–27
Blackbird	*Turdus merula*	13–14	13–14
Song thrush	*Turdus philomelos*	13–14	13–14
Robin	*Erithacus rubecula*	13–14	12–14
Starling	*Sturnus vulgaris*	12–16	20–22
House sparrow	*Passer domesticus*	12–14	about 15
Zebra finch	*Poephila guttata*	12	14–21
Cross bill	*Loxia curvirostra*	12–13	17–25
Gold finch	*Carduelis carduelis*	12–13	13–14
Chaffinch	*Fringilla coelebs*	11–13	13–14
Great tit	*Parus major*	13–14	18–20
Blue tit	*Parus caeruleus*	17–18	about 16
Canary	*Serinus canaria*	13–14	Fed by parents for 28 days

APPENDIX 12:
SCHEDULE OF WILD BIRD RELEASES BY JANE RATCLIFFE (1971–1984)*

Common name	Scientific name	Number received for treatment	Died or put to sleep	Unfit for release; retained for breeding	Number released	Number of short stay patients kept less than 3 months	†Number of long stay patients kept over 3 months	Number recovered after release and interval in months	Number sited and identified and interim in months
Kestrel‡	Falco tinnunculus	90	11	4	75	62	13	6 (0.3–9)	1(seen for many years in release area)
Merlin§	Falco columbarius	2	–	–	2	1	1	–	–
Peregrine¶	Falco peregrinus	3	–	3	–	–	–	–	–
Sparrow hawk**	Accipiter nisus	8	2	–	6	3	3	1 (7)	3 {36, 24, 16}
Buzzard††	Buteo buteo	7	1	1	5	4	1	2 (5)(4.5)	–
Barn owl‡‡	Tyto alba	26	2	1	23	13	10	8 (1–22)	–
Tawny owl§§	Strix aluco	40	6	1	33	27	6	4(1–14)(+1)	–
Short eared owl	Asio flammeus	7	3	–	4	2	2	–	–
Little owl¶¶	Athene noctua	13	2	2	9	4	5	–	–
Swift***	Apus apus	3	–	–	3	3	–	–	1 (seen for several weeks)

Common name	Scientific name									Notes
House martin***	*Delichon urbica*	2	1	—	1	1	—	—	—	—
Kingfisher	*Alcedo atthis*	1	1	—	—	—	—	—	—	—
Greater spotted woodpecker	*Dendrocopos major*	1	—	—	1	1	—	—	—	Visited bird table a number of times
Wood pigeon	*Columba palumbus*	2	—	—	2	1	1	—	—	1 seen in area 3 weeks later
Collared dove	*Streptopelia decaocto*	1	—	—	1	—	—	—	—	
Great crested grebe	*Podiceps cristatus*	1	1	1	—	—	—	—	—	
Red shank	*Tringa totanus*	2	2	—	—	—	—	—	—	
Lapwing	*Vanellus vanellus*	1	1	1	—	—	—	—	—	
Oyster-catcher	*Haematopus ostralegus*	1	1	1	—	—	—	—	—	
Dunnock	*Prunella modularis*	1	—	—	1	1	—	—	—	
Treecreeper	*Certhia familiaris*	1	1	1	1	1	—	—	—	Bred in nest box 4 months after release
Totals		213	32	12	169	123	42	21	9	

*Jane Ratcliffe is a naturalist resident in Cumbria. Many of these birds were initially examined and treated by the author and the table is given here as an indication of the level of success that can be achieved with adequate veterinary treatment combined with a high standard of nursing. All the birds were B.T.O. ringed before release so they could be subsequently identified.

†Some of the long-stay cases had damaged plumage and had to be retained until completely moulted.

‡ Some of these birds were recovered between 25 and 30 km away after an interval of 6–9 months. Approximately 42 of these kestrels had been held illegally captive and 8 were received with jesses on their legs. Ten were young birds that had fallen from the nest.

§ A merlin's nest was found in the release area 2 months after release and assumed to be that of the released bird because of the scarcity of the species in that area.

¶ All these birds were received weeks or months after injury when healing had started to take place. There was either gross malformation of the bone or severe soft tissue damage often together with infection.

** The one sparrow hawk recovered was found drowned 7 months after release. Of the three birds seen after release, they were seen for periods of between 16 months and 3 years in their particular territories after release.

†† Of the two birds recovered one was found shot 5 months after release, the other was hit by a train 8 weeks after release and 26 km away. This bird, a female, had been seen displaying with a male bird.

‡‡ Of the eight barn owls recovered 2 were found drowned in cattle troughs and 3 were involved in road accidents. The longest time after release was 22 months; most recoveries were within 3–5 months. One bird was recovered 40 km away. Fifteen of these birds were habituated to a barn before release and 3 pairs raised young.

§§ One of these tawny owls was recovered 8 years after initial release. It was known to have bred a number of times in a local nest box. After treatment a second time it was released.

¶¶ Two of these little owls bred in an aviary before release when young and parents were released together.

*** It is essential these insect feeders are hospitalised for the minimum time.

Of the total number of birds treated 44 had fractures and 21 of these were eventually released. Overall 61 were received in poor or emmaciated condition and only needed good nursing before release. The total number of illegally captive raptors received for retraining and release was 68.

APPENDIX 13:
GLOSSARY OF TERMS USED IN THE TEXT TOGETHER WITH THE MORE COMMON EXPRESSIONS USED BY FALCONERS AND OTHER AVICULTURISTS

Alcinae A family of short-winged marine diving birds, the auks, included in the infraorder Charadriides.

altricial nestlings Newly hatched birds born blind, helpless and without true feathers although they are covered in down. These chicks are nidicolous or nest attached and are entirely parent dependent.

Anseriformes The order of birds containing four families amongst which are the Anatidae (ducks, geese, swans).

Adeidae The family of birds containing the herons, egrets and bitterns.

ayre See **eyrie**.

bate, bating A falconer's term; fluttering or flying off the fist or an object.

bewits Short strips of leather by which bells are fastened to the legs.

block A cylindrical piece of wood to which the hawk is attached by a leash and upon which it can perch.

calling off Luring a hawk from an assistant at a distance.

casting Fur, feathers and bone being the indigestible part of a raptor's diet which are periodically ejected in the form of a pellet.

Charadriiformes The infraorder of birds containing fourteen families and subfamilies of aquatic birds, prominent amongst which are Haematopodidae (oyster catchers), Charadriidae (plovers and lapwings), Scolopacidae (sandpipers) and Laridae (gulls and terns).

cockatiel The smallest member of the sub-family Cacatuinae (cockatoos) group of parrots and a popular pet bird.

Ciconioidae A superfamily of birds including the storks and the New World Vultures.

Columbidae A large family of birds including the pigeons and doves.

Columbiformes The order of birds containing the Columbidae and the extinct dodos.

conspecific Of the same species.

coping A falconers' term meaning to cut off the sharp points of beak and talons.

covert feathers The smaller feathers which cover the base of the shaft of the main flight feathers.

Corvidae The family of birds included in the order of Passeriformes and which contains the crows, magpies and jays.

creance A falconers' term referring to long line attached to the swivel and used when 'calling off' (q.v.).

eyess or eyas A nestling hawk taken from the 'eyrie' or nest.

eyrie (Ayre) Nest of a bird of prey perched high up.

feake When a hawk wipes its beak on a perch after feeding.

fledgling The growing period of a young bird until it is able to fly.

frounce Trichomoniasis of the oropharanx of a raptor.

Galliformes An order of fowl-like birds including grouse, ptarmigan, pheasants, peacocks, partridges, quails, domestic fowl, turkeys and guinea fowl.

gallinaceous Pertaining to the order Galliformes.

graminivorous Grass and cereal eating.

granivorous Feeding on grain and seeds.

hack, flying at Young falcons recently taken from the nest are allowed to fly freely only coming back to the falconer to be fed.

hack back To train a captive hawk to hunt and sustain itself in the wild.

Haematopodini A tribe of seashore wading birds, the oystercatchers.

haggard A hawk which has been caught in the wild, after it has undergone its first moult and has got its adult plumage.

hardbills Birds that feed by cracking open seeds.

hood A leather hat placed over the head of a hawk to blindfold it and to make it more easy to handle.

hornbill Medium to large tropical bird with brightly coloured and large bill that is often surmounted by a large casque.

imping A falconer's method of repairing a broken flight or tail feather.

interremigial ligament An elastic ligament lying within the skin fold caudal to radius and ulna, carpus, metacarpus and digits of the wing. It unites the shafts of the primary and secondary feathers.

jack The male merlin (*Falco columbarius*).

jesses The short, narrow straps of leather fastened round the hawk's legs to hold it.

Laridae The family of birds containing the gulls and terns.

leash A long, narrow strip of leather attached via the swivel to the jesses (q.v.)

long-winged hawks The true falcons. The Falconidae including peregrine, saker, lanner, laggar, merlin and kestrel. See Appendix 10.

lure A falconer's apparatus for recalling a hawk. A bunch of feathers wrapped around a piece of meat and weighted. Sometimes two wings tied together. It is swung by a cord in a large arc around the falconer.

lutino A yellow bird (usually psittacine) with no other markings and red eyes.

macaw A group of South American parrots. These are mostly, but not all, fairly large, long-tailed birds with a patch of bare skin on each side of the face.

manning Taming a hawk.

Megapodiidae The family of robust ground dwelling birds resembling pheasants found in S.E. Asia and Australia. Also known as incubator birds.

Mergus A genus of sea ducks.

mews A place where hawks are kept to moult (Mew v. to moult).

mules Hybrid canaries produced by crossing the canary with other finches such as goldfinches and greenfinches.

musket The male sparrow-hawk.

mutes The faeces of a hawk (mute v. to void faeces). Short-winged hawks (e.g. sparrowhawk, goshawk) are said to 'slice', i.e. eject the mutes horizontally.

ostringer (austringer) A falconer who flies short-winged hawks (e.g. goshawk).

pannel A falconer's term meaning the stomach of a hawk.

parakeet A small parrot. In the USA usually refers to the budgerigar.

Passeriformes The order of birds containing the largest number of species grouped into 55 families. It contains all the birds that have three forward toes and one well developed hind toe – an adaptation to perching (see p. 12).

passerines Pertaining to the order Passeriformes.

Phalacrocoracidae The family of birds containing the cormorants and shags.

Picidae The family of birds containing the woodpeckers.

pin feathers First sign of a developing feather, still retained within its sheath.

precocial chicks Newly hatched birds born covered in downy feathers, active and able to find their own food. These chicks are nidifugous or nest leaving.

prepatagial (propatagial) Referring to the prepatagium, a membranous fold of skin between the shoulder and carpal joints forming the leading edge of the wing.

primary feathers The main flight feathers attached to the metacarpal bones and digits.

Psittaciformes The order of birds containing one family – the psittacidae or parrots.

psittacines Parrots and related species.

Psittacula **parakeets** A large genus of medium-sized, mostly Asiatic parakeets, including the popular plumheaded and ringnecked species.

Rallidae The family of birds known as rails including the coots, gallinules and moorhens.

Ramphastidae The toucans. S. American tropical birds with large brightly coloured bills.

raptor A bird with a hooked beak and sharp talons – a bird of prey.

redrump parakeet A species of small Australian parrot with red feathers over the base of the tail or rump.

remiges The main flight feathers of the wings (i.e. the primaries and secondaries).

short winged hawks Usually taken to mean the accipiters or bird hawks which include the goshawks and Cooper's hawk. Also refers to the broad winged birds – the buzzards.

soft bills Birds that feed on fruit or insects.

Spheniscidae The family of birds containing the penguins.

split A heterozygous bird carrying a recessive colour.

stoop The swift descent of a falcon on the quarry from a height.

Sulidae The family of birds containing the gannets and boobies.

swivel Used to prevent the jesses and leash (q.v.) from becoming twisted when the hawk is tethered to its perch.

tiercel (tercel) The male of any species of hawk. The female is known as the falcon, especially the peregrine.

tiring A touch piece of meat or tendon given to a hawk to help exercise the muscles of the back and neck.

Turdinae The subfamily of birds containing the thrushes and including such birds as the blackbird, the European robin and the nightingale.

Ulno carporemigial aponeurosis A triangular aponeurotic sheet of elastic tissue, lying on the ventral side of the wing, just caudal to the metacarpus and joining the bases of the shafts of the metacarpal primary feathers.

to wait on When a hawk soars above the falconer waiting for the game to be flushed.

to weather To place a hawk on a perch out in the open. Usually an area shielded from extreme weather is chosen.

weaver birds Small to medium sized passerine birds. Many species are gregarious and include the common house sparrow. Some species are popular aviary birds.

whydahs (Widow bird) A group of brood parasitic passerines (like cuckoos) allied to the weaver birds. The males usually have long tail feathers.

Further reading

Arnall, L. & Keymer, I.F. (1975) *Bird Diseases.* Bailliére Tindall, London.

Beynon, P.H., Forbes, N.A. & Lawton, M.P.C. (1996) *Manual of Psittacine Birds.* British Small Animal Veterinary Association, Cheltenham, Glos.

Cooper, J.E. (1978) *Veterinary Aspects of Captive Birds of Prey.* Standfast Press, Saul, Glos.

Cooper, J.E., & Eley J.T. (1979) *First Aid and Care of Wild Birds.* David & Charles, London.

Elkins, N. (1983) *Weather and Bird Behaviour* T.A.D. Poyser Ltd., Carlton.

Fowler, M.E. (1978) *Zoo and Wild Animal Medicine.* W.B. Saunders Co., Philadelphia/London.

Gordon, R.F. (1977) *Poultry Diseases.* Bailliére Tindall, London.

Harrison, G.J. & Harrison, L.R. (1986) *Clinical Avian Medicine and Surgery.* W.B. Saunders, Philadelphia.

King, A.S. & McLelland, J. (1984) *Birds: Their Structure and Function.* Bailliére Tindall, London.

Krautwald-Junghanns, M.E., Tellhelm, B., Hummel, G., Kostka, V. & Kaleta, E.F. (1992) *Atlas of Radiographic Anatomy and Diagnosis in Cage Birds.* Verlag Paul Parey, Berlin.

Mavrogordato, J.G. (1973) *A Hawk for the Bush.* 2nd edn Neville Spearman, London.

Petrak, M.L. (1969, 1982) *Diseases of Cage and Aviary Birds,* 1st and 2nd edns., Lea & Febiger, Philadelphia.

Ratcliffe, J. (1979) *Fly High, Run Free.* Chatto & Windus, London.

Redig, P.J., Cooper, J.E., Remple, J.D.& Hunter, D.B. (1993) *Raptor Biomedicine.* Chiron Publications, Keighley, Yorks.

Ritchie, B.W., Harrison, G.J. & Harrison, L.R. (1994) *Avian Medicine, Principles and Application.* Wingers Publishing, Lake Worth, Florida.

Ritchie, B.W. (1995) *Avian Viruses.* Wingers Publishing, Lake Worth, Florida.

Steiner, C.V. & Davis, R.B. (1981) *Caged Bird Medicine.* Iowa State University Press, Ames, Iowa.

Wallack, J.D. & Boever, W.J. (1983) *Diseases of Exotic Animals; Medical and Surgical Management.* W.B. Saunders, Philadelphia/London.

Woodford, M.H. (1960) *A Manual of Falconry.* A. & C. Black, London.

References

Ahlers, W. (1970) Report on the use of bisolvon in small animal practice. *Kleintier-Praxis*, **15**, 50–53.

Allwright, D.M. & van Rensburg, W.J.J. (1994) Botulism in ostriches (*Struthio camelus*). *Avian Pathology*, **23**, 183–186.

Altman, R.B. (1980) Avian Anaesthesia. *The Compendium on Continuing Veterinary Education*, **2**, 38–42.

Altman, R.B. (1982) In: *Diseases of Cage and Aviary Birds* 2nd edn, (ed. M.L. Petrak), p. 369, Lea & Fibiger, Philadelphia.

Altman, R.B. & Miller, M.S. (1979) The effect of Halothane and Ketamin anaesthesia on body temperature and electro-cardiographic changes of birds. *Proceedings of the American Association of Zoo Veterinarians*, Denver, Colorado, 61–62A.

Ar, A. & Rahn, H. (1977) Interdependence of gas conductance, incubation, length and weight of avian egg. In: 'Respiratory Function in Birds, Adult and Embryonic', a satellite symposium of the *27th International Congress of Physiological Sciences, Paris 1977* (ed J. Piper), pp. 227–236. Springer-Verlag, Berlin, Heileberg, New York.

Arañez, J.B. & Sanguin, C.S. (1955) Poulardization of native ducks. *Journal of the American Veterinary Medicine Association*, **127**, 314–317.

Ashash, E., Weisman, Y., Malkinson, M., Perl, S., Mechany, S. (1995) Borna disease in ostriches. *Proceedings 3rd Conference of European Committee of the Association of Avian Veterinarians*, Jerusalem, pp. 44–47.

Ashton, G. & Smith, H.G. (1984) *Psittacosis in Birds and Man*. The Unit for Veterinary Continuing Education, Vet 31, The Royal Veterinary College, London.

Bernier, G., Morin, M. & Marsolais, G. (1981) A generalised inclusion body disease in the budgerigar (*Melopsittacus undulatus*) caused by Papova-like agent. *Avian Diseases*, **23**, 1083–1093.

Berry, R.B. (1972) Reproduction by artificial insemination in captive American goshawks. *Journal of Wildlife Management*, **36**, 1283–1288.

Bird, D.M., Lague, P.C. & Buckland, R.B. (1976) Artificial insemination versus natural mating in captive American kestrels. *Canadian Journal of Zoology*, **54**, 1183–1191.

Blackmore, D.K. (1982) In: *Diseases of Cage and Aviary Birds* 2nd edn, (ed. M.L. Petrak), p. 484. Lea & Fibiger, Philadelphia.

Borland, E.D., Morgan, C.T., Smith, G.R. (1977) Avian botulism and the high prevalence of clostridium botulinum in the Norfolk broads. *Veterinary Record*, **100**, 106–109.

Bortch, A. & Vroege, C. (1972) Amputation of the wing under Rompun sedation and experimental sedation of the homing pigeon with Rompun. *Veterinary Review*, (**3/4**), 275.

Böttcher, M. (1980) Endoscopy of birds of prey in clinical veterinary practice. *Recent Advances in the Study of Raptor Diseases* (eds J.E. Cooper & A.G. Greenwood), pp. 101–104. Chiron Publications Ltd, Keighley, Yorks.

Bourne, W.R.P. (1989) The role of birds in the long-distance dispersal of disease. In: *Disease and threatened birds, 121. International Council for Bird Preservation Tech. Pub. No. 10*, (ed. J.E. Cooper), pp. 121–128. ICBP, Cambridge.

Boyd, L.L. (1978) Artificial insemination of falcons. *A Symposium of the Zoological Society of London*, **43**, 73–80.

Boyd, L.L. & Schwartz, C.H. (1983) Training imprinted semen donors. In: *Falcon Propagation, a Manual on Captive Breeding* (eds J.D. Weaver & T.J. Cade), p. 10. The Peregrine Fund, Inc. Ithaca, New York.

Brock, M.S. (1991) Semen collection and artificial insemination in hispaniolan parrot (*Amazonia ventralis*). *Journal of Zoo and Wildlife Medicine*, **22**(1), 107–114.

Brooks, N.G. (1982) Crop wall necrosis in a sparrowhawk. *Veterinary Record*, **3**(22), 513.

Brown, L. (1976) *Birds of Prey: Their Biology and Ecology*, p. 117. Hamlyn, London.

Burnham, W., Walton, B.J. & Weaver, J.D. (1983) Management and maintenance. In: *Falcon Propagation, a Manual on Captive Breeding* (eds J.D. Weaver & T.J. Cade), p. 11. The Peregrine Fund, Inc. Ithaca, New York.

Bush, M. (1980) *Animal Laparascopy* (eds R.M. Harrison and D.E. Wildt), pp. 183–193. Williams and Wilkins, Baltimore/London.

Bush, M. (1981) Avian fracture repair using external fixation. In: *Recent Advances in the Study of Raptor Diseases* (eds J.E. Cooper and A.G. Greenwood), pp. 83–93. Chiron Publishers Ltd, Keighley, Yorks.

Bush, M., Montali, R.I., Novak, R.G. & James, F.A. (1976) The healing of avian fractures. A histological xeroradiographic study. *American Animal Hospital Association Journal*, **12**(6), 768–773.

Bush, M., Neal, L.A. & Custer, R.S. (1979) Preliminary pharmacokinetic studies of selected antibiotics in birds. *Proceedings of the American Association of Zoo Veterinarians*, 45–47.

Bush, M., Locke, D., Neal, L.A. & Carpenter, J.W. (1980) Pharmacokinetics of Cephalin and Cephalexin in selected avian species. *American Journal of Veterinary Research*, **42**(6), 1014–1017.

Butler, E.J. & Laursen-Jones, A.P. (1977) Nutritional disorders. In: *Poultry Diseases* (ed. R.F. Gordon), p. 158. Bailliére Tindall, London.

Camburn, M.A. & Stead, C. (1966–1967) Anaesthesia of wild birds. *Proceedings of the Association of Veterinary Anaesthetists of Great Britain and Ireland*, **6**, 821.

Campbell, T.W. (1988) *Avian Haematology and Cytology*, pp. 3–17. Iowa State University Press, Ames, Iowa.

Campbell, T.W. (1994) In: Haematology. *Avian Medicine: Principles & Application* (eds B.W. Ritchie, G.J. Harrison & L.R. Harrison). Wingers Publishing, Lake Worth, Florida.

Campbell, T.W. & Dein, F.J. (1984) Avian haematology: the basics. In: Symposium on Cage Bird Medicine. *The Veterinary Clinics of North America*. **14**(2), 223–248.

Clubb, S.L. (1984) Therapeutics in avian medicine – flock vs. individual bird treatment regimens. *The Veterinary Clinics of North America* (ed. G.J. Harrison), **14**(2), 345–361.

Coffin, D.L. (1969) In: *Diseases of Parrots and Parrot-like Birds* (ed. the Duke of Bedford), p. 35. T.F.H. Publications, Inc., Hong Kong.

Coles, B.H. (1984a) Avian anaesthesia. *Veterinary Record*, **115**(12), 307.

Coles, B.H. (1984b) Some considerations when nursing birds in veterinary premises. *Journal of Small Animal Practice*, **25**(5), 275–288.

Cooke, S.W. (1984) Lead poisoning in cygnets. *Veterinary Record*, **114**(8), 203.

Cooper, J.E. (1970) The use of the hypnotic agent. Methoxymol in birds of prey. *Veterinary Record*, **87**, 751–752.

Cooper, J.E. (1974) Metomidate anaesthesia of some birds of prey for laparotomy and sexing. *Veterinary Record*, **24**, 437–440.

Cooper, J.E. (1978) *Veterinary Aspects of Captive Birds of Prey*, pp. 21, 28. Standfast Press, Saul, Gloucestershire.

Cooper, J.E. (1983) In: *Sonderdruk aus Verhandlungs bericht des 25 internationalen Symposiums über die Erkrankungen der Zootiere*. Wien Akademie Verlag, Berlin, 61–65.

Cooper, J.E. & Redig, P.T. (1975) Unexpected reactions to the use of C.T. 1341 by red-tailed hawks. *Veterinary Record*, **97**, 352.

Cooper, M.E. (1979) *Wild bird hospitals and the law in first aid and care of wild birds*, (eds J.E. Cooper and J.T. Eley), pp. 15–20. David & Charles Ltd, London.

Cribb, P.H. & Haigh, J.C. (1977) Anaesthesia for avian species. *Veterinary Record*, **100**, 472–473.

Crosta, L., Sironi, G., Rampin, T. (1995) An outbreak of avian pox in neophema parakeets. *Proceedings 3rd Conference of European Committee of Association of European Veterinarians*. Jerusalem 1995, pp. 23–25.

Dawson, R.W. (1975) Avian physiology. *Annual review of Physiology*, **37**, 441–465.

De Gruchy, P.H. (1983) Chlamydiosis in collared doves. *Veterinary Record*, **113**(14), 327.

Delius, J.D. (1966) Pentobarbitone anaesthesia in the herring and black-backed gull. *Journal of Small Animal Practice*, **7**, 605–609.

Dom, P., Ducateile, R., Charlier, G., de Herdt, P. (1993) Papilloma-like virus infections in canaries (*Serenius canarius*). *Proceeding of 1993 European Conference on Avian Medicine and Surgery*. The association of Avian Veterinarians and the Dutch Association of Avian Veterinarians. Utrecht, The Netherlands, pp. 224–231.

Donita, L.F., Jones, M.P. and Orosz, S.E. (1995). Pharmacokinetic considerations of the renal system in birds: anatomic and physiologic principles of allometric sealing, Part II Review of drugs excreted by renal pathways. *Journal of Avian Medicine and Surgery*, **9**(2), 92–104.

Dorrestein, G.M. (1996) Cytology and haemocytology. In: *The Manual of Psittacine Birds*, pp. 38–48. British Small Animal Veterinary Association, Cheltenham, Glos.

Duncan, J.S., Reid, H.W., Moss, R., Phillips, J.D.P., Watson, A. (1978) Ticks, louping ill and red grouse in Speyside, Scotland. *Journal of Wildlife Management*, **42**, 500–505.

Dunker, H.R. (1977) Development of the avian respiratory and circulatory systems; respiratory function in birds, adult and embryonic. *Satellite Symposium of the 27th International Congress of Physiological Sciences, Paris, 1977*, 267, Springer-Verlag, Berlin.

Dunker, H.R. (1978) Coelom-Gliederung der Wirbeltiere-Funktionelle Aspekte. *Verhandlungen der Anatomischen Gesellschaft.*, **72**, 91–112.

Durant, A.J. (1926) Caecal abligation in fowls. *Veterinary Medicine*, **21**, 14–17.

Durant, A.J. (1930) Blackhead in turkeys, surgical control by caecal abligation. *Research Bulletin University of Missouri College of Agriculture* No. **133**.

Durant, A.J. (1953) Removal of vocal cords of the fowl. *Journal of the American Veterinary Medical Association*, **122**, 14–17.

Elkins, N. (1983) *Weather and Bird Behaviour*, pp. 86–90. T.A.D. Poyser Ltd., Carlton.

Fedde, M.R. & Kuhlman, W.D. (1977) Intrapulmonary carbon-dioxide sensitive receptors: Amphibians to mammals. Respiratory function in birds, adult and embryonic. *Symposium of the 27th International Congress of Physiological Sciences, Paris* (ed. J. Piper), pp. 30–50. Springer-Verlag, Berlin.

Fiennes, T-W., R.N. (1969) Infectious diseases of bacterial origin. In: *Diseases of Cage and Aviary Birds* (ed. M.L. Petrak), pp. 361–369. Lea and Febiger, Philadelphia.

Fitzgerald, G. & Cooper, J.E. (1990) Preliminary studies on the use of Propofol in the domestic pigeon (*Columbia livia*). *Veterinary Science*, **49**, 334–338.

Forbes, N.A. (1984) Avian anaesthesia. *Veterinary Record*, **115**(6), 134.

Forbes, N.A. (1991) Wing tip oedema and dry gangrene of birds. *Veterinary Record*, **129**(3), 58.

Forbes, N.A. & Harcourt-Brown, N.H. (1991) Wing tip oedema and dry gangrene of raptors. *Veterinary Record*, **128**(24), 576.

Forbes, N.A. & Simpson, G.N. (1993) Pathogenicity of ticks on aviary birds. *Veterinary Record*, **133**, 21.

Forbes, N.A. & Simpson, G.N. (in press) A review and update of viruses affecting raptors in the United Kingdom. *Veterinary Record*.

Forbes, N.A., Simpson, G.N., Higgins, R.J. & Gough, R.F. (in press) Adenovirus in raptors. *Journal of Avian Medicine and Surgery*.

Forshaw, J.M. (1978) *Parrots of the World*. Illustrated by W.T. Cooper. David and Charles, Newton Abbot.

Fowler, Murray, E. (1978) *Zoo and Wild Animal Medicine*. W.B. Saunders, Philadelphia, London, Toronto.

Franchetti, D.R. & Klide, A.M. (1978) *Restraint and Anaesthesia in Zoo and Wild Animal Medicine* (ed. M.E. Fowler), p. 303, W.B. Saunders, Philadelphia.

Frith, H.J. (1959) Incubator birds. In: *Scientific American: Birds* (ed. B.W. Wilson), pp. 142–148. W.H. Freeman, San Francisco.

Galvin, C.E. (1978) Cage bird medicine. *Veterinary Clinics of North America*, **14**(2), p. 285.

Garcia del Campo, A.L., Puerta, M.L., Abelenda, M., Fernañdez, A., Monsalve, L. & Nava, M.P. *et al.* (1991) Haematology of free-living chicks of the Greater Flamingo. *Proceedings of First Conference of European Committee of Association of Avian Veterinarians*, Vienna, pp. 434–436.

Gassman, R. *et al.* (1981) Isolierung von Adenoviren bei Wellensittichen mit Zentralnervösen Ausfallserscheinungen II D.V.G.-Tagung, *Vogelkrankht, 1981*, München, pp. 44–47.

George, J.C. & Berger, A.J. (1966) *Avian Myology*. Academic Press, New York.

Gerlach, H. (1994) Viruses. In: *Avian Medicine: Principles & Application* (eds B.W. Ritchie, G.J. Harrison & L.R. Harrison). Wingers Publishing, Lake Worth, Florida.

Gerlach, S. (1991) Macaw wasting disease. *Proceedings of First Conference of Association of Avian Veterinarians*, Vienna, p. 273.

Gilbert, A.B. (1979) Female genital organs. In: *Form and Function in Birds* (eds A.S. King & J. McLelland), **1**, p. 331. Academic Press Inc. (London) Ltd.

Goldsmith, T.L. (1995) Documentation of passerine circoviral infection. *Proceedings Main Conference Association of Avian Veterinarians*, p. 349–350.

Gordon, R.F. & Jordan, F.T.W. (1977) *Poultry Diseases*, p. 219. Balliére Tindall, London.

Graham-Jones, O. (1966) The clinical approach to tumours in cage birds III: Restraint and anaesthesia of small cage birds. *Journal of Small Animal Practice*, **7**, 231–239.

Green, C.J. (1979) Animal anaesthesia. In: *Laboratory Animal Handbooks 8*, pp. 126–128. Laboratory Animals Ltd., London.

Green, C. & Simpkin, S. (1984) Avian anaesthesia. *The Veterinary Record*, **115**(7), 159.

Greenwood, A.G. (1992) Laparoscopic salpingectomy in a hybrid flamingo. *Veterinary Record*, **131**(15), 349.

Greenwood, A.G. & Barnett, K.C. (1980) The Investigation of the Visual Defects in Raptors. In: *Recent Advances in the Study of Raptor Diseases* (eds J.E. Cooper & A.G. Greenwood). Chiron Publications Ltd, Keighley, Yorks.

Greenwood, A.G. & Storm, J. (1994) Intestinal intussusception in two red-tailed hawks (*Buteo jamaicensis*). *Veterinary Record*, **134**(22), 578–579.

Grier, J.W. (1973) Techniques and results of artificial insemination with golden eagles. *Raptor Research*, **7**, 1–12.

Grier, J.W., Berry, R.B. & Temple, S.A. (1972) Artificial insemination with imprinted raptors. *Journal of the American Falconers Association*, **11**, 45–55.

Hagner, D., Prehn, H. & Krautwald-Junghanns, M.E. (1995) Ultrasonography of the avian urogenital tract. Physiology and pathological conditions. *Proceedings of 3rd Conference European Association of Avian Veterinarians*, Jerusalem, pp. 195–199.

Haigh, J.C. (1980) Anaesthesia of raptorial birds. In: *Recent Advances in the Study of Raptor Diseases* (eds J.E. Cooper & A.G. Greenwood), 61–66. Chiron Publications Ltd, Keighley, Yorks.

Harcourt-Brown, N.H. (1978) Avian anaesthesia in general practice. *Journal of Small Animal Practice*, **19**, 573–582.

Harcourt-Brown, N.H. (1995) *Diseases of the pelvic limb of birds of prey*. FRCVS thesis, Wellcome Library, Royal College of Veterinary Surgeons, London.

Harcourt-Brown, N.H. (1996) Pelvic limb problems. In: *Manual of Psittacine Birds* (eds. P. Beynon, N.A. Forbes & M. Lawton), pp. 126, 127. British Small Animals Veterinary Association, Cheltenham, Glos.

Harrison, G.J. (1984) New aspects of avian surgery. *Veterinary Clinics of North America*, **14**(2), 363–380.

Harrison, G.H. & Harrison, L.R. (1986) *Clinical Avian Medicine and Surgery*. W.B. Saunders, Philadelphia, London, Toronto.

Harrison, L.R. & Herron, A.J. (1984) Submission of diagnostic samples to a laboratory. *Veterinary Clinics of North America*, **14**(2), 165–172.

Hasholt, J. (1969) Diseases of the nervous system. In: *Diseases of Cage and Aviary Birds* (ed. M.L. Petrak). Lea and Febiger, Philadelphia.

Hawkey, C. & Gulland, F. (1988) Clinical haematology. In: *Manual of Parrots, Budgerigars and other Psittacine Birds* (ed. C.J. Price), pp. 35–47 & 113. British Small Animal Veterinary Association, Cheltenham, Glos.

Heck, R.W. & Konke, D. (1983) Incubation and Rearing. In: *Falcon Propagation, a Manual on Captive Breeding* (eds J.D. Weaver & T.J. Cade), p. 49. The Peregrine Fund, Inc., Ithaca, New York.

Hermandez, M. (1991) Raptor clinical haematology. *Proceedings of First Conference European Committee of Association Avian Veterinarians,* Vienna.

Hill, K.J. & Noakes, D.E. (1964) Cyclopropane anaesthesia in the fowl. In: *Small Animal Anaesthesia: Proceeding of B.S.A.V.A./U.F.A.W. Symposium* (ed. O. Graham-Jones), p. 123–126. Pergamon, Oxford.

Hochleithner, M. (1994) Biochemistries. In: *Avian Medicine: Principles & Application* (eds B.W. Ritchie, G.J. Harrison & L.R. Harrison) *Biochemistries.* Wingers Publishing, Lake Worth, Florida.

Hoop, R.K., Ossent, P., Gaby Pfyffer (1995) Mycobacteriosis genavense, a new cause of mycobacteriosis in pet birds. *Proceedings 3rd Conference of European Committee of Association of Avian Veterinarians,* Jerusalem, pp. 1–3.

Hurrel, L.H. (1968) Wild raptor casualties. *Journal of Devon Trust,* **19,** 806–807.

Ivins, G.K. (1975) Sex determination in raptorial birds – a study of chromatic bodies. *Journal of Zoo Animal Medicine,* **6,** 9–11.

Jalanka, H. (1991) Medetomidine-Ketamine and Atipamezine, a reversible method of chemical restraint of birds. *Proceedings First Conference of European Committee of Avian Veterinarians,* Vienna, 102–104.

Jericovà, Z., Hubálek, Z. (1993) Arboviral examination of free-living birds in the Czech Republic. *Proceedings of 1993 European Conference on Avian Medicine and Surgery.* Utrecht, The Netherlands, pp. 507–521.

Johnson, O.W. (1979) *Form and Function in Birds* Vol. I (eds A.S. King & J. McLelland). Academic Press, London.

Jojié, D. & Popovié, S. (1969) Artery vascularization of certain aerated bones of domestic hen and pigeon wings. *Acts Veterinaria (Belgrade),* **29,** 87–95.

Jones, C.G. (1980) Abnormal and maladaptive behaviour in captive raptors. In: *Recent Advances in the Study of Raptor Diseases* (eds J.E. Cooper & A.G. Greenwood). Chiron Publications Ltd., Keighley, Yorks.

Jones, D.M. (1977) The sedation and anaesthesia of birds and reptiles. *Veterinary Record,* **101,** 340–342.

Jones, D.M. (1979) The nutrition of parrots: the husbandry and medicine of the parrot family. *Proceedings of B.V.Z.S./Parrot Society Meeting* (eds J.E. Cooper & A.G. Greenwood), p. 31. Regent's Park, London.

Jones, R.S. (1966) Halothane anaesthesia in turkeys. *British Journal of Anaesthesia,* **38,** 656–658.

Kendeigh, S.C. (1970) Energy requirements for the existence in relation to size of birds. *Condor,* **72,** 60.

Kennedy, M.A. & Brenneman, K.A. (1995) Enteritis associated with a coronavirus-like agent in a rhea chick (*Rhea americana*). *Journal of Avian Medicine and Surgery,* **9**(2), 138–140.

Keymer, I.F. (1969) *Diseases of Cage and Aviary Birds* (ed. M.L. Petrak), 1st edn, p. 434. Lea & Febiger, Philadelphia.

King, A.S. & McLelland, J. (1975) *Outlines of Avian Anatomy,* **46,** pp. 6–7. Bailliére Tindall, London.

King, A.S. & McLelland, J. (1979) *Form and Function in Birds,* Vol. 1 (eds A.S. King & J. McLelland), pp. 74–79. Baillié Tindall, London.

King, A.S. & McLelland, J. (1984) *Birds: Their Structure and Function.* Bailliére Tindall, London.

King, A.S. & McLelland, J. (eds.) (1989) *Form and Function in Birds*, Vol. 4. Academic Press, London.

King, A.S. & Payne, D.C. (1964) Normal breathing and the effects of posture in *Gallus domesticus. Journal of Physiology*, **174**, 340–347.

Kirkwood, J.F. (1981) Recent advances in the study of raptor diseases. In: *Proceedings of the International Symposium on Diseases of Birds of Prey* (eds J.E. Cooper & A.G. Greenwood), pp. 153–157. Chiron Publications Ltd, Keighley, Yorks.

Klide, A.M. (1973) Avian anaesthesia. *Veterinary Clinics of North America*, **3**(2), 175–186.

Kock, M. (1983) Sexing birds. *Veterinary Record*, **112**(19), 463.

Korbel, R., Mlovanovic, A., Erhardt, W., Burike, S. & Hemke, J. (1993) Aerosaccular perfusion with isoflurane – an anaesthetic procedure for head surgery in birds. Proceedings European Conference Association of Avian Veterinarians, Utrecht, Netherlands. AAV, Lake Worth, Florida.

Kovách, A.G.B. & Szász, E. (1968) Survival of pigeons after graded haemorrhage. *Acta Physiologica*, **34**(301).

Kovách, A.G.B., Szász, E. & Pilmayer, N. (1969) The mortality of various avian and mammalian species following blood loss. *Acta. P.N. Acad. Sci.*, 35–109.

Krautwald-Junghanns, M.E., Reidel, V. & Neumann, W. (1991) Diagnostic use of ultrasonography in birds. *Proceedings Association of Avian Veterinarians Conference*, Chicago, pp. 269–275.

Krautwald-Junghanns, M.E., Tellhelm, B., Hummel, G., Kostka, V. & Kaleta, E.F. (1992) *Atlas of Radiographic Anatomy and Diagnosis in Cage Birds*. Paul Parey Scientific, Berlin and Hamburg.

Krautwald-Junghanns, M.E., Schulz, M., Hagner, D., Failing, K. & Redman, T. (1995) Transcoelomic two-dimensional echocardiography in the avian patient. *Proceedings 3rd Conference European Committee of the Association of Avian Veterinarians (Incorporating 1st E.C.A.M.S. Scientific Meeting)*, Jerusalem, p. 10.

Lack, D. (1975 *The Life of the Robin*, 4th edn. H.F. and G. Witherby, London.

Lasiewski, R.C. & Dawson, L.R. (1967) A re-examination of the relation between standard metabolic rate and bodyweight of birds. *Condor*, **69**, 13–23.

Lawton, P.C. (1984) Avian anaesthesia. *Veterinary Record*, **115**(3), 71.

Lawton, M.P.C. (1996) Anaesthesia. In: *Manual of Psittacine Birds* (eds P.H. Beynon, N.A. Forbes. & M.P.C. Lawton). British Small Animal Veterinary Association, Cheltenham, Glos.

Levinger, I.M., Kedem, J. & Abram, M. (1973) A new anaesthetic-sedative preparation for birds. *British Veterinary Journal*, **129**, 296–300.

Lewandowski, A.H., Campbell, T.W., Harrison, G.J. (1986) Clinical chemistries. In: *Clinical Avian Medicine and Surgery* (eds G.J. Harrison & L.R. Harrison), p. 195. W.B. Saunders, Philadelphia, London.

Lewis, J.C.M., Storm, J. & Greenwood, A.G. (1993) Treatment of wing tip oedema and dry gangrene of raptors. *Veterinary Record*, **128**(24), 578.

Lorenz, K. (1935) Companions as factors in the bird's environment. In: *Studies in Animals and Human Behaviour* (1970 edn, trans.) R. Martin), Vol. 1. Methuen, London.

Lorenz, K. (1937) The companions in the bird's world. *Auk*, **54**, 245–273.

Lorenz, K. (1965) Die 'Erfindung' von Flugmaschen in der Evolution der Wirbeltiere. In: *Darwin hat recht gesehen*. Neske Verlag.

Lumeij, J.T. (1987) *A contribution to clinical investigative methods for birds, with special reference to the racing pigeon* (Columba livia domestica. PhD thesis, Rijksuniversiteit, Utrecht.

Lumeij, J.T. & Overduin, L.M. (1990) Plasma chemistry references in Psittaciformes. *Avian Pathology*, *19*, 235–244.

Lumeij, J.T., Ritchie, B.W. & Blanco, J.M. (1993) Avian electrocardiography: a contribution for the practitioner. *Proceedings European Association of Avian Veterinarians*. Utrecht, pp. 137–154.

Lumeij, J.T., Ritchie, B.W. & Branson, W. (1994) Cardiology. In: *Avian Medicine: Principles and Application* (eds B.W. Ritchie, G.J. Harrison & L.R. Harrison), pp. 695–722. Wingers Publishing, Lake Worth, Florida.

McKeever, K. (1979) *Care and Rehabilitation of Injured Owls*, pp. 24–25, 92, 94. W.F. Rannie, Lincoln, Ontario, Canada.

McLelland, J. (1989) Anatomy of the air sacs. In: *Birds, Form and Function* (eds A.S. King & J. McLelland), pp. 258–273. Academic Press, London.

McMillan, M.C. (1982) *Diseases of Cage and Aviary Birds* (ed. M.L. Petrak), 2nd edn. Lea and Febiger, Philadelphia.

Mandelker, L. (1972) Ketamine hydrochloride as an anaesthetic for parakeets. *Veterinary Medicine/Small Animal Clinician*, **67**, 55–56.

Mandelker, L. (1973) A toxicity study of ketamine HCl in Parakeets. *Veterinary Medicine/Small Animal Clinician*, **68**, 487–489.

Mangilgi, G. (1971) Unilateral petagiectomy: A new method of preventing flight in captive birds. In: *International Zoo Year Book XI*, pp. 252–254.

Marley, E. & Payne, J.P. (1964) Halothane anaesthesia in the fowl. In: *Small Animal Anaesthesia Proceedings of a B.S.A.V.A./U.F.A.W. Symposium* (ed. O. Graham-Jones), p. 127. Pergamon, Oxford.

Martin, H.D., Bruecker, K.A., Herrick, D.D. & Scherpelz, J. (1993) Elbow luxations in raptors: a review of eight cases. In: *Raptor Biomedicine* (eds P.J. Redig, J.E. Cooper, J.D. Remple and D.B. Hunter), pp. 199–206. University of Minnesota Press, Minneapolis.

Martin, H.D. & Ritchie, W.B. (1994) Orthopaedic surgical technique. In: *Avian Medicine: Principles and Application* (eds W.B. Ritchie, G.J. Harrison and L.R. Harrison), pp. 1166–1168. Winger Publishing, Lake Worth, Florida.

Mavrogordato, J.G. (1960) *A Hawk for the Bush*, 2nd edn. Neville Spearman, London.

Murdock, H.R. & Lewis, J.O.D. (1964) A simple method for obtaining blood from ducks. *Proceedings of the Society for Experimental Biology and Medicine*, **116**, 51–52.

Murrell, L.R. (1975–76) A practical method of determining bird sex by chromosome analysis. *Annual Proceedings of the American Association of Zoological Parks and Aquariums*, 87–90.

Needham, J.R. (1981) Bacterial flora of birds of prey. In: *Recent Advances in the Study of Raptor Diseases* (eds J.E. Cooper and A.G. Greenwood), pp. 3–9. Chiron Publishers Ltd., Keighley, Yorks.

Newton, I. (1979) *Population Ecology of Raptors*. T.A.D. Poyser Ltd, pp. 81–94.

Olney, P.J.S. (1958/9) *Wild Fowl Trust Report 11*, p. 154. Slimbridge, Glos.

Pass, D.A. & Perry, R.A. (1984) The pathology of psittacine beak and feather disease. *Australian Veterinary Journal*, **61**(3), 69–74.

Peakall, D.B. (1970) Pesticides and reproduction of birds. In: *Scientific American: Birds* (ed. B.W. Wilson), pp. 255–261. W.H. Freeman, San Francisco.

Peiper, K. & Krautwald-Junghanns, M.E. (1991) Diagnosis of tuberculosis in pet birds with the help of radiology. *Proceedings of First Conference of European Committee of Association of Avian Veterinarians.* Vienna, p. 186.

Perman, V., Alsaker, R.D., Riis, R.C. (1979) *Cytology of the Dog and Cat.* American Animal Hospital Association, Indiana.

Perrins, C.M. (1979) *British Tits*, pp. 160, 260–261. Collins. London.

Petrak, M.L. (1982) *Diseases of Cage and Aviary Birds*, 2nd edn. Lea & Febiger, Philadelphia.

Philip, H.R.H. Prince (1984) *Address to General Assembly of the International Union for Conservation of Nature and Natural Resources.* Madrid.

Rahn, H., Ar, A. & Pagenelli, C.V. (1979) How birds breathe. In: *Scientific American: Birds* (ed. B.W. Wilson), pp. 208–217. W.H. Freeman and Company, San Francisco.

Raines, A.M., Kocan, A. & Schmidt, R. (1995) Pathogenicity of adenovirus in the ostrich (*Struthio camelus*). *Main Proceedings of Conference on Avian Veterinarians*, pp. 241–245. Association of Avian Veterinarians, Boca Raton, Fl.

Redig, P.T. (1978) Raptor rehabilitation: diagnosis, prognosis and moral issues. *Conference on Bird of Prey Management Techniques, Oxford.* (ed. T.A. Greer).

Redig, P.T. (1979) *First Aid and Care of Wild Birds* (eds. J.E. Cooper & J.T. Eley). David & Charles, Newton Abbot.

Redig, P.G. (1981) Aspergillosis in raptors. In: *Recent Advances in the Study of Raptor Diseases* (eds J.E. Cooper & A.G. Greenwood), pp. 117–122. Chiron Publications Ltd., Keighley, Yorks.

Redig, P.T. (1983) Anaesthesia for raptors. *Raptor Research & Rehabilitation Program*, Newsletter 4, 9–10.

Redig, P.T. & Duke, G.E. (1976) Intravenously administered ketamine and diazepam for anaesthesia of raptors. *Journal of the American Veterinary Medical Association*, **169**, 886–888.

Reece, R.L. (1982) Observations on the accidental poisoning of birds by organophosphate insecticides and other toxic substances. *Veterinary Record*, **111**(20), 453.

Reiser, M.H. & Temple, S.A. (1980) Effects of chronic lead ingestion on birds of prey. In: *Recent Advances in the Study of Raptor Diseases* (eds J.E. Cooper & A.G. Greenwood), pp. 21–25. Chiron Publications Ltd, Keighley, Yorks.

Reither, N.D. (1993) Medetomidine and Atipamezole in avian practice. *Proceedings European Conference Avian Medicine and Surgery*, Utrecht, pp. 43–48.

Remple, J.D. (1993) Raptor bumblefoot: a new treatment technique. In: *Raptor Biomedicine* (eds. P.T. Redig, J.E. Cooper, J.D. Remple & D.B. Hunter). Chiron Publications, Keighley, W. Yorks.

Richards, J.R. (1980) Current concepts in the metabolic responses to injury, infection and starvation. *Proceedings of the Nutrition Society*, **39**, 113.

Richardson, J.D. (1984) Avian anaesthesia. *Veterinary Record*, **115**(7), 154.

Riedel, V. (1991) Ultrasonagraphy in birds. *Proceedings First European Conference of Avian Veterinarians*, Vienna, pp. 190–198.

Ritchie, B.W., Harrison, G.J. & Harrison, L.R. (1994) Avian Medicine, Principles and Application. Wingers Publishing, Lake Worth, Florida.

Robinson, P. (1975) Unilateral patagiectomy. A technique for deflighting large birds. *Veterinary Medicine/Small Animal Clinician*, **70**(2), 143.

Rosskopf, W.J. & Woerpel, R.W. (1982) Abdominal surgery in pet birds. *Modern Veterinary Practice*, **63**(2), 889–890.

Rosskopf, W.J. & Woerpel, R.W. (1984) Clinical experiences with avian laboratory diagnostics. *Veterinary Clinics of North America*, **14**(2), 261.

Rosskopf, W.J., Woerpel, R.W. & Pitts, B.J. (1983) Surgical repair of a chronic cloacal prolapse in a greater sulphur crested cockatoo (*Cacatua galerita*). *Veterinary Medicine Small Animal Clinician*, **78**(5), 719–724.

Rupiper, D.J. (1993) Radial ostectomy in a barn owl. *Journal of the Association of Avian Veterinarians*, **7**(3), 160.

Samour, J.H., Jones, D.M., Knight, J.A. & Howlett, J.C. (1984) Comparative studies of the use of some injectable anaesthetic agents in birds. *Veterinary Record*, **115**(1), 6–11.

Samour, J.H., Baggott, G.K., Williams, G., Bailey, I.T. & Watson, P.F. (1986) Seminal plasma concentration in budgerigars (*Melopsittacus undulatus*). *Comparative Biochemistry and Physiology*, **84**(4), 735.

Schlotthauer, C.F., Essex, H.E. & Mann, F.C. (1933) Caecal occlusion in the prevention of blackhead (enterohepatitis) in turkeys. *Journal of the American Veterinary Medical Association*, **83**, 218.

Schöpf, A. & Vasicek, L. (1991) Blood chemistry in canary finches (*Serinus canaria*). *Proceedings of First Conference European Committee of Association Avian Veterinarians*, Vienna, p. 933.

Scott, D.C. (1968) Intramedullary fixation of a fractured humerus in a wild owl. *Canadian Veterinary Journal*, **9**, 98–99.

Scrollavezza, P., Zanichelli, S., Palestra, L., Stella, G. & Arus, A. (1995) Medetomidine-Ketamine association and Atipamazole in the anaesthesia of birds of prey. *Proceedings 3rd Conference of European Committee of the Association of Avian Veterinarians*. Jerusalem, p. 211.

Secord, A.C. (1958) Fractures in birds repaired with the Jonas splint. *Veterinary Medicine*, **53**, 655–656.

Sibley, C.G. & Ahlquist, J.E. (1990) *Phylogeny and Classification of Birds. A Study of Molecular Evolution*. Yale University Press, New Haven.

Simpson, V.R. (1991) Leucocytozoon-like infection in parakeets, budgerigars and a common buzzard. *Veterinary Record*, **129**, 30.

Simpson, V.R. (1996) Post-mortem examination. In: *Manual of Psittacine Birds* (eds P.H. Benyon, N.A. Forbes and M.P.C. Lawton), p. 70. British Small Animal Veterinary Association, Cheltenham, Glos.

Simpson, V.R. & Harris, E.A. (1992) *Cyathostoma lari* (Nematoda) infection of birds of prey. *Journal of Zoology* (London), **227**, 655–659.

Small, E. (1969) In: *Diseases of Cage and Aviary Birds*, (ed. M.L. Petrak), 1st edn, p. 354, Lea & Febiger, Philadelphia.

Smith, G.A. (1979) Parrot disease as encountered in a veterinary practice. In: *The Husbandry and Medicine of the Parrot Family – the proceedings of a B.V.Z.S./Parrot Society meeting, Regent's Park, London*. (eds A.G. Greenwood & J.E. Cooper).

Smith, G.A. (1982) *Magazine of the Parrot Society*, **16**(11), 340.

Stauber, E., Papgeorages, M., Sande, R. & Ward, L. (1990) Polyostotic hyperostosis associated with oviductal tumour in a cockatiel. *Journal of American Veterinary Medical Association*, **196**(6), 939–940.

Steiner, C.V. & Davis, R.B. (1981) *Caged Bird Medicine*, p. 136. Iowa State University Press, Ames, Iowa.

Strettenheim, P. (1972) The integument of birds. In: *Avian Biology*, Vol. II, (eds Farmer, King & Parks), 7, Academic Press, New York/London.

Stunkard, J.A. & Miller, J.C. (1974) An outline guide to general anaesthesia in exotic species. *Veterinary Medicine/Small Animal Clinician*, **69**, 1181–1186.

Sykes A.H. (1964) Some aspects of anaesthesia in the adult fowl in *Small Animal Anaesthesia – Proceedings of a B.S.A.V.A./U.F.A.W. Symposium, London, 1963* (ed. O. Graham-Jones), pp. 117–121. Pergamon, Oxford.

Tanzella, D.T. (1993) Ulna ostectomy in a pale-headed rosella (*Platycercus adscitus*) with multiple injuries. *Journal of the Association of Avian Veterinarians*, **7**(3), 153.

Taylor, M. (1994) Biopsy techniques. In: *Avian Medicine Principles and Application* (eds R.W. Ritchie, G.J. Harrison & L.R. Harrison). Wingers Publishing, Lake Worth, Florida.

Temple, S.A. (1972) Artificial insemination with imprinted birds of prey. *Nature*, **237**, 287–288.

Tiemeier, O.W. (1941) Repairing bone injuries. *Auk*, **58**, 350–359.

van der Hage, M.H. & Dorrestein, G.M. (1991) Flagellates in the crop of canary bird. Proceedings of First Conference of European Committee of Association of Avian Veterinarians, Utrecht, Netherlands, pp. 303–307. AAV, Boca Raton, Fl.

van der Hage, M.H., Dorrestein, G.M. & Zwart, P. (1984) Pancreatitis is associated with paramyxovirus III in some aviary birds (Neophemas and Passeriformes) *Proceedings Meeting of Veterinary Pathologists*, Utrecht, p. 28.

van der Hage, M.H., Dorrestein, G.M. & Zwart, P. (1987) Paramyxovirus infections in Psittaciformes and Passeriformes. *European Symposium over Vogelziekten*, Beerse, Belgique. Netherlands Association of Avian Veterinarians.

Von Becker, E. (1974) Schnabelschienung bel Afrikanischen Hornraben, *Praktische Tierärzt*, **55**(9), 492–494.

Wallack, J.D. & Boever, W.J. (1983) *Diseases of Exotic Animals: Medical and Surgical Management*. W.B. Saunders Co., Philadelphia.

Weaver, J.D. (1983) Artificial insemination. In: *Falcon Propagation, a Manual on Captive Breeding*, (eds. J.D. Weaver & T.J. Cade), pp. 19–23. The Peregrine Fund, Ithaca, New York.

Westerhof, I.N.A. (1996) Pituitary-adrenocortical function and glucocorticoid administration in pigeons (Columbia livia domestica). PhD thesis. University of Utrecht.

Wilgus, H.S. (1960) Reserpine for tranquillising geese. *The 2nd Conference on the Use of Reserpine in Poultry Production*. The Institute of Agriculture, Minnesota, St. Paul, Minnesota, 54–56.

Wilkinson, J.S. (1984) A.I. Work in France. *Journal of the Welsh Hawking Club*, 9–13.

Wilkinson, R. & Birkhead, T.R. (1995) Copulation behaviour in vasa parrots *Coracopsis vasa* and *C. nigra. Ibis*, **37**(1), 117–119.

Woerpel, R.W. & Rosskopf, W.J. (1984) Clinical experience with avian laboratory diagnostics. In: Symposium on caged bird medicine. *The Veterinary Clinics of North America*, **14**(2), 249–286.

Yeisey, C.L. (1993) Surgical correction of valgus carpal deformities in water-fowl. In: *Proceedings of the Association of Avian Veterinarians Annual Conference*. Lake Worth, Fl.

Index